Textbook of
Veterinary Anaesthesia

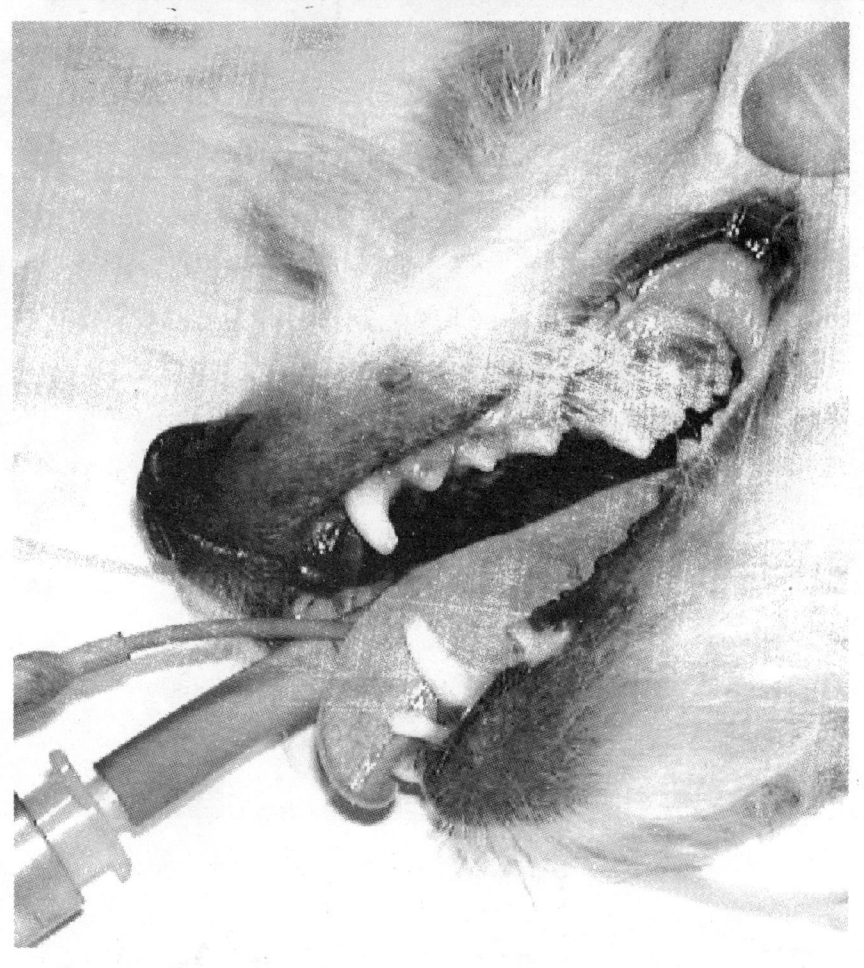

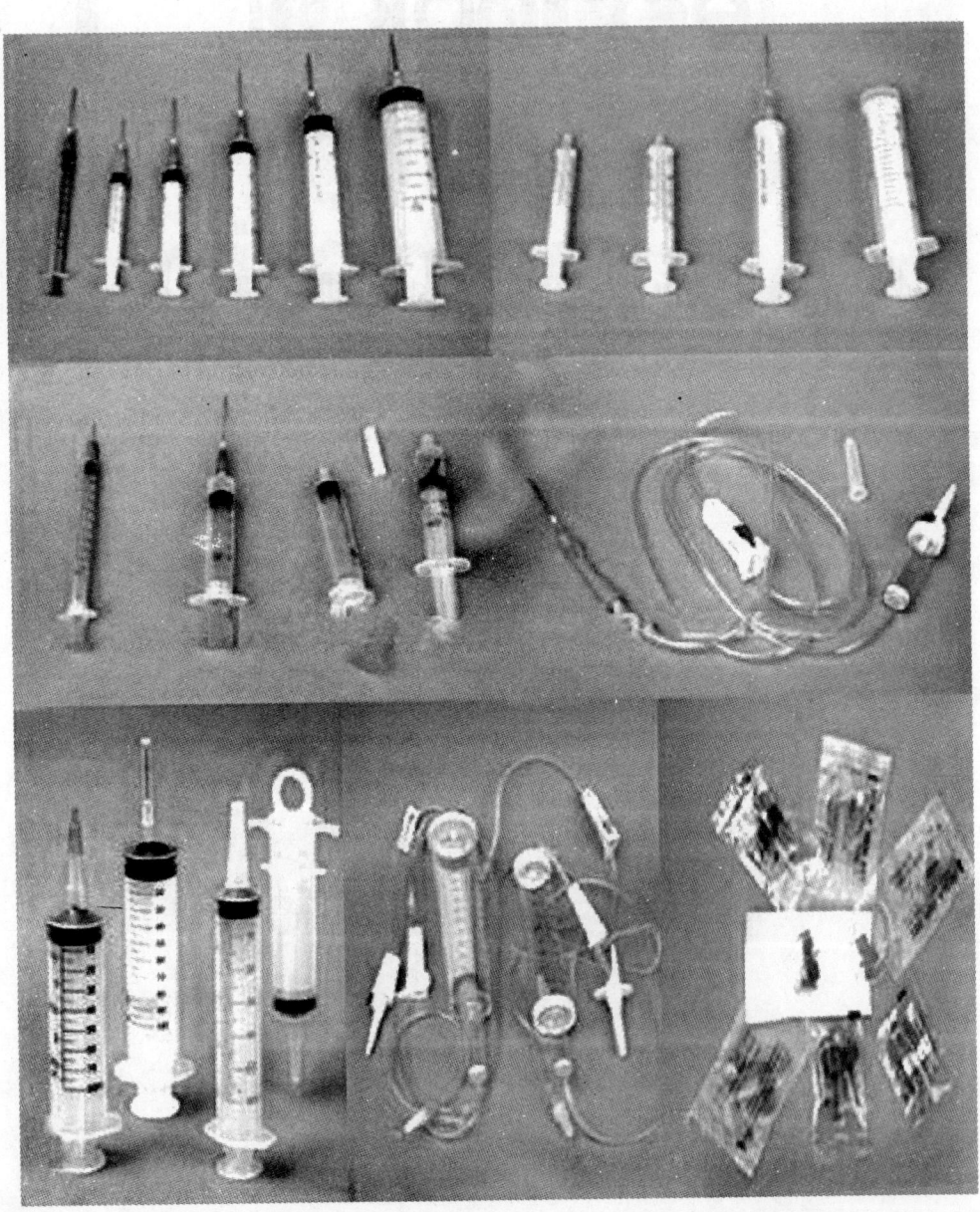

Textbook of
Veterinary
Anaesthesia

Pramod Kumar

Senior Professor and Head
Department of Anaesthesiology
Government Medical College and
Medical Superintendent, Sir T. Hospital, Bhavnagar, Gujarat

Former Faculty

MP Shah Medical College, Jamnagar
Institute of Medical Sciences, Banaras Hindu University, Varanasi
Mahatama Gandhi Institute of Medical Sciences, Wardha
SSIHMS, Prasanthi Gram

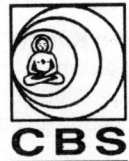

CBS

CBS Publishers & Distributors Pvt. Ltd.

New Delhi • Bengaluru • Chennai • Kochi • Kolkata • Mumbai
Hyderabad • Nagpur • Patna • Pune • Vijayawada

Textbook of
Veterinary
Anaesthesia

ISBN: 978-81-239-1772-6

First Edition: 2009
Reprint: 2018

Copyright © Author & Publisher

Published by **Satish Kumar Jain** and produced by **Varun Jain** for
CBS Publishers & Distributors Pvt. Ltd.,
4819/XI Prahlad Street, 24 Ansari Road, Daryaganj, New Delhi - 110002
delhi@cbspd.com, cbspubs@airtelmail.in • www.cbspd.com
Ph.: 23289259, 23266861, 23266867 • Fax: 011-23243014

Corporate Office: 204 FIE, Industrial Area, Patparganj, Delhi - 110 092
Ph: 49344934 • Fax: 011-49344935
E-mail: publishing@cbspd.com • publicity@cbspd.com

Branches:
• *Bengaluru:* 2975, 17th Cross, K.R. Road, Bansankari 2nd Stage,
  Bengaluru - 70 • Ph: +91-80-26771678/79 • Fax: +91-80-26771680
  E-mail: cbsbng@gmail.com, bangalore@cbspd.com
• *Chennai:* No. 7, Subbaraya Street, Shenoy Nagar, Chennai - 600030
  Ph: +91-44-26681266, 26680620 • Fax: +91-44-42032115
  E-mail: chennai@cbspd.com
• *Kochi:* Ashana House, 39/1904, A.M. Thomas Road, Valanjambalam,
  Ernakulum, Kochi • Ph: +91-484-4059061-65
  Fax: +91-484-4059065 • E-mail: cochin@cbspd.com
• *Kolkata:* 6-B, Ground Floor, Rameshwar Shaw Road, Kolkata - 700014
  Ph: +91-33-22891126/7/8 • E-mail: kolkata@cbspd.com
• *Mumbai:* 83-C, Dr. E. Moses Road, Worli, Mumbai - 400018
  Ph: +91-9833017933, 022-24902340/41 • E-mail: mumbai@cbspd.com

Representatives:
• Hyderabad: 0-9885175004   • Nagpur: 0-9021734563
• Patna: 0-9334159340   • Pune: 0-9623451994
• Jharkhand: 0-9811541605   • Uttarakhand: 0-9716462459

Printed at: J.S. Offset Printers, Delhi (India)

to

the great god

Bhagwan Pashupatinath

for his invisible inspiration and guidance

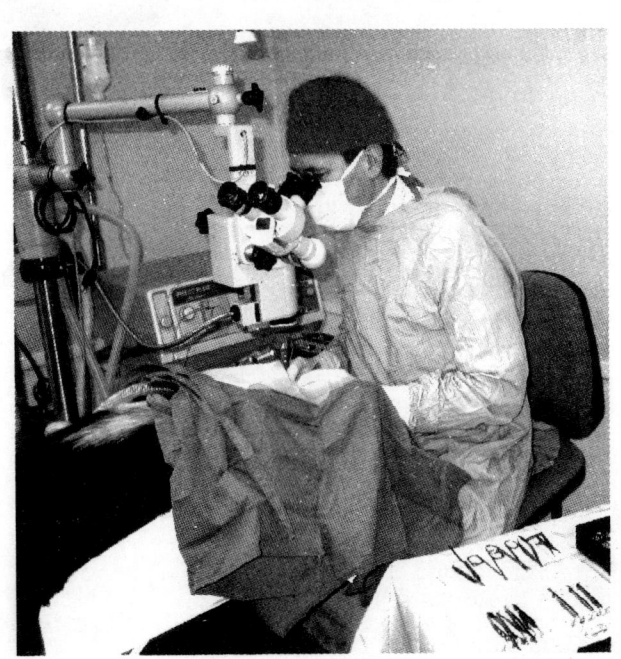

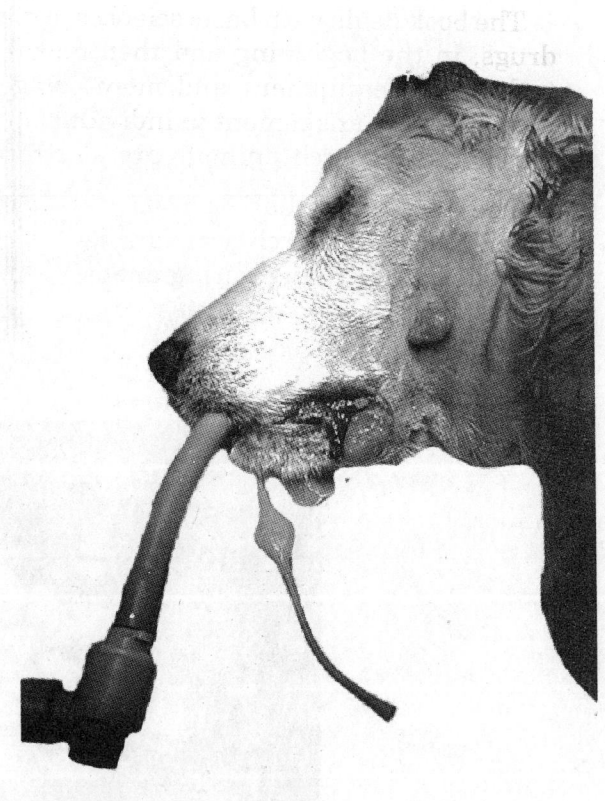

Preface

In India the practice of veterinary anaesthesia is primitive and borders on the crudeness, rudeness and inefficiency. There has been a wide gap in the available books on anaesthesia in our country. One or two books on the subject are from the UK. There is a priority about anaesthesia for horses in the Western books. While in India priority is cows, buffaloes and bulls. The district veterinary officers cater to above population mostly. Then there is a town-based practice in domestic animals, e.g. dogs and cats. In this book the contents are selected according to priority.

The book deals with basic sciences, e.g. physiology and pharmacology of anaesthetic drugs, in the beginning and then moves on to a section about various anaesthetic techniques, equipment and monitoring. The next section of the book deals with anaesthesia management in individual animals. Anaesthesia in animals in zoological parks and research animals are also discussed.

The last section has been written to increase the scope of this textbook so as to cater to the research workers in various scientific projects. Emergencies and complications arising during anaesthesia has been discussed to increase the margin of safety in veterinary anaesthesia.

I do hope this book will increase the awareness of students and practitioners of veterinary sciences.

Pramod Kumar

Acknowledgments

I would like to express my thanks to Dr Gunjan Sharma, Dr Ratan Kr. Choudhary, Dr Praveen Kumar, Dr Venkatesh, Dr Umesh, Dr Sunil, Dr Nirav, Dr Kirubahar and Dr Kannu Bhut (all Residents) for their kind support.

Parmod Kumar

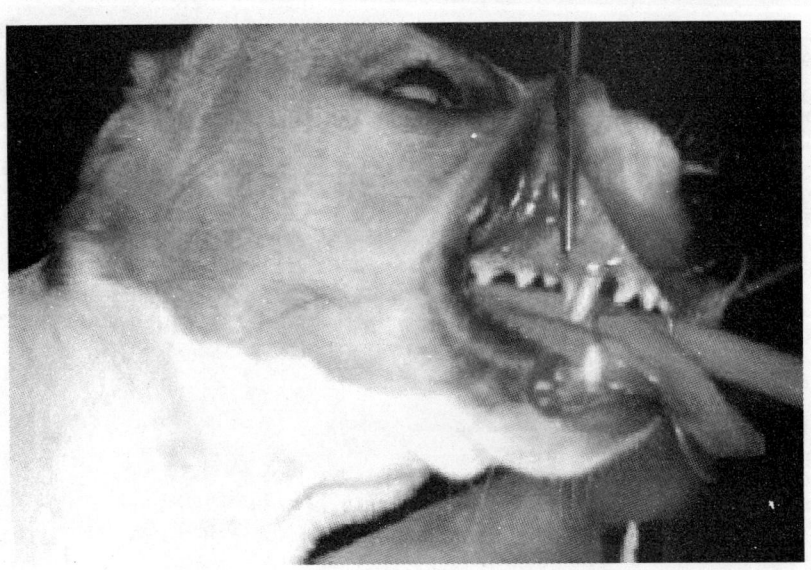

Contents

Section 2 — TECHNIQUES OF ANAESTHESIA   75

Section 3   ANAESTHESIA FOR INDIVIDUAL SPECIES   173

Section 1

Basics of
Anaesthesiology

1. Basic Mechanisms
2. General Anaesthesia
3. Inhalational Agents
4. Intravenous Induction Agents
5. Hypnotics, Sedatives and Anticonvulsants
6. Neurolept Analgesics and Narcotic Antagonist
7. Nonsteroidal Anti-inflammatory Drugs
8. Local Anaesthetics

Basic Mechanisms

ANAESTHESIA

The Greek philosopher Dioscorides first used the term *anaesthesia* in the first century AD to describe the narcotic like effect of mandragora. Bailey's dictionary in 1721 described it as a defect in sensation.

Anaesthesia can be defined as an reversible loss of sensation of part or whole of the body with or without loss of consciousness.

> *General anaesthesia is defined as an altered physiological state characterised by reversible loss of consciousness, analgesia of the entire body, amnesia and some degree of muscle relaxation.*

Basic Mechanisms of Action of Anaesthetics

The wide diversity of chemical structures, physical and physiological action of inhaled anaesthetic drugs suggest that they do not interact directly with a single specific receptor site. An effort is made to correlate their potency with physiochemical properties, e.g. lipid solubility. Various theories have been proposed for the mechanism of action of anaesthetics, e.g. hydrophobic sites, lipid solubility, hydrophilic sites, and membrane transmission on the basis of experimental studies.

Physiochemical actions: The anaesthetics may act at several gross (e.g. spinal cord reticular activating system) or microscopic (e.g. pre and postsynaptic) sites. There is a varied nature of these sites. The depression of presynaptic neurotransmitter release and blockade of current flow through the postsynaptic membrane may arise from anaesthetic perturbation at an identical molecular site, even if their geographic location is different. This lead to the concept that anaesthetics may have a common mode of action on a specific molecular structure which is called unitary theory of narcosis. The effort was made to correlate the anaesthetic potency with their physical properties. The correlation of minimal alveolar concentration (MAC) with lipid solubility (Fig. 1.1) mediated that site of action in hydrophobic site.

Hydrophobic Site (The Meyer-Overton Rule)

The physical property which correlates best with anaesthetic property is lipid solubility,[1] termed as the Meyer-Overton rule. The partial pressure of anaesthetic (inhalation) and its oil gas partition coefficient varies little over 100,000 fold range (Tables 1.1 and 1.2) within a given species of animal the product of partial pressure and oil gas partition coefficient varies only slightly (Table 1.1). This led to the unitary molecular site and suggests that anaesthesia results when a specific number of anaesthetic molecules occupy a hydrophobic site in the brain.[2]

Meyer-Overton postulated that it is the number of molecules dissolved at the site of action and not the type that produces anaesthesia. The MAC value of one agent has the same action as that of the other agent as seen in experimental studies,[3] with a little/slight variation occasionally.

Exceptions to Meyer-Overton Rule

Isomers: Enflurane and isoflurane are structural isomers with same oil/gas partition coefficient yet requirement for enflurane is 45 to 90% greater than that for isoflurane (Fig. 1.1). This suggests that potency of an agent depends on factors other than lipid solubility.

The isoflurane like other inhalation agents exist as mixture of two stereoisomers, which are mirror image of each other and not superimposable with similar physiochemical properties except for the direction in which they rotate polarized light. The isoflurane (+) isomer is 17 to 53% more potent than (−) isomer in rats.

Table 1.1: Oil gas partition coefficients and potency of inhaled anaesthetics in humans

	O/G coefficient	MAC
Methoxyflurane	970	0.0016
Halothane	224	0.0074
Enflurane	96.5	0.0168
Isoflurane	90.5	0.0115
Desflurane	18.7	0.070
Diethyl ether	65	0.0192
Fluroxene	47.7	0.034
Sevoflurane	47.2	0.0205
Cyclopropane	11.8	0.092
Xenon	1.9	0.71
Ethylene	1.26	0.67
Nitrous oxide	1.4	1.04

Convulsant gases: Complete halogenations of alkanes and ethers, e.g. fluorothyl agents tend to decrease the anaesthetic potency while enhancing their convulsant activity.[5] Convulsant halogenated ethers have different physical properties from anaesthetic halogenated ethers[8] because convulsant have low solubility parameters and have different effects on synaptic transmission on GABA receptors.

Cut-off effect: While highly lipid soluble paraffin hydrocarbon n-decane was nonanaesthetic, the less soluble homologue n-pentone caused anaesthesia. This decrease in potency in the higher members of a homologous series is called cut-off effect, which is due to the delivery of the larger alkanes due to decreasing volatility. The perfluro alkanes (Cfu) produce anaesthesia despite being soluble in hydrophilic solvents and tissues. An observation contrary to Meyer-Overton rule.

Non-anaesthetics: Certain polyhalogenated agents that are more lipid soluble lack anaesthetic properties, neither they lower MAC for conventional anaesthetics. These drugs called non-immobilizers quickly reach brain, cause excitability and convulsions, but do not produce anaesthesia[7] in the relation to their MAC value.

Hydrophilic site: Pauling suggested that anaesthesia might be caused by the ability of anaesthetics to produce hydrate crystals, which are cage-like structures of water surrounding a central anaesthetic molecule. These hydrate microcrystals can alter the transmission of electric charge through a neuron. However, there is a poor correlation between the ability of anaesthetics to form hydrates and their anaesthetic property.[1]

Hydrogen bond disruption: Another hypothesis is that certain inhaled anaesthetics act by disrupting hydrogen bond.[9] However compounds like argon and xenon are anaesthetics but do not form hydrogen bonds. It was suggested that

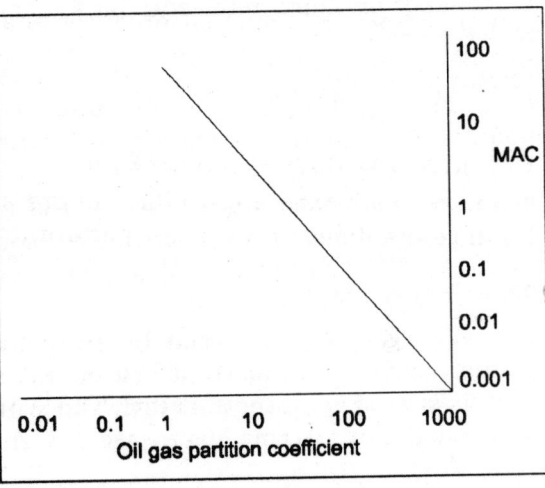

Fig. 1.1 Correlation of MAC with lipid solubility

general anaesthetics target sites have; in addition to an overall hydrophobicity, a polar component that is relatively poor hydrogen bond donor but that accepts a hydrogen bond as well as water. If hydrogen bonds are important in anaesthesia, then substitution of hydrogen for atoms in anaesthetic molecules might alter the hydrogen binding capabilities and change in anaesthetic potency, which is not the case.

Volume expansion by inhaled anaesthetics: Although Meyer-Overton postulates that anaesthesia occurs when a certain number of molecules dissolve at site, it does not explain why anaesthesia results. Mullin's hypothesis that anaesthesia occurs when absorption of anaesthetic molecules expand the volume of a hydrophobic region beyond a critical volume and obstruct ion channels or alter the electrical properties of neurons. The compression of the expanded hydrophobic region did reverse the effects of anaesthetic in vivo.[10] This is a useful model for estimating the interaction between pressure and inhaled anaesthetics, in spite of the non-linear pressure antagonism for some anaesthetics.

Measurement of Anaesthetic Potency

The anaesthesia is a complex behavioral phenomenon with several end points like hypnosis, amnesia, analgesia, depression of autonomic reflexes and immobility in response to a noxious stimulus. The last is the most common and desirable end point measured by minimal alveolar concentration (MAC), a vapor phase concentration. It prevents response of 50% of subjects to anxious stimulus and can be easily applied to experimental animals.[11]

MAC awake was introduced in relation to hypnosis and was more sensitive to movement in response to mechanical stimulation. MAC awake is defined as the concentration of inhaled anaesthetic at which 50% patients fail to respond to verbal command. It is related to learning and memory, which reside in brain, compared to MAC, which is mainly mediated by anaesthetic action on spinal cord. The use by volume of a volatile anaesthetic unit of anaesthetic potency is faulty as energy consumed to dissolve the molecule, reducing its potency as in case of ethanol. The halothane, which has a more chemical potential (ratio of its vapor pressure to the standard vapor pressure of pure liquid at same temperature), which remains same in all phases of matter, is more potent than ethanol, which has a high % vapor pressure. Many anaesthetics achieve MAC at the same chemical potential, thus, making it a more reliable unit of potency. All the anaesthetics which interact additively have different shapes and volumes of their molecules, requires that either the sites be flexible or there are many sites occupancy of any of them in additive. For a rapid action of onset within a few seconds of reaching the brain, the anaesthetics require a rapid reversal meaning a low affinity for their receptor sites.

Sites of Anaesthetic Action

The electrical activity (transfer of ions) changes by anaesthetics occur at neuronal membranes, which consist of hydrophobic/amphipathic components. There are lipid and protein sites of anaesthetic action. The latter is demonstrated by inhibitory action of many anaesthetics on enzyme hici furase,[12] whose potency for inhibition is for a wide variety of compounds.

The electrophysiological studies reveal the depressant effect of anaesthetics on the flow of sodium and potassium ions through selective membrane channels.[13] In contrast to this, anaesthetic enhance the conductance of chloride ions enhancing the inhibitory response produced by GABA[14] and of potassium ions by producing a marked hyperpolarization of cell membrane thus preventing firing of action potential.[15] However, the anaesthetic effects on resting membrane potential are voltage dependent and agent specific and not a universal feature of all anaesthetic action on CNS neurons. The action of anaesthetics on ion flow through plasma membrane to a membrane site of action. The calcium accumulation in mitochondria is altered by anaesthetics leading to intracellular free calcium, which in turn alters conductance of excitable membrane and presynaptic release of neurotransmitters.

The biological membranes consist of a cholesterol-phospholipid bilayer matrix of 4 mm thickness. Peripheral proteins are bound to external hydrophilic membrane while integral proteins are deeply embedded in or pass through the lipid bilayer (Fig. 1.2). So anaesthetic can act on lipid or protein component of the membrane.

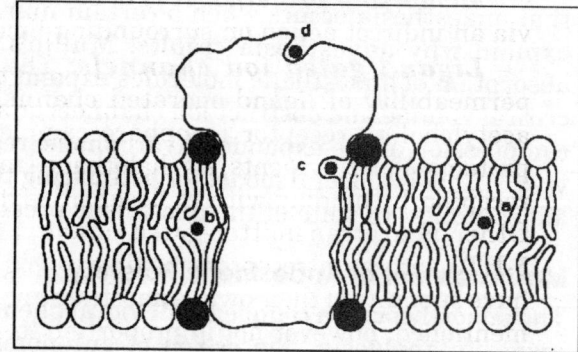

Fig 1.2: Possible sites for inhalational agents. Anaesthetics molecules in a neuronal membrane (a-lipid bilayer, b-lipids at interface, c-protein site bound by lipid, d-protein site exposed to aqueous environment)

Lipid membrane sites: The solubility of inhalational agents in membrane lipids tends to correlate with their anaesthetic potencies.[15] The temperature decrease increases the partitioning of anaesthetics into the phospholipid membrane. Though anaesthetics penetrate all depths of lipid bilayer, there is a preference for membrane interface near the aqueous environment, which may be responsible for response to noxious stimulation of anaesthetics while amnesia is related to penetration into the nonpolar bilayer.[16]

Mode of action on lipid membrane can be explained by the following

1. The anaesthetics may increase the flow of protons across lipid vesicles, collapsing the pH gradient required to retention of catecholamines in their charged form and thus depressing the neurotransmission by releasing catecholamines from synaptic storage.[17]

2. Lipid monolayer adsorbs inhaled agents, resulting in an increase in lateral pressure of the monolayer in proportion to anaesthetic potency.

3. The anaesthetics increase the mobility of membrane components by fluidizing the lipid bilayer. Even a sudden change in fluidity can produce a profound membrane function change.

4. There is other hypothesis about anaesthetic action on lipids such as alterations in membrane electrical properties or membrane pressures.

Interaction of inhaled agents with proteins. The inhalational agents act on specific neuronal membrane proteins that permit the translocation of ions during membrane excitation, either by disrupting ion flow through indirect action on lipids or via a second messenger or by a direct specific binding to channel proteins.

Distinct anaesthetic binding sites have been identified in several soluble proteins, including hemoglobin, myoglobin and albumin, in case of halothane when anaesthetics move rapidly between their binding sites in soluble proteins and the surrounding aqueous solvent and bind to albumin with an average life span of about 200 microsec[18] leading to changes in enzyme activity.

Membrane proteins: It is debatable whether inhalational agents act on ion flow or via an indirect action on surrounding lipids.

Ligand gated ion channels: The binding neurotransmitter alters membrane permeability of ligand-operated channels to specific ions. The muscle type nicotinic acetylcholine receptor ionophore complex is one of the examples of these membrane proteins. Volatile agents, e.g. halothane stabilize one of the subunit of acetylcholine complex receptor, by binding with it, desensitize it and inactive closed channel state is reached.[19] Other neurotransmitter-gated channel is $GABA_A$, glycine, ionotropic glutamate and 5-HT3 serotonin receptors having considerable overlap with acetylcholine receptor and have subunits of their own. Anaesthetic may enhance the function of some of these proteins mentioned; however not in proportion to their potency.

Voltage gated ion channels: The flux of ions through these is controlled by electric field across the membrane. The[4] pharmacological effects on a partial channel may vary from tissue to tissue or among channel subtypes as seen with calcium, sodium and potassium currents experimental animals; acted upon at a protein site.[20]

G proteins: Metatropic receptors coupled to G protein evoke changes in neuronal excitability as seen with halothane, which inhibits muscarinic signaling activated by acetylcholine. This may be a variable effect suggesting side effects anaesthetics. G proteins are potential membrane sites where anaesthetic exerts their functional effects rather than immobility component.[21]

Role of membrane enzymes and transporters: The enzyme Ca^{2+}–APPase is inhibited by halothane (20–39%) at 1 MAC. The inhaled agents may compete directly with ligand known to have direct binding sites on proteins.[22] The Na^+, K^+, and Cl^- cotransporter is inhibited by halothane but not by other agents possibly because it contains a hydrophobic pocket of circumscribed dimensions that allow binding of halothane only.[23] Protein kinase is another enzyme modulating transmitter that release and conduct ions through membrane channels. Protein kinase C inhibitor may lower anaesthetic requirements playing a role in anaesthesia. The research is presently being done to find specific site of anaesthetic action by structural analysis of ion channels, molecular modeling to define properties of binding and defining important receptors with transgenic mice.

Role of neurochemical composition and anaesthetic potency: A correlation between changes in anaesthetic requirements and a structural change in the nervous system might indicate critical properties of anaesthetic site of action.

Dietary studies: Mice fed diets of different fatty acid composition (saturated v/s unsaturated) from birth have large alterations in certain synaptic membrane fatty acid components in the brain and correlated with altered anaesthetic potency.

The fat deprived mice exhibited a 10–33% decrease in MAC for methoxyflurane, halothane, isoflurane and cyclopropane as compared with control mice,[24] which can be reversed by supplementing them with linoleic acid. The alterations in anaesthetic potency are correlated with brain arachidony-phosphatidylinositol content might alter the ability of neurotransmitters to synthesize chemical second messengers, thus altering neuronal excitability and anaesthetic requirements.[25]

Tolerance studies: Chronic tolerance —inhaled anaesthetic requirements can be measured by the chronic exposure of mice to sub-anaesthetic levels of N_2O after 2 weeks and disappears within 6 days of removing the mice from sub-anaesthetic environment. This is same in the case of cyclopropane, isoflurane.[26] This continuous exposure to anaesthetic alters the physical state of neuronal membranes to which the animal adapts by adjusting lipid composition of neuronal membrane. However, such changes do not occur in mice tolerance to N_2O. The prolonged exposure of rats to nitrous alters brain neurotransmitter level or receptors, e.g. opiate receptors, which may account for the tolerance to analgesic action of nitrous oxide.

Acute tolerance: A rapidly developed tolerance to N_2O is seen in mice, associated with withdrawal symptoms when removed from anaesthetic environment. This involves calcium channels as suggested by the ability of a calcium entry blocker to prevent N_2O tolerance and withdrawal seizures.

Genetic studies: Genetic approaches to anaesthetic mechanisms involve the development of mutants that are markedly sensitive or resistant to anaesthetics. The development of physiologic and molecular changes in these animals explain their altered anaesthetic sensitivity as in nematodes and fruit flies whose genomes are well mapped. However, the behavioral assays used to assess anaesthetic potencies in these simpler organisms may be different to relate to the anaesthetic induced immobility and amnesia in patients during anaesthesia.

Table 1.2: Possible site of anaesthetic action

CNS, brain, spinal cord	Anaesthetics disrupt the transmission throughout the CNS. Decerebration does not alter MAC
Axons vs. synapses	Higher concentrations of anaesthetics required to disrupt axonal synaptic transmission
Excitatory vs. inhibitory synapse	Anaesthetic may alter presynaptic release of neurotransmitter (via Ca^{++}) and modify flow of ions through postsynaptic channels
Presynaptic vs. post synaptic	Mayer-Overton rule implies a hydrophobic site of action. Critical volume hypothesis propose anaesthetic action through membrane expansion. Possible membrane aqueous interface.
Membrane	
Lipid vs. protein	Lipid fluidization theories cannot account for the production of the anaesthetic state. Evidence accumulating for direct binding of anaesthetics to excitable membrane proteins.

ACTIONS OF INHALED ANAESTHETICS IN THE CNS

Brain: Inhaled anaesthetics act by altering neuronal activity in the selected regions of the CNS. Brainstem reticular formations also play an important role as it alters the state of consciousness alertness and regulate motor activity, depending upon the agent and the neuronal. There might be alteration of spontaneous and evoked activity in cerebral cortex and by hippocampus. The inhaled anaesthetics may depress excitability of neurons or enhance excitability and influence inhibitory postsynaptic potentials. The transfer of sensory information from the thalamus to cortical region pathways is particularly sensitive to anaesthetics through inhibitory and excitatory components.[29]

Spinal cord: Both excitatory and inhibitory neurotransmission in spinal cord may be altered by anaesthetics, depending upon its concentration and also on the particular spinal cord pathway examined. Inhaled anaesthetics after response to the spinal dorsal horn (sensory) to both noxious and non-noxious stimuli, along with depression of spinal motor neurons by decreasing F-wave amplitude in rats. Thus a reduction in sensory processing and inhibition of motor neuron excitation, along with a alteration of tonic inputs received from descending modulator systems from the brain.[29]

Since anaesthesia is defined as amnesia and immobility in response to noxious stimuli, there must be two separate anatomical sites. Supraspinal involved in amnesia and spinal site involved in preventing movement to noxious stimuli. This had lead to experiments on neurons at various levels, e.g. peripheral receptors and synapses.

Peripheral receptors: Anaesthetics do not depress or affect the peripheral receptors as seen by non-alteration of cutaneous responses, e.g. touch. They can sensitize and promote excitation of nociceptors in mammalian A and C fibers. These may exist exquisitely sensitive cells with their firing activity, expressed by agents like halothane even at 1 MAC, producing amnesia.[29]

Axonal and synaptic transmission: The lower concentrations of anaesthetics altering synaptic transmission have a small effect on axonal transmission. However in clinical concentrations there is alteration of transmission through axons and partial effect on synaptic transmission. This effect at synapse may reflect depression of axonal transmission. The inhaled anaesthetics depress unmyelinated fibers. The frequency at which axons transmit impulses may alter potency. At low impulse frequency there is constant level of action potential block while at high frequencies conduction block increases progressively.

Synapses: Anaesthetics may depress transmission by interfering with release of neurotransmitter from presynaptic nerve terminals into the synaptic cleft by altering later's release, uptake and binding to receptor sites on postsynaptic membrane or by influencing conduction following activation of postsynaptic receptor.

Neurotransmitters: Neurotransmitters involved in anaesthesia production are: Acetylcholine, which is the classic transmitter and its concentrations turn over is decreased by anaesthetics in specific brain nuclei. The anaesthetic impair synthesis by inhibiting choline uptake. The effect is reversed by ventricular injection of hemi choliniam-3, which reduces synaptic acetylcholine in mice in case of isoflurane. In case of catecholamines, while noradrenaline content in most brain remain unchanged by anaesthetics, it may be elevated in nucleus accumbens, locus circuleus and central gray catecholamine areas. A change in noradrenaline availability certainly influences anaesthetic requirements as shown by using drugs, which increase or decrease noradrenaline levels. In contrast, dopamine brain levels are inversely related to anaesthetic requirements as seen by the use of levodopa (increased dopamine levels) and chemical destruction of dopaminergic neurons (lowers it) in case of halothane. Alpha-2 adrenergic agonists markedly lower anaesthetic MAC.

Serotonin: Administration of adenosine or adenosine analogue decreases halothane MAC by about 50%, probably by decreasing CNS noradrenergic transmission, a response that is not seen with small alterations in endogenous adenosine concentrations.

GABA: Anaesthesia may alter GABA levels in selected areas of brain, e.g. cerebral cortex by inhibiting the metabolism and levels of GABA, without altering its release and uptake, thus decreasing the synaptic transmission and contribute to anaesthetic state.

Excitatory amino acids: The anaesthetics depress glutamate-induced transmission, an action reversed by administering inhibitors of excitatory amino acid transmission.

Cyclic nucleotides: Their production is influenced by neurotransmitters and anaesthetics and they may serve as second messengers in altering neurotransmission as seen in case of cAMP in rodents in particular brain regions only. The cAMP may effect (via phosphorylation) macromolecules that are important in neurotransmission.

Calcium: Calcium is a neuroregulator as it is acted upon by anaesthetics through intracellular content changes and neuronal excitability through a calcium dependent release of neurotransmitter.

Endogenous opiates: Inhaled anaesthetic may work through opiate receptors as seen by former's decreased requirements and partial reversal of action by naloxone in high doses. There may be a release of endogenous opiates related to proenkephalin as seen with a mixture of nitrous and halothane, reversed by naloxone without elevation of opiate peptide in cerebrospinal fluid.

Nitric oxide: Nitric oxide is a neuro-modulator playing a role in mediating consciousness. This action may occur via production of cAMP and various other neurotransmitter pathways.

It can be concluded from above that predominant effects of inhaled anaesthetics cannot be explained by depletion, production or release of a single neuro-modulator in the CNS. There may a balance required between many different neuro-modulator systems.

Factors altering anaesthetic requirements[29]

1. *Temperature:* The MAC decreases (2–5%) with decreasing body temperature per degree, depending from agent to agent, with associated increase in anaesthetic solubility in aqueous phase.
2. *Pressure:* The increasing hydrostatic pressure increase anaesthetic requirements, exhibiting a pressure reversal in some species.
3. *Age:* In humans, MAC of volatile agents are maximal in infants at 6 months of age, while MAC in old age of 80 year is approximately one half that in the infant. The increase in potency and decrease in MAC with increasing age is seen for all anaesthetics and averages 6% change per decade of age.
4. *Ion concentration:* Hypernatremia increases sodium proportionally in CSF and increases halothane MAC by 43% and conversely hyponatraemia dilutes CSF sodium and reduce halothane MAC. Hyperkalemia does not alter CSF potassium or MAC. Calcium infusions increase serum and CSF levels without influencing MAC. However, calcium entry blockers in high doses increase the potency of anaesthetics. Magnesium levels affect potency only at very high plasma levels (10 times). While intravenous infusion of hydrochloric acid or soda bicarb have no effect, intrathecal injection of blockers of chloride transport increase the MACs of isoflurane and halothane in rats.

References and Bibliography

1. Franks N.P., Lieb W.B., *What is the Molecular Nature of General Anaesthetic Target Sites?* Trends Pharmacol, Sci. p 987, 8:109.
2. Miller K.W., Paton N.D.M., Smith E.B. et al., *Physicochemical Approaches to the Mode of Action of General Anaesthetics,* Anesthesiology, 36:339, 1972.
3. Eger E.I. II, Does 1+2=2?, Anaesth. Analg. 68:551., 1989.
4. Eger E.I. II, Ksblin D.D., Laster M.J. et al., *Minimum Alveolar Anaesthetic Concentration Values for the Enantiomers of Isoflurane Differ Minimally.* Anaesth. Analg, 85: 188, 1997.

5. Kablin D.D., Eger E. I. II; Johnson B.H. et al.. *Are Convulsant Gases Also Anaesthetics?* Anesth. Analg. p. 54:318, 1981.

6. Liu J., Laster M.J., Koblin D.D. et al., *A Cut Offin Anaesthetic Potency Exists in the Perfluroalkanes,* Anesth. Analg, 84, 1974.

7. Eang J., Laster M.J., Copong D. et al., *Convulsant Activity of Non-anaesthetic Gas Combinations,* Anesth. Analg, 84:634.

8. Pauling L. A. *Molecular Theory of General Anaesthesia,* Science. 1961; 134:15.

9. Abraham M.H., Lieb W.B., Franks N.P., *Role of Hydrogen Bonding in General Anaesthesia.* J Pharma Sci, 80:719, 1991.

10. Wann K.T., Mac Donalds A.G., *Actions and Interactions of High Pressure and General Anaesthetics,* Prog. Neurobiol, 30:217, 1987.

11. Rehberg B., Xiao Y.H., Duch D.S., *Central Nervous System Sodium Channels are Significantly Suppressed at Clinical Concentrations of Volatile Anesthetics,* Anesthesiology, 84:1223, 1996.

12. Kendig J.J., Trudell J.R., Cohon E.N., *Halothane stereoisomers: Lack of Stereospecificity in Two Model Systems,* Anesthesiology, 39:518–24, 1973.

13. Curry S., Lieb W.R., Franks N.P., *Effects of General Anaesthetics on the Bacterial Luciferase Enzyme from Vibrio Harvey; An Anaesthetic Target Site with Differential Sensitivity.* Biochemistry, 29:464–52, 1990.

14. Fanelign D.L., Kosek P., Moely H.I. et al. *The Role of Gaba$_a$ Receptor / Chloride Channel Complex in Anaesthesia.* Anesthesiology, 1993; 78:757.

15. Franks N.P., Lieb W.R. *Volatile General Anaesthetics Activate —A Novel Neuronal K^+ Current,* Nature, 333:662, 1985.

16. Koblin D.D., Eger E. I. II, Johnson B.H. et al., *Minimal Alveolar Concentrations and Oil/Gas Partition Coefficients of Four Anaesthetic Isomers,* Anesthesiology, 54:314, 1981.

17. Eggers E.I. II, Koblin D.D., Harris R.A. et al. *Hypothesis—Inhaled Anaesthetics Produce Immobility and Amnesia by Different Mechanisms at Different Sites,* Anesth Analg, 84:915, 1997.

18. Bengham A.D., Mill M.W., *The Proton Pump Leak Mechanism of Unconsciousness,* Chem Phys lipids, 40:189, 1986.

19. Xu Y, Tang P., Firestone L. et al., *19F Nuclear Magnetic Resonance Investigation of Stereoselective Binding of Isoflurane to Bovine Serum Albumin,.* Biophys J. 70:532, 1996.

20. Raines D.E., Rankin S.E., Miller K.W., *General Anaesthetics Modify the Kinetics of Nicotinic Acetylcholine Receptor Desensitization at Clinically Relevant Concentrations,* Anesthesiology, 82:108, 1995.

21. Hall A.L., Lieb W.R, Franks N.P. *Insensitivity of P Type Calcium Channels to Inhalational and Intravenous General Anaesthetics,* Anaesthesiology, 81:117, 1994.

22. Frank J.J., Horn J.L., Janicki P.K. et al., *Halothane, Isoflurane, Xenon and Nitrous Oxide Inhibit Calcium Atpase Pump Activity in Rat Brain Synaptic Plasma Membranes,* Anesthesiology 82:108, 1995.

23. Tas P.W.L., Kress H.G., Koschel K., *General Anaesthetics can Competitively Interfere with Sensitive Membrane Proteins,* Proc Nati Acad Sci, USA, 84:5972, 1987.

24. Evers A.S., Elliot W.J., Lef Kowith J.B. et al., *Alteration of Synaptic Membrane Fatty Acid Composition and Anaesthetic Requirement. Manipulation of Rat Brain Fatty Acid Composition Alters Volatile Anesthetic Potency.* J. Clin. Invest 77:1028, 1986.

25. Koblin D.D., Egers E.I. II, Smith R.A. et al., *Chronic Exposure of Mice to Subanaesthetic Doses of Nitrous Oxide,* In: Progress in Anesthesiology, Vol. 2, Molecular Mechanisms of Anaesthesia, New York, Raven, 159–164, 1980.

26. Smith R.A., Winter P.M., Smith M. et al., *Tolerance to and Dependence on Inhalational Anaesthetics,* Anesthesiology, 50:5.5., 1979.

27. Smith R.A., Winter P.M., Smith M. et al., *Rapidly Developing Tolerance to Acute Exposures to Anaesthetic Agents,* Anesthesiology, 59:494, 1979.

28. Dolin S.J., Little H.J., *Effects of Mitrendipine on Nitrous Oxide Anaesthesia, Tolerance and Physical Dependence,* Anesthesiology, 70: 91, 1989.

29. Koblin D.D., *Mechanism of Action,* In: Anaesthesia, Miller R.D., (ed), Vol. 1st, 5th edition, Churchill-Livingstone, New York, 2000.

2

General Anaesthesia

Induction of inhalation anaesthesia can be difficult. Anaesthetic gases are irritating to eyes and nasal passages. Animals may resist as they begin to lose consciousness or they may stop breathing temporarily. For this reason induction using a mask or nose cone held over the animal's nose can only be performed on smaller or non-fractious animals. In smaller animals gas can be delivered into an induction chamber large enough to contain the entire animal. Induction via a nose cone or chamber requires delivery of the anaesthetic gas at 2–3 × MAC. Frequently an injectable anaesthetic is used to induce anaesthesia and the inhalation agent is used for maintenance.

Maintenance of inhalation anaesthesia is normally accomplished by delivering approximately 1.2 MAC to an animal via a mask or nose cone, or directly into the lungs via an endotracheal tube. Intubation is recommended whenever possible, particularly when a procedure will be prolonged. Endotracheal access is essential to provide ventilation support.

GAS DELIVERY SYSTEMS

The most complicated aspect of using inhalant anaesthesia is the delivery system. A delivery system must provide the anaesthetic gas to the animal at a known and constant rate. It must also ensure that animals receive adequate oxygen. There are several types of delivery systems typically used in laboratory animals. A more complete discussion of anaesthetic delivery systems is available here.

Drop System

The drop system is the most basic type of anaesthetic delivery system. It involves application of the anaesthetic gas to an absorbent material that is then placed in the bottom of an anaesthetic chamber or nose cone device. The gas mixes with the air in the chamber until it reaches a concentration equal to the vapour pressure of the gas. For this reason drop systems have been traditionally used with low vapour pressure anaesthetics such as methoxyflurane or with slow acting drugs like ether. Some success has been achieved by mixing high vapour pressure drugs such as Halothane or Isoflurane at a concentration of 15% by volume with mineral oil and using this mixture in the drop system.

Problems with a drop system and how to deal with them

- The concentration of the gas being delivered to the animal is largely unknown
  - Place animals in the chamber. Remove them as soon as they lose consciousness (i.e. they lay down and do not respond to a gentle stimulus)

- There is a limited ability to adjust the concentration
  - For anaesthetic maintenance (after animals lose consciousness) place absorbent material soaked with anaesthetic in the bottom of a nose cone or empty syringe case
  - Move the cone closer to or further away from the animal's face to adjust the concentration
  - If a closed chamber is used, there is a danger that the animal will not receive adequate oxygen
  - Do not leave animals in a closed chamber after they have lost consciousness

- Significant waste gas is produced. To minimize waste:
  - Perform anaesthesia in a fume hood or other well-ventilated area
  - Use a chamber with a tight-fitting cover
  - Use a chamber with the smallest diameter mouth possible
  - Keep the lid on except when the animal is being placed into or removed from the chamber
  - Add anaesthetic to the absorbent material only in a fume hood.

Apparatus for Rodent Anaesthesia (Fig. 2.1)

Left: a non-rebreathing nose cone that can be used with a large animal anaesthetic machine. Middle: a typical drop system closed anaesthetic chamber. Right: a gas scavenging system that can be used with a drop system.

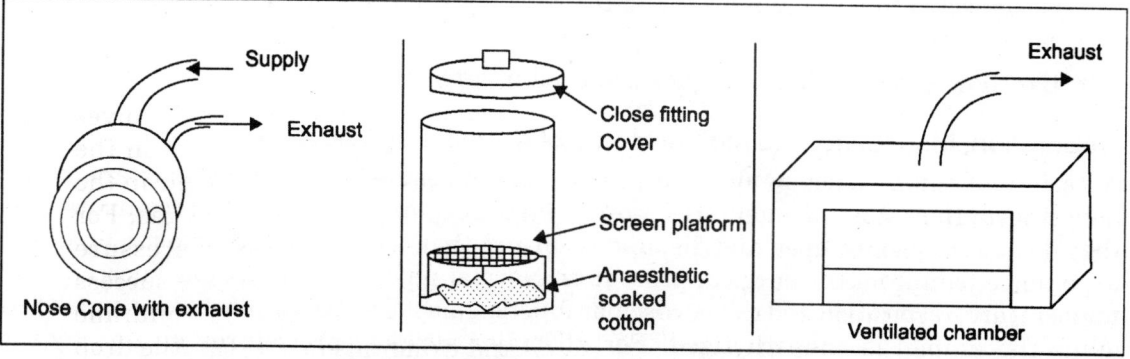

Fig. 2.1: Apparatus for rodent anaesthesia

ANAESTHETIC MACHINE

The best method of delivering an inhalant anaesthetic is with an anaesthetic machine. These machines precisely mix the gas with air or oxygen and can be easily adjusted. Machines can vary in construction and design. Anaesthetic machines typically require more training to learn to operate.

- Anaesthetic concentration is accomplished by sets of mixing valves or a precision vaporizer. Vaporizers are easier to use but are very expensive. Vaporizers are calibrated for the specific anaesthetic gas to be used.

- Anaesthesia circuits can be rebreathing or non-rebreathing.

  - Rebreathing circuits include typical circle systems used in large animals. The gas/oxygen mixture is delivered to the animal via a one-way valve. When the animal breathes out, the gas passes out through another valve attached to a Y-piece. This is passed over a carbon dioxide absorbent and then back into the system. Additional gas and oxygen are continuously delivered to replace that lost.

  - Rebreathing circuits conserve anaesthetic gas and the animal's body heat. The CO_2 absorbent must be replaced regularly.

  - Non-rebreathing circuits are primarily used for smaller animals that cannot cycle the gases in a rebreathing system. With newer machines non-rebreathing circuits are normally only necessary for rodents and birds. In older machines with metal valves a non-rebreathing circuit may be necessary for rabbits and cats as well. A Bain system is the most common non-rebreathing circuit available.

  - The non-rebreathing circuit is attached to the same anaesthetic supply as used for a rebreathing system. However, the exhaust line is connected directly to the waste gas scavenging system.

  - Non-rebreathing circuits depend on gas and oxygen being delivered at a higher pressure than is present in the exhaust line. This tends to increase anaesthetic usage and can increase body heat loss in the patient.

- Anaesthesia machines must have a waste gas scavenging system. Normally the exhaust line on a non-rebreathing system or the pop-off valve on a rebreathing system is connected to a vacuum line or to the building exhaust. Other scavenging systems can be used.

- Low-flow anaesthetic techniques are used in large animals.

Preparation, Monitoring and Maintenance of Normal Physiology

A variety of things must be done to prepare for anaesthesia. Once animals are under anaesthesia they must be monitored closely while they are anaesthetized to ensure that they do not become too deep and die, and to ensure that they do not become too light and experience pain from the surgical procedure. Normal physiologic functions such as body temperature, respiration and cardiovascular function must also be monitored and supported while the animal is anaesthetized. For all major surgical procedures on non-rodent mammals, an intraoperative anaesthesia record must be kept and included with the surgeon's reports as part of the animal's record. The anaesthetist must be prepared to handle emergencies if they occur.

Preparation

- **Withhold food and water** from large animals for 12 hour prior to anaesthesia and from small animals for 2 hour to prevent regurgitation and aspiration. It is not necessary to withhold food and water from rodents prior to anaesthesia. Prolonged food or water deprivation is distressful to animals and are rarely necessary.

- **Have all drugs and equipment ready** before the animal is anaesthetized. You may not have time to look for things once the animal is under anaesthesia.

- **Have an assistant**. Anaesthesia takes time to perform and monitor. A person should be available to assist so that the surgeon does not have to break sterility to monitor the animal or administer medications.

- **Premedication** with atropine or glycopyrrolate (anticholinergics) may reduce the respiratory tract secretions in some animals.

- **Protect** the eyes from drying out using an ophthalmic ointment and protect them from being contaminated with surgical scrub solutions. Also protect pressure points, such as bony protrusions, from pressure necrosis or peripheral nerve damage by providing padding between the animal and the table.

Respiration

Most anaesthetics cause direct depression of the respiratory center in the brain and reduce ventilation. This is complicated by other factors that may interfere with respiration. When an animal is in lateral recumbency the lung that is down is being compressed by the rest of the body. Likewise, animals in dorsal recumbency may experience compression of the diaphragm by abdominal viscera. The airway may be compromised by regurgitated food or pharyngeal and tracheal secretions that normally would be removed by reflex swallowing or coughing. These reflexes are lost during anaesthesia. There are several ways to monitor and support the ventilation of an anaesthetized animal.

- **Intubate** the trachea whenever possible, even if injectable anaesthetics are being used. Intubation can be achieved on animals as small as a rat. This will prevent aspiration pneumonia and allow you to assist respiration if the animal stops breathing.

- **Assist respiration** during the procedure. This can be done with a mechanical ventilator. However, mechanical ventilation is rarely needed (unless a thoracotomy or diaphragmectomy is being performed) and can be detrimental to the animal if over-done. Attaching an AMBU bag to the endotracheal tube or using an anaesthetic machine's rebreathing bag will allow one to administer a deep breath every 2–5 min during the procedure. This will inflate all areas of the lungs and improve gas exchange. If the animal is not intubated, ventilation can be performed using a nose cone or face mask.

- **Monitor** respiratory function throughout the procedure and recovery.

- Monitor respiratory rate and depth (compare to normal for this species. One can expect them to be slightly decreased). Observe chest movement, or use a stethoscope or oesophageal stethoscope.

- Monitor the color of the mucous membranes (gums, conjunctiva, and vulvar mucosa). A bluish color means the animal is not getting enough oxygen —ventilate.

- Red-tinged foam present in the airway along with dyspnea (difficulty breathing) may indicate pulmonary oedema. This can result from overventilation or overhydration. A diuretic like furosemide can be administered, but prognosis is poor.

- Sophisticated respiratory monitoring can be achieved by measuring blood gasses, or expired oxygen and carbon dioxide concentration or by use of a pulse oximeter.

FLUID THERAPY/CARDIOVASCULAR SUPPORT

Many anaesthetics have direct effects on the heart or vasculature, decreasing cardiac output and blood pressure. This is further complicated by increased fluid requirements during anaesthesia and surgery that may result in hypovolemia. Fluid requirements are increased because: breathing dry, cold oxygen (if inhalant anaesthesia is used) increases respiratory fluid loss; the animal has not received its normal fluid intake since it was fasted; fluid may be lost through hemorrhage or exposure of moist viscera to room air; many anaesthetics are metabolized in the kidney (creating a slight diuresis minimizes renal toxicity).

To minimize the effects of surgery and anaesthesia on hydration

- Place an **intravenous catheter** whenever possible to provide access for fluids and medications.

- **Supplement fluids**, intravenously if possible; otherwise intraperitoneally or subcutaneously.
  - Fluid should be supplemented at the rate of 5–10 ml/kg/hour during anaesthesia
  - **Monitor** the hydration status. **Overhydration** results in frequent urination and pulmonary oedema, **underhydration** results in sticky mucous membranes, loss of skin elasticity, the eyes sinking into the orbit, decrease in blood pressure and increase in heart rate.
  - **To replace blood loss** with saline or lactated ringers, administer 3X the volume of blood lost by slow IV drip. Monitor the hematocrit. If it drops below 20%, whole blood replacement may be necessary.

- **Monitor cardiovascular function** by monitoring one or more of the following:
  - Mucous membrane color and capillary refill time (the time it takes for the mucous membranes to regain their normal color after pressure is applied).
  - Heart rate and rhythm —stethoscope or oesophageal stethoscope.
  - Pulse rate and pressure —using your fingers.
  - Blood pressure- arterial catheter or Doppler cuff required.
  - ECG.

If the animal has pale mucous membranes, the capillary refill time is greater than 2 seconds, or if the other cardiovascular parameters are out of normal range (determine normal for the species you are using!) you may have a cardiovascular emergency. Increasing the rate of intravenous fluid administration will improve cardiac output temporarily. However, the depth of anaesthesia will need to be reduced and if there is a primary cardiac problem it will require specific treatment. Consult with an expert veterinarian for more information on anaesthetic emergencies.

Thermoregulation

Animals frequently become hypothermic during anaesthesia because of inhalation of cold gases, exposure of body cavities to the room air, and loss of normal thermoregulatory mechanisms and behaviors. Hypothermia depresses all physiologic functions, including respiration and cardiac function, slows the metabolism of anaesthetics and results in prolonged recoveries. All of these can contribute to anaesthetic death. Hyperthermia is less common, but may occur because of excessive application of heat, hot surgery lights or malignant hyperthermia in genetically predisposed animals. To thermoregulate your patient:

- **Monitor the body temperature** frequently using a thermometer during the procedure and during anaesthetic recovery. While animal normally vary from species-to-species, in general, when body temperature drops below 99° F, an animal is considered hypothermic. Below 95–96° F an animal cannot regain normal body temperature without supplementation.

- **Prevent heat loss** by insulating cold surfaces with a blanket.

- **Prevent heat loss** during gas anaesthesia by utilizing low flow techniques that conserve heat.

  - **Supplement heat** with a thermal blanket (keep blanket temperature below 40° C to prevent burns!) or with pre-warmed fluids (Fig. 2.2).

  - **Treat hyperthermia** by administering intravenous fluids or applying water to foot pads or exposed skin. Only use an ice bath as a last resort, as it may cause cardiovascular shock.

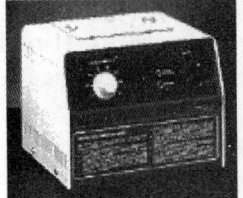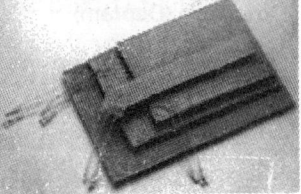

Fig. 2.2: Water blanket and heater

Monitoring Anaesthesia

The depth of anaesthesia must be monitored carefully. Animals that are too light will experience pain and may move during the procedure. Animals that are too deep run the risk of experiencing cardiopulmonary arrest. If an animal is too light the anaesthesia should be supplemented, if too deep, animals on gas anaesthesia can be turned down. Animals given injectable anaesthetics cannot be lightened directly. Instead respiratory and cardiovascular support must be administered until the anaesthetic is metabolized and the animal begins to lighten on its own.

To monitor the depth of anaesthesia, perform the following

- **Reflexes**: These reflexes disappear as the animal becomes deeper in the following order:
  - *Palpebral reflex*: Touching the eyelids causes blinking. The animal is light if it is blinking.
  - *Toe pinch reflex*: Pinching the toe or foot web will cause a pain response. If the animal withdraws the toe it is not deep enough. If it does not, it is not sensing pain.
  - *Corneal reflex*: Touching the cornea of the eye with a tuft of cotton results in a blink. Once the animal has lost its corneal reflex, it is too deep.
- **Muscle tone** increases as the depth of anaesthesia decreases, unless the animal is receiving a cataleptic drug like ketamine in the absence of a sedative. Test muscle tone by pulling on the lower jaw or a limb. Rigid tone indicates inadequate depth of anaesthesia.
- ***Monitor cardiopulmonary function and body temperature:*** As an animal becomes too deeply anaesthetized, respiration and cardiac output decrease, resulting in poor blood oxygenation and tissue perfusion and decreased blood pressure and temperature. Likewise, elevations in heart rate and blood pressure may be indications that an animal may be feeling pain and is anaesthetized too lightly. Monitor as previously described.

Emergency anaesthetic drugs are given in Table 2.1.

Table 2.1: Emergency anaesthetic drugs

Anesthetic emergency dose	Drugs (mg/kg)	Indications
Doxopram (Dopram)	1–5 IV (10x in farm animals)	Respiratory stimulant, for complete respiratory arrest only, use with CPR
Furosemide (Lasix)	2–IV, IMP	For pulmonary edema. Administer as needed
Naloxone (Narcan)	0.04 IV	For reversal of narcotic sedation or respiratory depression
Yohimbine	0.1–0.15 IV	Reversal of xylazine or detomidine sedation
Atropine	0.02–0.04 IV	For bradycardia
Epinephrine (1:1000)	0.1 ml/kg IV, IT, IC, IMP	For cardiac arrest only. Administer IV, intratracheal or intracardiac and perform cardiac massage
Lidocaine	2, IV (0.5 mg/kg in cats)	For diagnosed ventricular tachy-cardia only. Administer to effect and monitor.

POSITIONING LARGE IMMOBILIZED ANIMALS

The weight of the upper lung and heart will compress the lower lung and compromise its circulation and aeration. The larger the animal the more significant the effect (because of the greater weight of the upper lung and heart). It is very important to roll every immobilized animal to the opposite side every 5–10 minutes to prevent problems.

Secretions of saliva are increased in ruminants and felids with some immobilizing agents, i.e. ketamine and telazol. This is not seen in black bears. Atropine can be used to reduce these secretions but animals should still be positioned in a way to prevent these from entering the airway. In animals with long necks, like deer and elk, elevate the "Adam's Apple" (pharynx) by putting a rolled up jacket or backpack under the neck. The nose should then be allowed to rest slightly below the level of the pharynx. This allows saliva to flow out of the mouth not into the airway and makes it a little harder for stomach contents to be forced uphill, over the backpack, and if they do; they will hopefully run out the mouth or nose and not into the airway. Short necked animals like bison and bears, position on a slight downhill angle in hopes of keeping the airway clear. Do not position any animal on too much of a downhill grade or the weight of the abdominal contents will prevent the proper movement of the diaphragm.

In ruminants, the fermentation of the rumen's contents continues to produce gas during immobilization (up to 1 liter per minute in elk and bison). The only way for them to expel this gas is by belching (eructation). If the immobilization procedure will last more than 30 minutes you may have to pass a special floating stomach tube to suction off the gas. A regular stomach tube will get plugged with rumen contents. Even small amounts of this gas may force rumen contents up the esophagus and they may then gravitate into the airway. Inhalation pneumonia is very serious and frequently fatal. If very large amounts of gas build up, the pressure in the rumen may even begin to prevent blood from flowing through the vessels in the rumen wall and other vessels in the abdomen. These animals are hugely distended and if you thump them like a melon on their left side they will ping like an inner tube. This is a grave situation. Give them the reversing agent right away intravenously. Get them onto their chest and lift their head. If you can get them to eructate soon enough and fast enough, they might live.

Again, in short necked animals, the chest should only be slightly (10°) downhill from the abdomen. The weight of the abdominal contents will make it harder for the diaphragm to pull back. This will lessen ventilation.

During any immobilization: Work quickly, be efficient. Use reversible agents when possible so you can get these animals onto their feet when you are done. Remember: *Anesthesia is the controlled poisoning of an animal*.

STAGES OF GENERAL ANAESTHESIA

Stage 1: Stage of Voluntary Excitement or Stage of Analgesia

It is most characteristic of stage 1. It includes struggling and ataxia by the patient. To reduce the struggling by animals, preanesthetics are employed that minimize its response.

- Rapid acting anaesthetics are given to avoid the excitatory response of the animals.

- Pupils dilate and urine, feces may be voided due to fear.

The lower one half of its stage is characterized by the presence of analgesia.

Stage 2: Involuntary Excitement (Delirium)

- It begins with loss of consciousness and voluntary control. It characterizes CNS excitation.
- Selective blockade of reticulospinal inhibitory pathways is the basis for this stage. Intravenous induction by rapid acting agents should be done.
- Some anaesthetics like halothane, barbiturates bypass stage 2 and directly produce surgical anaesthesia.
- Anaesthetics which produce stage 1 and stage 2 and do not produce stage 3 are ketamine, N_2O, phencyclidine, enflurane, chloralose, trichloroethylene. During this stage pulse is rapid and strong and respiration is irregular.
- Reaction of eye to light reflex is retained.

Table 2.2 gives principal characteristic of stages and planes of ether anaesthesia in dog.

Grouping of anaesthetics according to induced stages

Drugs	Stages
Diethyl ether	1–4
N_2O	1–2
Trichloroethylene	
Ketamine	
Phencyclidine	1–2-Seizures
Alfachloralose	
Enfulrane	
Barbiturate	1–3–4
Halothane	
Methoxy flurane	

Stage 3: Surgical Anaesthesia

During this stage depressant action of the anaesthetic is extended from the cortex and midbrain to the spinal cord. Consciousness, pain as well as many neuromuscular reflexes are abolished, muscular relaxation occurs and coordinated movements disappear. All surgical procedures are done in this stage.

It is divided into four different planes

Light surgical anaesthesia: Nystagmus or oscillation of eyeball occurs but slower than the stage 2. Eyeball activity following induction and maintenance has been observed in cattle.

Table 2.2: Principal characteristics of stages and planes of ether anaesthesia in the dog

Stages of anaesthesia	Depression of CNS	Mucous membrane colour	Skeletal Muscle tone	Respiration	Pulse and blood pressure (BP)	Reflexes present					
						Lid	Corneal	Skin	Swallowing	Cough	Pedal
I–Analgesia (stage of voluntary movement)	Sensory cortex	Normal flushed		Rapid and irregular	Rapid pulse and elevated BP	+	+	+	+	+	+
II– Delirium (stage of involuntary movement)	Motor cortex DRS	Flushed		Very irregular (erratic)	Rapid pulse and elevated BP	+	+	+	+	+	+
III–Surgical											
Plane 1	Midbrain and spinal cord	Flushed, normal		Slow and regular	Normal pulse and normal BP	+	+	–	–	–	–
Plane 2	Spinal cord (increased depression)	Normal pale		Delayed thoracic, chiefly abdominal	Rapid weak pulse and fall in BP	–	–	–	–	–	–
Plane 3	Spinal cord (increased depression)	Normal pale		Delayed thoracic, chiefly	Rapid pulse and fall in BP	–	–	–	–	–	–
Plane 4	Slight medullary depression	Pale		Abdominal (shallow)	Rapid weak pulse and fall in BP	–	–	–	–	–	–
IV–Paralysis (death follows)	Medullary paralysis	Cyanosis	None	None	Shock level	–	–	–	–	–	–

- When inhalational anaesthesia is initiated in the cattle eyeball moves dorsally or upwards until cornea is partially observed by upper eyelid. As depth of anaesthesia is increased eyeball moves in vertical direction. Palpebral reflex can be elicited. This will be stage 2 plane 2 anaesthesia.
- With advancement of depth of anaesthesia the eyeball rotates dorsally until the cornea is centered within the palpebral opening.
- Major surgical procedures can be maintained at this depth of anaesthesia with 1.5–2.5 gm halothane with N_2O and oxygen.
- With continuance of plane 1 anaesthesia the cornea and palpebral reflexes are still present in dog but slow to respond to stimulation.
- Pedal reflex disappears almost at the onset of stage 3 in dog.
- Palpebral reflex is abolished at the end of plane 1 in all animals except cat.
- In rabbit, medium surgical anaesthesia is presented when palpebral reflex is lost following use of barbiturates.
- Loss of corneal reflex is dangerous or deep anaesthesia.
- In horse corneal reflex may be elicited under deep surgical anaesthesia with most anaesthetics up to the point of respiratory failure or beginning of stage 4.
- Lacrimation is increased in plane 1 and 2 in ruminants and is observed to persist longer than in other species.
- Corneal surface sometimes loses its sheen and has a glazed appearance when lower plane 3 or 4 is reached.
- Effect on enflurane on eye of dog is different than that seen with other anaesthetics.
- Pupillary constriction occurs despite of prior administration of atropine.
- Swallowing reflex disappears in the dog at the termination of stage 2 or upon entry into plane 1.
- In cat swallowing reflex is not abolished till early plane 2.
- Skeletal muscle tone decreases as a result of depression of ordinary postural reflex.

If relaxants are used in conjunction with anaesthetic agents assessment of depth of anaesthesia can not be done. Therefore photomotor reflex is checked. Both pupils react to a unilateral stimulus. In horse, the tail becomes lean and the penis often protrudes from the sheath. Cutting of the muscle or skin does not produce contraction. Laryngospasm is more readily encountered in cat during induction than any other species. Histamine release from mucus membrane induced by barbiturate anaesthesia may be responsible.

Spasm may occur from mechanical stimulation of larynx or pharynx under light anaesthesia or an attempt to intubate the trachea. Local anaesthetic sprays can minimize this.

DEEP SURGICAL ANAESTHESIA

In deep surgical anaesthesia, reflexes such as palpebral, corneal and pedal are completely depressed in most species by inhalant anaesthetics.

- *Skeletal muscle tone disappears:* Arterial pulse is rapid and weak. Diaphragmatic respiration is regular but shallower. Intercostal respiration is depressed early in plane 3.

- *Pupils are maximally dilated:* Most surgeries are performed in lighter planes of anaesthesia in large animals.

Stage 4: Medullary Paralysis

- Paralysis of vital regulatory centers in the medulla and death soon ensues if resuscitative measures are not taken.

- Respiratory arrest and fall in arterial BP are most characteristic of stage 4.

- Heart usually beats for a short time after respiration ceases. There is complete absence of all reflexes and complete dilatation of pupil. Anal and urinary sphincters are relaxed.

EEG

Stage 1: Activate pattern with higher frequencies.

Stage 2a: Intermittent bouts of high amplitude 2.5 Hz waves

Stage 2b: Continuous bizarre waves.

Stage 2c: 1.5 Hz slow waves with occasional spiking.

Stage 3: Mixture of 10–12 Hz spindle like bursts and irregular high amplitude slow waves.

Components of Balanced Anaesthesia

a. Sensory blockade (afferent).
b. Motor blockade (efferent).
c. Reflex blockade.
d. Mental blockade or awareness blockade.

Bibliography

1. Altura B.M., Carella B.T., et al., Fed Proc, 39:1584, 1980.
2. Borison H. L., Pharmacol Ther, 3:377, 1978.
3. Franc G.B. and Ohta M., Br J Pharmacol, 42:328, 1971.
4. Mc Donell.W., Mod. Vet. Pract., 53;31, 1972.
5. Smith R.A., Winter M. et al., Pharmacol Ther, 4, 1979.

3

Inhalational Agents

Inhalation of highly volatile agents was method of general anaesthesia. Ether and chloroform were the first general anaesthetics to be used.

Inhalation anaesthesia is superior to most injectable forms of anaesthesia in safety and efficacy. It is easy to adjust the anaesthetic depth. Because the anaesthetics are eliminated from the blood by exhalation, with less reliance on drug metabolism to remove the drug from the body, there is less chance for drug-induced toxicity. Inhalation anaesthetics are always administered to effect, because the dosage can vary greatly among individual animals and different animal species (Table 3.1). The disadvantages to inhalant anaesthesia are the complexity and cost of the equipment needed to administer the anaesthesia, and potential hazards to personnel. All inhalant drugs are volatile liquids. They should not be stored in animal rooms because the vapors are either flammable or toxic to inhale over extended periods of time. In particular, ether must be stored in a proper hood or cabinet for flammable materials.

Table 3.1: Inhalant agents

Drug	MAC	Response	Toxicity	Comments
Ether	3.2	Slow	Liver	Pre-medication with an anticholinergic may be necessary to reduce excessive respiratory secretions. Induction and recovery can be rough. Flammable and can become explosive with prolonged storage. Ether must be used according to appropriate safety guidelines.
Chloroform				A hazardous agent (carcinogenic) and cannot be used at U of M.
Methoxyflurane	0.2	Slow	Nephrotoxicity is potentiated by tetracyclines	It has good analgesic activity, but there is significant metabolism, ++ respiratory depression and + cardiac depression. This drug is not currently being manufactured. For a replacement, consider ether or diluted isoflurane.

Drug	MAC	Response	Toxicity	Comments
Halothane	0.9	Moderate	Hepato- and nephrotoxicity if the animal is hypotensive	++ cardiopulmonary depression, and a risk of malignant hyperthermia in some breeds/strains
Isoflurane	1.5	Fast	None	++ respiratory depression and + cardiovascular depression
Enflurane	2.0	Fast	None	++ cardiopulmonary depression and minimal respiratory depression
Nitrous oxide	180	Very fast	Hepatotoxic	Cannot be used as a sole anaesthetic agent. Do not exceed a 50% mix with oxygen and other inhalant agent to prevent hypoxia. Moderate analgesia is provided by nitrous oxide. In general, use of nitrous oxide in animals is discouraged.
Carbon dioxide (CO_2)	50–70	Very fast	Cerebral anoxia	Can be used as an anaesthetic for brief procedures and as a euthanasia agent. It has antinociceptive activity and causes unconsciousness prior to hypoxia. It is necessary to monitor carefully and work quickly, as animals die quickly (1–2 min) after losing consciousness, and likewise they wake up quickly when exposed to room air. Appropriate for quick procedures such as tail snipping, ear marking and orbital bleeding. Poses minimal hazard to personnel and can be used in laboratories or animal room

MAC: This is the % concentration of the drug needed to anaesthetize 50% of animals. It does vary somewhat by species and by individual. 1.2 X MAC is an approximate vaporizer setting for maintenance of anaesthesia. Induction generally requires 2–3 X MAC. MAC listed here is for rats (ether), mice (CO_2), goat (enflurane) and dogs (all others).

Response: This refers to how rapidly concentrations in the blood change when the lung alveolar concentration is changed. Slow anaesthetics have slow induction and recovery times.

Toxicity: Drugs that are metabolized by the body can cause toxicity, especially if a pre-existing organ dysfunction exists.

METHOXYFLURANE: (METOFANE, PENTHANE)

2, 2, dichloro1, 1 difluroethyl methyl ether.

Boiling point 104.8°C. It has fruit like odour and is non-explosive and non-inflammable at 20ºC.

Systemic Actions

a *CNS:* Anaesthesia induced in large animals by inhalation within 4 to 11 mins. Stage 2 is bypassed which produce excellent anaesthesia. In the cows uninterrupted tremors have been seen throughout all stages of anaesthesia.

b. *Pulmonary system:* Respiratory activity is gradually depressed until respiratory arrest occurs. Tidal volume reduces by 50%.

c. *CVS:* Heart rate does not change appreciably during anaesthesia in horse. Moderate tachycardia is observed in cattle. Cardiac arrthymias may occur occasionally but respond to atropine. Epinephrine and norepinephrine during methoxyfurane anaesthesia is well tolerated. Cardiac output is decreased by 25 to 40%. Arterial blood pressure is reduced considerably especially as depth of anaesthesia increases.

d. *Liver and kidney:* Its not hepatotoxic. Hepatotoxic effects of steroids and phenothiazine derivatives are increased. Renal functions altered because of decreased renal blood flow. Vasoconstriction metabolism of methoxyflurane may cause renal damage.

e. *Muscle:* Relaxes smooth and skeletal muscles.

f. *Fetus:* As labour analgesia.

Advantages

- In small and large species
- Non inflammable.
- Good analgesia and relaxation.

Disadvantages

- High blood solubility makes it difficult to change depth of anaesthesia.

Contraindications

- None. Use with caution in hepatic and renal impairment.

Clinical Use

- Used in combination with barbiturate anaesthesia, N_2O and ether.
- Compatible with large number of preanaesthetic and anaesthetic agents
- Large animals maintenance of anaesthesia.
- In small animal for induction as well as maintenance.

Halothane (fluthane)

$C_2HBrClF_3$

B.P–50.2°C

Sweetish odour and non-explosive or inflammable.

Effects on Systems

CVS: Myocardial depressant. As myocardial depression increases, the CVP rises. Marked increase in CVP seen in horse.

Marked arterial hypotension in horse and mean arterial pressure decreases. It influences myocardial performance by affecting on calcium dependent mechanism. In subhuman primates unlike dog the addition of N_2O to halothane O_2 anaesthesia results in less depression of cardiovascular junction than using halothane O_2 alone.

- In horse halothane decreases cardiac output, stroke volume and left ventricular work.
- Cardiac arrhythmias observed during the induction.
- Epinephrine and norepinephrine are contraindicated during induction due to risk of arrthymias.
- Use of halothane in mice, dogs and monkeys indicate that it has a low margin of safety.

Thermoregulatory functions: Thermoregulatory function of hypothalamus is depressed during halothane anaesthesia. It may trigger malignanat hyperthermia.

It is treated by dantrolene

- *Liver:* Hypercapnia enhance the toxicity of halothane upon liver functions similarly to that of chloroform. Microsomal enzymes inducing agents such as Phenobarbital or other inducers must precede exposure to halothane.
- *Kidney:* Reduction in renal blood flow. Blood urea increases but returns to normal after recovery from anaesthesia.
- *Skeletal muscles:* If additional relaxation over halothane is needed, succinylcholine or pancuronium can be used.
- *Fetus:* Tone decreases
- *Endocrine:* Gonadotropins and steroid hormone's concentration decreases.

Advantages

1. Smooth maintenance of anaesthesia in large animals.
2. Recovery is rapid.

Disadvantage

Cardiac depression.

Contraindication

1. Should not be used in animals with recently received aminoglycosides.
2. Animals receiving phenobarbital should not be given halothane.
3. Animals with chronic heart failure.
4. Pregnant animals.

Use

1. Induction and maintenance of anaesthesia with or without assistance.
2. Large and small animals both can be given this.
3. Very effective in cattle anaesthesia.

N$_2$O

- Colorless non-irritant, slightly sweetish smelling, non-inflammable, heavier than air.
- It supports combustion. When nitrous oxide is used in conjunction with halothane or methoxyflurane, the concentration of these gases can be reduced for maintenance of anaesthesia.
- It is incapable of inducing depth of anaesthesia greater than stage 2. It must be used in combination with O$_2$ so that severe hypoxia does not occur during induction or maintenance of anaesthesia. It induces effect on the hemopetic and reticuloendothelial system.
- Under no circumstances should N$_2$O be given for maintenance of anaesthesia in humans be more than 70%.

CARDIOVASCULAR SYSTEM

Mean arterial pressure, mean pulmonary arterial pressure, heart rate, cardiac output, stroke volume, total peripheral resistance and left ventricular works increase in the dogs when 75% N$_2$O is added to halothane anaesthesia during spontaneous breathing.

- It is mild alfa adrenergic stimulant.
- Vital functions of the body are not significantly altered if hypoxia is not permitted to develop.
- Cardiopulmonary function is not affected.

Contraindication

In animals with trapped air pocket such as seen in pneumoperitonium or pneumothorax nitrogen diffuses from an air pocket into blood plasma much more slowly than N$_2$O enters it from the blood plasma during equilibration. Consequently the trapped gas will increase.

Clinical Use

It usually can not be used alone in maintenance of anaesthesia.

It has been used to maintain anaesthesia in the horse, pig, ruminants, dog ,cat and rabbit. It should be supplemented with an anaesthetic that is relatively insoluble in blood (halothane) to attain high alveolar tension. Use of nitrous following premedication with fentanyl, droperidol in the dog appears to be effective. It enhances ketamine by reducing the total dose of ketamine by 39% and shortening the recovery period by 64%.

Ether (Ethyl ether, diethyl ether)

Colorless highly volatile liquid with characteristic odour and burning sweetish taste.

B.P–35° C: It should be stored in cool place but not refrigerator.

Nervous system: The anaesthetic potency of ether is less than that of halothane or methoxyflurane. Cortical action potential activity is suppressed by ether anaesthesia and is not affected when sensory fibers in the sciatic nerve are stimulated.

Respiratory system: Alkalosis or hypocapnia results in irregular respiration.

During deep surgical anaesthesia respiratory centers are depressed progressively until the level of anaesthesia approaches stage 4 where breathing is absent. Ether vapors are irritating to respiratory tract and stimulate profuse secretion of mucus.

Cardiovascular system: It has a little effect on heart in anaesthetic concentrations.

Heart rate and blood pressure are increased during the excitement of induction due to release of epinephrine.

Cardiac output during light surgical anaesthesia is increased by about 20%. Deep surgical anaesthesia causes a progressive fall in blood pressure as result of drop in cardiac output and progressive depression of the vasomotor centers with peripheral vasodilatation.

Kidneys: Urine output is probably decreased by antidiuretic hormone of the pituitary.

Liver: Prolonged etherization on successive days produces no demonstrable pathology in livers of dogs.

GIT: Depresses the tone and motility of the GIT.

Skeletal muscle: Profound relaxation is achieved partly by its depressant effect upon the extrapyramidal and pyramidal pathways of the CNS. An adverse interaction of ether and neomycin resulting in death has been reported in human.

Endocrine: Increase the plasma corticosterone level significantly.

Metabolism: The general level of metabolism is decreased.

Advantages

Most popular volatile anaesthetic used in rodents. It is a low cost anaesthetic.

Disadvantage

Its vapours are flammable and it boils at a low temperature. It irritates mucus membranes.

CHLOROFORM

CHCl$_3$: It is a clear colourless volatile liquid having a characteristic odour and a burning sweet taste.

Respiratory system: During the induction of anaesthesia, respiration is accelerated and deepened because of struggling. It progressively depresses respiration. Bronchial musculature is relaxed.

CVS: It is 25 to 30 times as poisonous as ether on direct contact with the mammalian heart. It sensitizes the myocardium to the catecholamine thus increasing the risk of serious cardiac arrthymias and or ventricular fibrillation.

Kidney: It depresses kidney functions. Anuria may occur after recovery and albuminuria is often quite marked.

Metabolism: It is decreased by chloroform anaesthesia.

Hyperglycemia results from the decreased tissue metabolism of blood sugar and also from increased conversion of liver glycogen into blood glucose after release of epinephrine during induction.

Liver: It decreases liver efficiency as measured by dye excretion and other liver function tests. It has been suggested that metabolism of chloroform may result in formation of free radicals.

Advantages

- Inexpensive
- Easily stored
- Potent
- Nonflammable

Applicable by open drop technique and provides prompt induction.

Use of chloroform for brief periods of anaesthesia in large animals and also for emergency anaesthesia in many species under a variety of conditions.

Isoflurane: It is chemically 1-chloro-2,2,2-trifluroethyl diflouromethyl ether. Isoflurane and enflurane are structural isomers. It does not interact chemically with sodalime and is unaffected by natural light.

Cardiovascular system: It depresses cardiovascular function in horses to a lesser degree than enflurane. It is essentially equivalent to halothane as a depressant of CVS

In dogs it depresses cardiovascular function to a lesser degree than enflurane.

Respiratory system: Isoflurane and enflurane like halothane are potent depressors of ventilation in horses.

In experimental ponies following two hour anaesthetic period, recovery is shortest after isoflurane followed by enflurane, halothane and methoxyflurane.

However, the standing position is achieved more rapidly after enflurane than isoflurane. The smoothest recovery occurs after isoflurane anaesthesia followed by methoxyflurane, halothane and enflurane.

Desflurane

- It is fluorinated methyl ethyl ether. It contains no chlorine or bromide and therefore should not deplete the ozone layer.
- It has pungent odour, irritating.
- Boiling point–22.8 °C.

It cannot be administered using the standard vaporizer. A new vaporizer has been developed in which the anaesthetic agent is converted to gas by heating it to a constant temperature and maintaining it at constant pressure about 200 kpa.

Its blood gas solubility coefficient is 0.42, lowest of all the inhalational agents.

Central nervous system: Effects of desflurane on the EEG is similar to isoflurane. Both produce a dose dependant suppression. Desflurane causes dose dependant cerebral vasodilatation and dose dependant reduction in cerebral metabolism. It also impairs cerebral autoregulation to the same extent as isoflurane. It increases lumbar CSF pressure in normocapnic patients without an intracranial mass lesion.

Respiratory system: It is unsuitable for an induction because of extreme irritability to the airway. Concentration of 6% or more have been shown to cause coughing, breath holding and laryngospasm in children and the adults. It is a potent respiratory depressant. It causes a dose dependent decrease in the tidal volume and an increase in respiratory rate with an overall reduction in minute alveolar ventilation. $PaCO_2$ increases and the ventilatory response to CO_2 is increased.

The intrapulmonary shunt fraction and physiological dead space are also increased.

Cardiovascular system: It causes a dose dependant tachycardia in humans that is associated within a depression in myocardial contractility and a decrease in the SVR resulting from peripheral vasodilatation.

In ventilated patients the cardiac index remains unchanged and the systemic blood pressure fall. Studies in dogs suggest splanchnic that blood flow is well preserved.

Clinical Uses

It is a cardiostable drug and can be used in the patients needing safe anaesthesia and rapid recovery.

It is a potent depressant of neuromuscular functions, augmenting neuromuscular block due to muscle relaxants requiring less doses. It is however pungent smelling and irritating to awake patients, making it unsuitable for anaesthesia induction by face mask. Desflurane requires special vaporizer for administration which is expensive unless lower flow rates are used.

SEVOFLURANE

- It is a newer and safer anaesthetic to a greater degree than with halothane.
- It abolishes the hypoxic pulmonary vasoconstriction in a dose dependant manner in isolated perfused rabbit lungs.
- It is also an effective bronchodilator. It is as effective as isoflurane in attenuating bronhcospasm in antigen induced anaphylaxis in dogs.

Cardiovascular Effects

It can cause tachycardia and has a minimal effect on heart rate. Animal studies have suggested that it can cause a direct depressant effect on heart through action on calcium channels. It decreased cardiac output which causes a decrease in the systemic blood pressure.

- It also causes a reduction in pulmonary arterial pressure which is not dose dependant.
- Hepatic and renal blood flows are well preserved.
- Sevoflurane does not sensitize heart to the effect of epinephrine. It does not cause sympathetic mediated cardiovascular stimulation associated with a rapid increase in end tidal concentration that is seen with desflurane and isoflurane.

Neuromuscular Effects

Dose dependant muscle relaxation. At deeper planes it provides sufficient relaxation to allow tracheal intubation.

It prolongs train of four response, when monitored with a peripheral nerve stimulator, when compared with fentanyl droperidol combination with halothane.

TOXICITY

Metabolism of sevoflurane results in the production of inorganic fluoride ions and HFIP.

- It can cause nephrotoxicity in humans involves degradation product called compound A. When Sevoflurane is exposed to sodalime or barylime it is absorbed and degraded to a variety of compounds of which compound A and compound B are produced in significant amounts.
- The addition of water to soda lime and use of partially exhausted soda lime seem to reduce production of compound A during low flow anaesthesia.

Clinical Uses

Lower blood gas solubility, so induction and recovery are slightly quicker. It offers a good hemodynamic stability. It contains no chloride ions and therefore its environment friendly.

Pleasant to inhale and therefore suitable for inhalational induction.

Bibliography

1. Hasting S.G. Booth N. H. and Hopwood M.L., In L.K. Bustad and R.K. McClellan, ed., *Swine in Biomedical Research,* p.679, 1966.
2. Healey E. G., In O. Graham Jones, ed., *Small Animal Anesthesia,* p.59, 1964.
3. Szabuniewicz M. Davis R. H., Jr., and Wiersig D.O., *Veterinary Anaesthesia,* 1st ed. 1975.
4. Occupational Safety and Health Administration. New Publication of National Institute of Occupational Safety and Health (NIOSH). Washington DC. US Govt. Printing Office, 1992.
5. P. Kumar, *Textbook of Anaesthesiology,* 1st ed., Paras Med. Publishers, Hyderabad, 2008.
6. Soma L.R., *Textbook of Veterinary Anaesthesia,* p. 621, 1971.
7. M.C. Donell W. *Modern Veterinary Practice,* 53, 31, 1972.

4

Intravenous Induction Agents

THE PERFECT ANAESTHETIC DRUG

The perfect anaesthetic is a drug that produces no heart or lung depression, provides adequate analgesia, provides excellent muscle relaxation, is not metabolized by the patient, is not toxic, and is readily reversible. Although the general anaesthetics in use in veterinary anaesthesia today are great improvements compared to the anaesthetics of yesteryear, they still fall far short of the perfect agent.

Probably, the most desirable general anaesthetic for a young, healthy dog is the one, veterinarian is most familiar with. There are a great many anaesthetic drugs available to today's practicing veterinarian, however most practitioners use a few carefully chosen anaesthetics with which they have the most experience and the most confidence. A veterinarian's experience in the use of a certain anaesthetic drug often will more than offset one or two undesirable properties of a general anaesthetic agent.

General

Some of the drugs listed here do not possess all three criteria for an anaesthetic and must be used in combinations to achieve full anaesthesia or may be administered individually for restraint, sedation or analgesia. Often injectable drugs are used in combinations. These drugs tend to have synergistic effects. Mixing them can significantly reduce the dosage needed for any individual drug.

As with inhalation anaesthesia, injectables are titrated to a given effect. Dosages listed are just the guidelines. Effects may vary among individuals. If a drug is scheduled by the Controlled Substances Act, licenses are required to purchase them, and written records must be kept of their use. Anaesthesia policy outlines these requirements. Anaesthetic drugs that have exceeded their expiration date may not be used, even for terminal procedures.

Injectable anaesthetics are, in general, metabolized by the liver and excreted by the kidneys. Animals with liver or kidney disease should not be anaesthetized with these agents. Inhalation anaesthetics are safer for use in sick or debilitated animals, because there is minimal metabolism, the amount of anaesthetic administered can be controlled and one can cease administration as the sit uation dictates. Injectable anaesthetics offer the advantage of requiring less expensive equipment.

Phenothiazine and Buterophenone Sedatives

These sedatives include acepromazine, chlorpromazine, droperidol (Innovar-Vet) and azaperone (Stresnil). These drugs have excellent sedative properties, as well as muscle relaxation, antiemetic and antiarrhythmogenic effects. They have no analgesic activity, but when administered with other anaesthetics can potentiate their effect. Acepromazine is the most commonly used. It is recommended as a sole sedative in dogs and as an anaesthetic premedication to improve both induction and recovery (it is long acting) in all species. Droperidol is usually used in combination with the narcotic, fentanyl and has been associated with aggressive behavior in dogs.

Disadvantages of these sedatives are that they are alpha adrenergic blockers and cause peripheral vasodilation which can lead to hypothermia. They may have prolonged activity in hounds. Acepromazine and chlorpromazine decrease seizure threshold, and are contraindicated in animals with CNS lesions. Because these sedatives lack analgesic activity it is important to realize that any painful stimulation of the animal may cause it to emerge rapidly from the sedated state.

Thiazines

The thiazine derivatives include xylazine and medetomidine. These two drugs are very similar. They are alpha-2 adrenergic agonists. They cause CNS depression resulting in sedation, emesis and mild analgesia. They also cause hypotension, second degree atrio-ventricular block and bradycardia. Occasionally, aggressive behavior changes have been seen in dogs. They are very useful in combination with other drugs, like ketamine for anaesthesia in rodents and swine. They are best avoided in dogs, cats and nonhuman primates, primarily because their significant side effects can be avoided by using other drugs. They can be used alone for minor procedures in ruminants. *It is important to note that the dose for these drugs in ruminants is 1/10 of that used in other species.* The effects of the thiazine derivatives can be reversed with yohimbine or atapimazole. Use of these drugs with the reversal agent shortens anaesthetic recovery and greatly expands the safety and utility of these drugs. Xylazine is a potent analgesic in frogs appropriate for relief of post-surgical pain.

Opiates

The opiates, sometimes referred to as narcotics, are a large class of drugs that exert their effects on the opiate receptors in the central nervous system. Depending on the receptors a drug is active against, and the type of action it has on the receptor, the effects of narcotics can be primarily analgesic, as with buprenorphine, pentazocine and nalbuphine, or a mixture of analgesia and euphoria with sedation as with butorphanol, fentanyl (innovar-Vet), morphine, meperidine or oxymorphone. Opiates have little effect on the myocardium. However, there can be significant respiratory depression, as well as other sideeffects such as nausea and vomiting, delayed gastric emptying, hypotension, and bradycardia. Some species may develop hyperexcitability if given certain opiates. These sideeffects are seen more with the mixed effect opiates than the pure analgesics. Naloxone is a opiate antagonist that can be used to reverse the effects of other narcotics. Other opiates, like buprenorphine, nalbuphine and nalorphine, have mixed agonist-antagonist effects and may interfere with the effects of concurrently administered narcotics. All opiates are controlled substances and their use requires special record keeping. These drugs can be given alone as a post-procedural analgesic or in combination with other agents to provide balanced anaesthesia, restraint with analgesia for minor procedures, or can be used to decrease the dose of an anaesthetic that is needed to provide a surgical plane of anaesthesia.

Barbiturates

The barbiturates are an acid ring molecule with various ring substitutes that imparts the drug with different properties. Barbiturates are also considered narcotics.

- Phenobarbital is the longest-acting of the barbiturates. Its use is limited primarily to sedation or as an anticonvulsant.

- Pentobarbital is a short-acting oxybarbiturate. It is usually used as a sole anaesthetic agent, or is supplemented with an analgesic.When given intravenously, about 50–75% of the calculated dose is administered. Within several minutes the animal will lose consciousness, although it may experience a brief period of excitement. When the jaw muscle tone is relaxed, the animal should be intubated. If given intraperitoneally, usually the entire dose of pentobarbital is given and surgery can be performed when the animal no longer reacts to a toe pinch. Anesthesia from pentobarbital can last from 45–120 min, depending on the dose given. Additional drug can be supplemented as needed, being careful not to cause overdose.

- Thiopental and thiamylal are thiobarbiturates that are considered ultrashort acting. Similar to these is methohexital which is an oxybarbiturate. Because of the extremely short duration of activity (up to 10 min with methohexital, up to 15–20 min with thiopental or thiamylal) of these drugs, they are usually used as an intravenous anaesthetic induction agent to allow intubation prior to use of inhalant anaesthesia. Use is similar to that described for pentobarbital. However, when low doses are given IV, there may only be several minutes of anaesthesia before the animal begins to waken. This is desirable as an induction agent. If higher doses are given for longer effect, care must be taken not to overdose. Longer anaesthesia may be seen when these drugs are used intraperitoneally in rodents.

- *Effects and side effects:* In general the barbiturates cause generalized central nervous system depression, which can be dosed to provide sedation or general anaesthesia. The drugs also have an anticonvulsant effect. Analgesia provided by the barbiturates is poor and a relatively deep plane of anaesthesia is required for surgery, unless used in combination with analgesics. The barbiturates have significant cardiopulmonary depression, with apnoea and hypotension commonly seen. Anaesthetic death is common in animals that are not receiving supportive care. The barbiturates induce hepatic microsomal enzymes and may increase the metabolic rate of other drugs. Tolerance to the barbiturates develops with repeated use and doses may have to be adjusted accordingly.

Precautions

- Barbiturates are poorly water soluble and are only available in intravenous preparations, although they are frequently administered intraperitoneally to smaller animals with limited venous access. Because of their acidic properties, barbiturates can be irritating when administered intraperitoneal, or if any leak from the intravenous injection site. Perivascular barbiturates can result in significant tissue necrosis and skin sloughing. If any barbiturate leaks (a visible swelling is seen during injection), the best thing to do is to infuse the area with sterile saline at several times the volume of the original leak. Some people recommend mixing the saline with 2% lidocaine to prevent pain and subsequent self-trauma.

- The barbiturates redistribute rapidly into all body tissues, including fat. Redistribution is one way that the drug is eliminated from the blood and obese animals may require higher doses of barbiturates to induce anaesthesia. However, once the fat becomes saturated with the drug, metabolism becomes the primary means of elimination. Because metabolism is much slower, a common problem in administering barbiturates is overdosing with prolonged anaesthetic recoveries (up to several days). Because of this problem it is best to titrate the dose carefully rather than administer large boluses. For obese animals, alternative anaesthetics might be considered, although to a greater or lesser extent, most anaesthetics share this problem when administered to obese animals. Prolonged anaesthetic recovery can also be a problem when barbiturates are used in older animals or other animals with compromised hepatic and renal function which decreases metabolism of the drugs.

- Barbiturates are also controlled substances and their use requires special record keeping.

- Despite these disadvantages, the barbiturates are perhaps the most commonly used anaesthetics in laboratory animals. Overall, they are a relatively easy to use anaesthetic.

DISSOCIATIVE ANAESTHETICS

The dissociative anaesthetics include ketamine (Ketalar, Ketaset) and tiletamine (Telazol). These drugs are easy to use and have a wide margin of safety for most laboratory species. They are cyclohexamine compounds, chemically related to piperazine and phencyclidine. The dissociative anaesthetics uncouple sensory, motor, integrative, memory and emotional activities in the brain, providing there is a functional cerebral cortex. The state induced by high doses of ketamine is best described as catalepsy and is not accompanied by central nervous system depression. There is depression of respiratory function, but cardiovascular function is maintained. Muscle relaxation is very poor.

Ketamine and telazol are supplied in a solution of 100 mg/ml. Telazol is a 50–50 mixture of tiletamine and zolezepam, a benzodiazepine. These drugs can be injected intramuscularly (IM), intraperitoneally (IP) or intravenously (IV). IP and IM injections of the dissociative anaesthetics can be painful, as the drug is very acidic. Induction time for IM administration is three to five minutes; peak effect lasts about 20 min in most laboratory species. IP induction times are longer than with IM administration and recovery may be prolonged. Because the volumes needed are very small, in small animals there is no real advantage to IP injection and IM injection should be used whenever possible. Induction time following IV administration is rapid with only about 10 min of anaesthesia provided.

Approximately 1/2 of the dose should be given when dosing IV. The drug can be supplemented as needed.

The swallowing reflex is often preserved in animals receiving dissociative anaesthetics. This may help prevent aspiration pneumonia if the animal regurgitates. However, this is not 100% and fasting and intubation are still recommended when using these anaesthetics. The animal's eyes will usually remain open and the corneas should be protected with a layer of ophthalmic ointment. These drugs have poor analgesic activity, especially for visceral pain, and should be used in conjunction with an analgesic for abdominal, intracranial, orthopedic, ophthalmic or thoracic surgery.

Other Anaesthetics

Propofol is a sedative/hypnotic that can be used for induction or maintenance of general anaesthesia. Analgesic effect is poor and addition of an analgesic to the anaesthetic regimen is necesssary for surgery. The drug comes as an emulsion that must be mixed and used within several days. The advantages of propofol are that it has rapid induction and recovery times. It can be easily titrated and given to effect for prolonged periods without resulting in prolonged recovery. The disadvantages are that it must be given intravenously, it is expensive, it may result in apnoea and it can cause bradycardia and hypotension.

Alpha chloralose or **chloral hydrate** is a mild hypnotic drug that does not produce complete anaesthesia because of its poor analgesic properties. Chloral hydrate is shorter acting (1– 2 h) than alpha chloralose (8–10 h). The primary advantage of these drugs is the minimal cardiopulmonary depression seen at the normal doses (high doses can cause severe respiratory depression). The disadvantage is that they can only be used alone for non-painful procedures. In addition, the drugs are very irritating to the GI tract, causing a dynamic ileus if given IP and ulcers if given orally. Therefore IV use is the only route recommended. These drugs should not be used if any other alternative is available.

Tribromoethanol is a short-acting anaesthetic used in rodents for surgeries. The drug has rapid induction and recovery (15 min of surgical anaesthesia and up to 90 min for complete recovery). The effect on animals is reported to be quite variable. Tribromoethanol was commonly used in the past but its use is now discouraged. Abdominal adhesions caused by IP administration have been reported to cause high post-procedural mortality, however, other studies have not demonstrated this. Tribromoethanol is not available commercially and must be prepared. Sterile preparation procedures are essential. The drug must be stored in the dark at 4°C to prevent degradation.

Urethane is a long-acting (8–10h) anaesthetic with minimal cardiopulmonary depression. The drug is used for long procedures in rodents. However, it is carcinogenic and is only allowed to be used with special justification and only for terminal (acute) procedures.

Non Steroidal Anti-inflammatory Drugs (NASIDs)

Analgesics are pain relievers most often given after a surgery. Narcotic analgesics have already been described above. Nonsteroidal antiiflammatory drugs (NSAIDs) may also be used for their analgesic effect. The NSAIDs consist of drugs like aspirin, ketoprofen, acetaminophen, flunixin and ketorolac. There are a large number of these drugs available, however, relatively few are used in animals. NSAIDs are, in general, less potent analgesics than are the narcotics. However, in specific instances they can have similar activity.

The advantages of the NSAIDs are that they do not cause sedation nor are they addictive as are the narcotic analgesics. There are no special recordkeeping requirements. In addition, they are more effective against pain caused by inflammation, such as is seen with tissue repair, orthopedic surgery, infection and injury.

The NSAIDs have several sideeffects related to their pronounced antiprostaglandin (anti-cyclooxygenase and in some cases lipooxygenase) activity. This is peripheral with most drugs, but is primarily central with acetaminophen. These effects can alter immune function, platelet function and can cause gastrointestinal ulceration. In addition, the NSAIDs all have the potential to cause nephro- and hepatotoxicity. This is variable among species. Cats, in particular, are sensitive to the NSAIDs. Acetaminophen is contraindicated in cats due to risk of methemoglobinemia.

- Acetaminophen is a mild analgesic, antipyretic, no effect on platelet function/bleeding time.
- Aspirin is a mild analgesic, antipyretic, antiinflammatory, affects platelet function/bleeding time.
- Carprofen is a nonsteroidal antiinflammatory drug with antiinflammatory and analgesic effects and lower risk for toxicity in animals than other NSAIDs.
- Flunixin meglumine (Banamine) is a potent analgesic, antiinflammatory, antipyretic. Has potential for GI ulceration, hepato and nephrotoxicity.
- Ketoprofen is a moderate potency analgesic, antiinflammatory, antipyretic and has potential for GI ulceration, hepato- and nephrotoxicity, affects platelet function/bleeding time.
- Ketorolac (Toradol) is a potent analgesic, antiinflammatory, antipyretic has potential for hepato- and nephrotoxicity, less potential for GI ulceration than other NSAIDs, affects platelet function/bleeding time.

Acetaminophen: Alternative to acetaminophen in rats and mice.

Anaesthetic drug combinations: In general, by mixing anaesthetic and analgesic drugs, the dose required for each individual drug is reduced, sometimes quite dramatically. Start at the low end of the dose range listed; can always give more if needed! Drugs not listed below can be mixed using the same concepts, mix a sedative or hypnotic with an analgesic. Do not mix drugs in the syringe until it is determined that they are compatible when mixed. If in doubt administer separately.

Ketamine/diazepam: Mix drugs 1:1 by volume and administer 0.1 ml/kg IV for restraint, anaesthetic induction or for non-painful procedures. This gives excellent muscle relaxation, has minimal respiratory or cardiovascular depression and the animals wake up smoothly and quickly (within 10–15 min). Visually, these drugs do not appear to mix completely. When combined and administered as described, the dose is 5 mg/kg ketamine and 0.25 mg/kg diazepam.

Ketamine/acepromazine: Mix 10 mg acepromazine (1 ml) with 1 g (10 ml) ketamine and give 0.1–0.3 ml/kg mixture IM or IV (up to 0.6 ml/kg in rodents and rabbits). Good for restraint, but not for painful procedures. When combined and administered as described, the dose is 0.09–0.27 mg/kg acepromazine and 9–27 mg/kg ketamine.

Acepromazine/butorphanol: Mix drugs 1:1 by volume (using 10 mg/ml butorphanol) and administer at 0.01–0.02 ml/kg IV or IM. Creates a hypnotic state that is good for restraint and minor procedures that cause some pain. When combined and administered as described, the dose is 0.05–0.1 mg/kg butorphanol and 0.05–0.1 mg/kg acepromazine.

Ketamine/acepromazine/butorphanol: Mix 10 mg acepromazine (1 ml), 10 mg butorphanol (1 ml) with 1 g (10 ml) ketamine and give 0.1–0.3 ml/kg of mixture IM or IV (up to 0.6–0.8 ml/kg in rodents and rabbits). Good for restraint and moderately painful procedures. More cardiac and respiratory depression will be seen with this mixture than with ketamine alone. When combined and administered as described, the dose is 8–25 mg/kg ketamine, 0.08–0.25 mg/kg acepromazine, and 0.08–0.25 mg/kg butorphanol. For rodents and rabbits, the dose is 50–67 mg/kg ketamine, 0.5–0.7 mg/kg acepromazine, and 0.5–0.7 mg/kg butorphanol.

Ketamine/xylazine: Good for restraint and painful procedures. Administer IM, IP, or IV. More cardiac and respiratory depression will be seen with this mixture than with ketamine alone. Use 100 mg/ml ketamine and 20 mg/ml xylazine to create any of the mixtures listed in Table 4.1.

Do not use this cocktail of ketamine-xylazine for cattle, sheep, goats, or other ruminants. Giving ketamine and xylazine simultaneously is not recommended for horses.

Table 4.1: Ketamine-xylazine combination doses

Species	Ratio by volume (ket:xyl)	Vol to give (ml/kg)	Dose (per kg body weight)	Sedation insufficient? May redose once
Mouse	mix 2:1	1.5	100 mg Ket + 10 mg Xyl	At 1/2 original volume
	mix 8:3	2.75	200 mg Ket + 15 mg Xyl	*Not recommended*
Rat	mix 3:2	1.25	75 mg Ket + 10 mg Xyl	At 1/3 original volume
Rabbit	mix 4:3	0.6	34 mg Ket + 5.2 mg Xyl	At original volume
Dogs, cats,	mix 1:1	0.1–0.3	5–15 mg Ket to 1–3 mg Xyl	See applicable range

Ketamine/midazolam/butorphanol: Mix 0.4 ml each ketamine and midazolam with 0.01 ml of 10 mg/ml butorphanol and administer 0.8 ml/kg. This provides good muscle relaxation and surgical anaesthesia in rodents. When combined and administered as described, the dose is 40 mg/kg ketamine, 2 mg/kg midazolam, and 0.1 mg/kg butorphanol.

Telazol/xylazine: *For pigs:* reconstitute powdered telazol (tiletamine and zolazepam) with 5 ml of xylazine instead of saline. For pigs < 50 kg, use 20 mg/ml xylazine to make the cocktail. For pigs > 50 kg, use 100 mg/ml xylazine. Administer at 0.05–0.1 ml/kg IV or IM. When combined and administered as described, the dose is 2.5–5 mg/kg tiletamine, 2.5–5 mg/kg zolazepam, and either 1–2 mg/kg xylazine (if 20 mg/ml xylazine was used) or 5–10 mg/kg xylazine (100 mg/ml xylazine). For rats, use 20 mg/ml xylazine and administer up to 0.4 ml/kg IM. Here, the dose can be as high as 8 mg/kg xylazine, 20 mg/kg tiletamine, and 20 mg/kg zolazepam. More cardiac and respiratory depression will be seen with this mixture than with telazol alone. Reversal with yohimbine 0.1–0.15 mg/kg (IM or IV) or atipamezole at 0.25 (IM) or 0.2 (IV) mg/kg is recommended to shorten recovery times.

Precaution: Do not use this cocktail of telazol-xylazine for mice, rabbits, or ruminants such as cattle, sheep, or goats. Giving telazol and xylazine simultaneously is not recommended for horses.

ANAESTHETIC INDUCTION AND MAINTENANCE

Injectable Anaesthesia

Anaesthetic induction using injectable anaesthetics is fairly simple. It involves admininsistration of the drug and monitoring the depth of anaesthesia. Supportive care may be needed. Maintenance of injectable anaesthesia can be through repeated bolus doses of the drug or through a constant infusion. Infusion rates are calculated based on the clearance time of the drug. Bolus dosing is simpler. Typically, 1/2 of the original dose is given for repeat doses.

Injectable anaesthetics can be administered by various routes depending upon the specific compound. The most frequently used routes of administration in laboratory animals are intraperitoneal, intramuscular and intravenous. Less frequently used routes, among others, are intrathoracic, oral and rectal. Techniques are described below.

Intravenous (IV)

Procedure: An appropriate vein must be selected. For large animals, the saphenous, cephalic or jugular veins are best. For rodents, the tail veins are best. For rabbits and swine, ear veins may be used. The vein is held off proximal to the venipuncture site. The vessel may be stroked with a finger to stimulate blood flow into it. The needle is inserted at a 30–45° angle to the vessel. Then the needle is lowered to align with the longitudinal axis of the vessel and advanced slightly. Draw back. If blood appears in the hub of the needle, the drug may be injected. If not, try redirecting the needle (before you pull it out of the skin) and repeat. You may need to try several times while learning. Using a new, sharp needle for each stick, even if it is the same animal, will improve your chances for success. Once the needle is withdrawn, it is necessary to put pressure on the vessel to prevent bleeding.

Advantages: Rapid delivery of drug, ability to titrate dose, irritating substances may be given IV.

Disadvantages: Small veins are hard to access (i.e. small animals), restraint is critical, developing skill in venipuncture takes experience.

Intramuscular (IM)

Procedure: Insert the needle into a large muscle mass. Draw back slightly. If blood is aspirated, you are in a blood vessel. Redirect the needle. When the needle is placed correctly, inject the drug. The best muscle masses to use for small animals are the caudal thigh muscles. For larger animals, the lateral dorsal spinal muscles or the cranial or caudal thigh muscles may be used. When administering into thigh muscles, inject from the lateral aspect, or if from the caudal aspect, direct the needle slightly lateral. This will help avoid injecting into the sciatic nerve.

Advantages: Fairly rapid absorption, technique is simple.

Disadvantages: IM injections are painful, small volumes are necessary, the animal may try to bite or escape.

Intraperitoneal (IP)

Procedure: The animal is usually restrained in dorsal recumbency. The drug may be injected anywhere in the caudal 2/3 of the abdomen. However, it is best to try to avoid the left side in rodents and rabbits because of the presence of the cecum. After the needle is inserted, draw back. If anything is aspirated, you have likely hit the viscera. Withdraw and get a new needle before trying again. If the needle is placed correctly the drug may be injected.

Advantages: Relatively large volumes may be injected (0.5 ml in mice, 2 ml in rats, etc.)

Disadvantages: Technique is more difficult than IM injections, drug may be administered into the viscera resulting in no effect or in a complication.

Subcutaneous (SC)

Procedure: Pinch an area of loose skin. Inject into the center of the "tent" created by pinching.

Advantages: Technique is the simplest of any, large volumes may be given (basically as much as the tent of skin will hold that does not cause discomfort to the animal).

Disadvantages: Irritating substances cannot be given this way, absorption is slow.

Bibliography

1. Amand, W.B. In R.W. Kirk ed., Current Veterinary Therapy, 6th ed., p.705 1977.
2. Clifford, D. In L.R. Soma ed., Textbook of Veterinary Anaesthesia, p. 385, 1971
3. Heath R.B. Colo State Univ Clin Sci News l 1, No.10, 1977.
4. Soma L.R. Textbook of Veterinary Anaesthesia, p.621, 1971.
5. Stoliker, H.E. In D.C. Sawyer ed., Experimrntal Animal Anaesthesiology p.158: USAF School of Aerospace Medicine, 1965.

5

Hypnotics, Sedatives and Anticonvulsants

HYPNOTICS AND SEDATIVES

Barbital Sodium

It is primarily used as a sedative and hypnotic. It is highly shorter duration of action than phenobarbitone.

Dose: 180–200 mg/kg SC, LD 250 mg/kg SC.

Oral sedative dose 150–1000 mg daily.

When injected IV barbital tends to paralyze the vital medullary center.

Barbital have exceptionally long period of action in the cat. In the rat the plasma level of barbital has a biological half life of 19.3 hrs after an intraperitoneal inj. of 200 mg/kg.

Phenobarbital Sodium

It was the second barbiturate acid derivative of clinical importance to be developed. Hepatic microtonal enzyme activity is accelerated by phenobarbital.

- The major site of metabolism of phenobarbitone is in the liver.
- It is metabolized by oxidative hydroxylation to form hydroxyl phenobarbital.

This metabolite has weak anticonvulsant activity. It is rapidly eliminated from blood by conjugation with glucuronide and excretion in urine of the dog. Alkalinization of urine accelerate excretion of phenobarbital.[2]

Dosage: Oral dose 30–300 mg in dog, 15–60 mg in cat.

- Sedative dose in a 7–11 kg dog is 15 mg orally every 6 hrs.
- LD 30 mg/9 kg in the dog, maintenance dose every 6–24 hrs.

Amobarbital Sodium

5-ethyl-5-isoamylbarbiyuric acid.

It is metabolized by oxidation to form a 3'-hydroxy metabolite. About 40% of a hypnotic dose of amobarbital is excreted in urine within 2 days as hydroxylated metabolite.

Since it is an intermediate acting barbiturate, it is not suitable as a general anaesthetic agent in mammals.

Secobarbital Sodium

Sodium 5-allyl-5-[1-methylbutyl] barbiturate.

It is used as a short acting hypnotic and sedative in veterinary medicine. The oral dose varies from 30–200 mg in dogs and cat.

Pentobarbital Sodium

Oral sedative dose is 4.4 mg/kg , 1–1.5 mg/kg iv.

Chloral Hydrate

It is one of the oldest sedative. It is also used for its hypnotic and anaesthetic effect.

ANTICONVULSANTS

Phenobarbital Sodium

It depresses the motor centers of cerebral cortex. It has a widest spectrum of activity. It is the anticonvulsant choice in cat. It can be given by oral, iv IM route. It is the least toxic of all antiepileptic drugs.

Doses: 30–300 mg iv in dog, 4 mg/kg orally every 12 hrs and 15–60 mg iv in cat

Side effects: Polyphagia, polyurea, polydypsia.

Phenytoin Sodium

It depresses the motor area of cortex without depressing sensory areas. It is a hydantoin derivative. Oral preparations are available in suspension capsule and tablet form.

Phenytoin and phenobarbital are used in combination for treatment of epilepsy in both humans and dog. Prolongation of effect occurs with chloramphenicol, phenylbutazone and phenothiazine. In vitro inhibition of phenytoin metabolism is seen with diazepam and proposyphene.

Side effects: Transient incoordination, oversedation polyphagia, polydypsia, polyurea

Uses: In dogs for control of convulsion and in treatment of grandmal, psychomotor, focal seizures.

Primidone

5-phenyl-5-ethylhexahydropyrimidine-4,6-dione.

Approximately 60–80% of an oral dose of primidone is rapidly absorbed from the GIT, in humans. Half life is 12 +/– 6 hrs. In animals it is oxidized to phenobarbital and phenylethylmalondiamide. These metabolites have anticonvulsant activities in animals.

It is more potent in protection of animals against maximal seizures. It is more toxic in cats and rabbits than rats or mice; it is not recommended for therapeutic use in cats.

Side effects: Ataxia, polydypsia, polyphagia.

Toxicity: It is less neurotoxic in mice and rats than phenobarbital. It may induce nystagmus, nausea, drowsiness. Megaloblastic anaemia is one of the more serious adverse effects of primidone in humans. Primidone may induce hepatic microsomal enzymes that increase the metabolism of vitamins.

Benzodiazepines

The benzodiazepines include diazepam (valium), midazolam and zolazepam (telazol). These drugs are anti-anxiety and anticonvulsant drugs with good muscle relaxation. They have minimal cardiovascular and respiratory effects. Sedation is minimal in most species, except for swine and nonhuman primates. The primary use of these drugs in anaesthesia is in combination with other drugs. Ketamine-diazepam, midazolam-narcotic, and tiletamine-zolazepam (telazol) combinations can be very useful for induction of general anaesthesia and for short procedures. These drugs are regulated by the Controlled Substances Act and require special record keeping.

Bibliography

1. Kay, W.J. and Fenner, W.R. In R.W. Kirk, ed, *Current Veterinary Therapy,* 6th ed., p.853. W.B. Saunders, Philadelphia, 1977.
2. Kumar Pramod, *Textbook of Anaesthesia,* 1st ed., Paras Med. Publishers, Hyderabad, 2008.

6

Neurolept Analgesics and Narcotic Antagonist

The analgesic drugs play an important role in the practice of veterinary medicine and have increasing importance in laboratory medicine. Guidelines issued Jan 1975 by the US Department of Agriculture (USDA) which has responsibility for enforcing the US Animal Welfare Act to assure appropriate use of pain relieving drugs by biomedical research laboratories.

Since the 1960s new analgesic agents such as fentanyl, oxymorphone, etorphine, and others have been introduced for use in animals.

NEUROLEPT ANALGESIC

The neurolept analgesia is derived from two words 'neurolepsia' and 'analgesia'. The term came into use when the combination of droperidol and fentanyl was first administered in human to induce psychomotor sedation and analgesia.

Droperidol–Fentanyl Citrate (Insofar –Vet)

It is classified as a neuroleptic, tranquilizer or psychotropic agent. The combination of droperidol : Fentanyl is in a 50:1 ratio. Each ml contains 20 mg of droperidol and 0.4 mg of fentanyl. The pH is adjusted to 3.1+/–0.4.

Fentanyl Citrate

It is an analgesic with a potency about 100 times that of an equivalent quantity of morphine sulphate. It binds with the opiate receptors? It does not produce analgesia but is a potent neurolepsia agent. Each compound in the droperidol-fentanyl mixture exert its own action. Droperidol enhances the analgesic potency of fentanyl. The primary objective of neurolepsia analgesia is to provide a method of anaesthesia for major operation and avoid the severe CNS, CVS and metabolic depressant effects of conventional anaesthetics. In veterinary medicine the combination of droperidol and fentanyl has been approved by the US Food and Drug Administration (FDA) for use only in the dogs for various clinical procedures. Fentanyl has been used illegally as a CNS stimulant in racehorse. The intravenous administration in thoroughbreds increases spontaneous locomotion 15-fold within a few mins; this effect can last upto 1 hour. Limb movement is well controlled and coordinated. The horse rarely stumbles or bumps into objects. This motor activity occurs from dopaminergic receptor activation. However, it is more likely to be the result of an action of fentanyl upon noradrenergic cerebral function resulting in an increased release of norepinephrine. Fentanyl (2.2 mcg/kg) has been used for its analgesic action in horse; the drug is used intramuscularly or slowly by the IV route. The peak effect attained in 5 min. duration is about 1 hr.

Side effects: Adverse effects of droperidol and fentanyl are dose related and encountered most frequently at maximum therapeutic or high dosages. Bradycardia and respiratory depression with occasional tachypnea, salivation and defecation frequently observed within 10 mins of intramuscular administration are induced by fentanyl component of the combination. Atropine sulphate (0.045mg/kg) can be used to treat this condition. If the droperidol and fentanyl combination is used alone in the dog, the animal can be aroused at any time during a minor surgery. Loud noises often elicit an involuntary startled movement when the dog has not received adjunctive general anaesthesia. Occasionally an animal may exhibit convulsive seizures at higher doses. Other side effects include nystagmus like activity of the eyes. Some discomfort occur following IM injection due to the low pH of droperidol-fentanyl combination.

In the guinea pigs, Leash and associates reported that swelling, lameness and self mutilation of the injected leg develops several days to 1 week later in 33% of the animals. The dose that produces this effect is 0.88 ml/kg; despite the excellent anaesthesia IM injection of the drug into guinea pigs at this dosages can not be recommended.

Droperidol-fentanyl combination with ketamine hydrochloride and with pentobarbital sodium has been used successfully for various surgical procedures in pigs.

A condition referred to as "woody chest syndrome" occurs in dogs and humans following rapid IV administration of droperidol-fentanyl. The syndrome has not been seen in swine. Woddy chest syndrome is attributed to the fentanyl fraction of the drug combination and reversed by use of naloxone hydrochloride or muscle relaxants and mechanical ventilation.

Contraindication

Must not be used in food producing animals. Because of its undesirable central nervous stimulant effects in cats, horses and ruminants droperidol and fentanyl is not recommended. In cesarean section it is recommended that droperidol-fentanyl not be used with barbiturates because of hazardous effect to the neonate.

Clinical Use

Dogs: In a clinical study by Franklin and Reid (1965), which included most of the major breeds of dogs varying in age from 6 weeks to 16 years and in wt from 1.4 to 68 kgs, IM doses of fentanyl-droperidol of 0.11 ml/kg and in a few instances, 0.146 ml/kg or 0.055 ml/kg were used in 567 animals. The drug combination was used either alone or in conjunction with local or general anaesthesia (Table 6.1).

Table 6.1: IM doses of droperidol-fentanyl for induction of neurolept analgesia in laboratory animals

Species	Doses (ml/kg)
Mouse	0.002–0.005
Rat	0.016–0.02
Guinea pigs	0.66–0.88
Rabbit	0.22
Hamster	0.01–0.016
Primates	0.0275–0.22
Opossum	0.22–0.5

Table 6.2: The dose of droperidol and fentanyl recommended in the dog for analgesia and tranquilization

Route	Weight	Dose
IM	6.75–9	1 ml
IV	10.25–27	1 ml

When the neurolept analgesic preparation is used with either thymlal sodium or methoxyflurane, induction is smooth, muscular relaxation is marked and recovery time is shortened and free of an excitatory phase. Use of droperidol in cesarean section does not produce neonatal depression in puppies when used alone or with 1% procaine. Tables 6.2 and 6.3 give useful information.

Table 6.3: The doses recommended for general anaesthesia in the dog

Route	Dose	Follow-up
IM	1 ml/18 kg	after 10 min give IV pentobarbital (6.6 mg/kg)
IV	1 ml/10.25–27 kg	within 15 sec give IV pentobarbital (6.6 mg/kg)

Nitrous oxide 50–70% with oxygen is considered an excellent anaesthetic for concurrent administration with droperidol-fentanyl.

ETORPHINE AND NEUROLEPTIC COMBINATION

The combination has been used on an experimental basis in the pig. A combination of 2.45 mg/ml etorphine and 10 mg/ml acepromazine was used in 116 pigs ranging in age from 8–17 weeks and in 10 adult pigs. The dose range of the mixture used in the young pigs was less than 0.375 ml/kg to over 0.625 ml/50kg. The average dose was 0.515ml/50kg. The characteristics effects produced after an IM injection is an unsteady gait after about 1 min with a twitching movement of the legs. Soon after pigs loses the control and sits down. About 2 min after injection animal resumes sternal recumbency. Slight involuntary movement of the head, neck and limbs are also seen in most pigs. Five mins after administration of the drug the animals can be placed in lateral recumbency without resistance. Fully immobilized peaks are usually unaffected by sternal stimuli however some responds to noise and others move their ears and heads slightly in response to stimuli. There were 15 deaths in this study.

Sheep: Effects of etorphin-acepromazine upon oesophageal and ruminal motility had been studied in three sheep. IV doses of 0.05 ml to 0.1 ml of etorphin and acepromazine were administered. Body weights of the animal were not given. The drug mixture induces immediate cessation of oesophageal and ruminal movements. Following IV administration of a narcotic antagonist these movements reappear at normal amplitude and frequency within one minute. Passive resuscitation in sheep may be avoided if the head of animal is lowered following use of etorphin-acepromazine. Excessive salivation does not appear to pose any difficulty if duration of anaesthetic recumbence is not prolonged. Sufficient information is lacking regarding the safety and efficacy of this combined drug preparation in sheep.

Other domestic animals: Etorphin in combination with triflupromazine hydrochloride has been evaluated in the goat. Doses of etorphin (0.07 ± 0.018 mg/kg) and triflupromazine (1.98 ± 0.396 mg/kg) were administered intramuscularly and supplemented with local anaesthesia (2% lignocaine). Upon completion of surgery diprenorphine (0.140 ± 0.025 mg/kg) was administered to reverse the action of etorphin. Onset of immobilization occurred in 1–8.5 minutes and duration was 60–120 minutes. Reversal of immobilization from etorphin by the antagonist was complete within 2–25 minutes. There will undoubtly be more combination of neurolepsia and analgesic agents developed in the future. Many referred to in this chapter will in all probability fall by the way side as more effective combinations are developed.

Horse and cattle: 1 ml/100 kg IM given contains 24.5 mcg/kg etorphin and 100 mcg/kg acepromazine.

Contraindication: Domestic animal should be controlled and restrained prior to IV and IM administration to avoid accidental self injection. Because it causes serious respiratory depression and coma of a veterinary assistant and leading to death. In the event of an accidental injection warnings include immediate iv or IM injection of naloxine saloon (0.8 mg) and is to be repeated at five minutes interval if symptoms are not reversed. If saloon is unavailable nalorphine should be administered iv or IM in a dose of 10 mg and can be repeated at five minutes interval if necessary upto a total 4 mg. In the event neither saloon or nalorphine is available diprenorphine is recommended in a dose of 0.3 mg imp and repeated until respiratory depression is reversed. Adequate cardio pulmonary activity and or resuscitation must be maintained until emergency medical assistance arrives.

Analgesics (Opium Alkaloids)

It was recommended for relief of pain in the papyrus Ebers written about 1500 B.C. Opium has been widely used by the physicians throughout the world.

Source and composition: Opium is the air dried milky exudates obtained from the incised unripe seed capsules of the poppy plant – papaver somniferum which is indigenous to Asia Minor. Pharmacologically the active constituents of the opium are alkaloids. Opium contains about 24 alkaloids but only two morphine and codeine have much clinical use. The principal alkaloid of opium is morphine.

Morphine sulfate: Chemistry, the morphine molecule consists of partially hydrogenated phenanthrene nucleus an oxide link and a nitrogen containing structure. In addition two hydroxyl groups are important in maintaining the pharmacological integrity of morphine molecules Table 6.4.

Table 6.4: Natural and semisynthetic opioids

Drug	Phenolic position	Alcoholic position
Morphine	H	H
Methyl morphine	CH_3	H
Hydromorphone	H	O
Diacetyl morphine (heroin)	$COCH_3$	$COCH_3$
Oxymorphone	H	O

OPIATE RECEPTORS, ENKEPHALINS AND SUBSTANCE P

Specific opiate receptors have been identified within the brain, spinal cord and myenteric plexus of the GI tract, heart, kidney and adrenal glands. These receptors bind in a stereospecific manner with morphine, fentanyl, etorphine, mepridine, methadone and other opiate agonist. Upon combining with the receptor, the agonist apparently induce conformation change in the receptor leading to biochemical alteration in the neuron containing the receptor. α-Endorphine in particular induces analgesia and contains a pentapeptide referred to as methionine encephalin. Of the encephalins, methionine encephalin is the dominant pentapeptide in swine. The pig brain contain methionine encephalin four times more than leucine-encephalin; in the cattle ratio is reversed. A relationship occur between encephalin pain pathways. The best example of this is in the spinal cord. A pathway projecting efferently from the brainstem activates encephalonergic neurons; this suppress pain at the first relay path.

Pharmacological actions: Brain and spinal cord: the action of the morphine is irregular. The basis of the irregular action attributable to morphine can be better understood now. The different types of opiate receptor have been identified. The major pharmacologic action of morphine is produced almost exclusively by (−) enantiomer or isomer. The unnatural (+) enantiomer of morphine induces only minimal activity.

Early CNS effects of morphine administration in animals include changes in behavior. CNS depression is seen in dog, monkey, and human, while CNS stimulation or excitatory behavior is elicited in the cat, horse, goat, sheep, pig and cow following systemic administration of morphine. In an effort to ascertain whether the species difference in behavior induced by morphine is a reflection in the distribution pattern of opiate binding site in the brain. Simon investigated binding of radiolabeled etorphine various region of the brain in a number of species. There is reasonably good reproducibility of binding level for any given anatomical region in dog, monkey, human, sheep, cows and cat. The only areas of CNS that show consistent differences are amygdale and frontal cortex. These regions are atleast two times higher in receptor level for species that show CNS depression than for the species that shows CNS excitation to opioids. The amygdale and frontal cortex are component of limbic system where most of the areas of opiate binding in dog, monkey and human are located. Interestingly monkeys become placid following bilateral amygdalactomy where as cat shows sustained aggression and ferocity. Consequently amagdalactomy resembles the effects seen in subcutaneous morphine administration in this two species. Considerable controversy has existed regarding whether morphine should be used in the cat because of its inability to produce sedation. The excitatory response frequently observed in cat may be the effect of overdoses of morphine. When doses of 5, 10 and 20 mg/kg are injected intraperitoneally a manic response is observed. This can be prevented by pretreatment with CNS catecholamine depletes or central dopaminergic receptor blocker which also have α receptor blocking action. The CNS excitation effect induced by morphine in cat may occur from alteration in functioning of brain dopaminergic or noradrenergic system. Brain concentration of homovanilic acid, a metabolite of dopamine, increases following morphine suggesting that an increase in catabolism occurs in brain dopamine. Conversely morphine depresses noradrenergic activity in the locus cerulus of rat due to unavailability of norepinephrine at the receptor sites. It is possible that stimulatory action of morphine and related compounds like fentanyl is due to noradrenergic cerebral functions. These explain the inhibitory effect of reserpine on stimulatory action of morphine and fentanyl. Reserpine decreases the rate of synthesis of norepinephrine. Increased locomotor activity due to morphine is due to release of norepinephrine and not dopamine as stated. Swine, sheep, goat, cattle and horses are generally stimulated by morphine, however effects in horse and ox are somewhat irregular. It may be due to increase turnover of dopamine or increase release of norepinephrine following morphine administration. CNS depression does not necessarily need to occur prior to or concomitantly with development of state of analgesia. Morphine is capable of producing a high degree of analgesia without accompanying CNS or respiratory depression in animals such as hamster.

In addition to analgesic effect of intracerebral morphine, long lasting electrographic seizures occur in most animals. Seizures are accompanied by myoclonic twitches, catalepsy, muscular rigidity and wet dog shakes and are blocked by prior administration of naloxone. This suggest that analgesia and seizures are mediated by opiate receptors located in different regions of brain. Morphine is strictly contraindicated in treatment of strychnine poisoning and control of epilepsy in dogs and cats.

The dogs shows a brief preliminary period of central excitement marked by restlessness, fainting, salivation, nausea, vomiting, urination and defecation. This symptoms gradually disappear and are followed by stupor indicating depression of cerebral cortex. Morphine is preferred for premedication in dog because it facilitates induction of general anaesthesia.

Information on effectiveness of morphine in relieving pain comes from use of drugs in human patients. Morphine will relieve pain without blocking motor activity of consciousness. Anxiety and alarm disappear. Sleep may be produced. These observations give some indication to effectiveness of morphine in animals.

Emetic Centre

Both dogs and cats will respond to central and long acting emetics; however cat requires higher doses of morphine or apomorphine. Within 5–10 mins after SC injection of morphine most dogs will vomit profusely unless stomach is empty. The act of vomiting is preceded by salivation and nausea and accompanied by defecation. A trace of morphine applied directly to the floor of 4th ventricle will produce stimulated vomiting in dogs from which the entire GI tract has been removed. This effect would seem to exclude gastric irritation as a causative factor.

Cough Centre

The cough centre appears to be more susceptible to morphine than other medullary centres. Morphine is an excellent cough sedative and where it not for its addictive properties to dogs as well as humans. The drug probably would be most widely used for dry nonproductive cough. Morphine is used in those patients for whom codein was ineffective.

Thermoregulation

A variation in effect on body temperature is seen in different species following administration of morphine. Hypothermia occurs in rabbits, dog and monkeys while hyperthermia occurs in cats, goats, cattle and horses. In guinea pigs, rats and mice, low doses elicit hyperthermia while higher doses induce hypothermia. In monkeys and rats, not only the hypothermic response of morphine is reduced following repeated administration but hyperthermia becomes dominant response, morphine induced hypothermia is abolished following serotonin depletion with parachlorophenyl alanine. The administration of 5-hydroxytryptophane to animals pretreated with para-chlorophenylalanine restores the typical hypothermic response to morphine, meperidine and methadone.

Iris

Morphine produces a variable effect upon the size of the pupil in animals. The pupillary size of the cat, sheep and horse increases after morphine; it causes pinpoint pupil in dog rats and humans. The iris of the bird is not affected as it contains nonresponsive skeletal muscle. Adrenalectomy or administration of phenoxybenzamine antagonizes the mydriasis induced by release of catecholamine in the cat.

Respiratory System

The respiratory system of the dog is initially stimulated; panting is seen and is attributable to the initial rise in body temperature. As body temperature declines and CNS depression increases, respiratory activity is depressed by morphine, resulting in decreased minute volume of respired air. The threshold of response to carbon dioxide stimulation is increased and the alveolar CO_2 concentration is higher, respiration becomes slower and shallower. In deep sedation Cheyne-Stokes type respiration may occur. Bronchoconstriction occur following an IV dose of 1 mg/kg and more marked effect is produced following a dose of 2.5 mg/kg.

Cardiovascular System

In the conscious dog morphine administered IV induces coronary vasoconstriction, reduces coronary blood flow and increases coronary vascular resistance. In anaesthetized dog morphine administered IV induces transient drop in arterial pressure and increase in heart rate. As arterial pressure return to normal, heart rate decreases from increased pressoreceptor activity as well as from vagotonic effect of morphine.

Urinary Tract

The initial effect of morphine may also include urination. As the effect progresses morphine decrease urine secretion in dog to 10% or less of normal by liberating excess of ADH from pituitary gland. Morphine increases muscular tone of bladder which may make urination difficult. Conversely animals seems to be less affected and have less difficulty in this respect than humans.

GI Tract

Emptying GI tract in the dog's first response to morphine causes constipation of the dog and other animals. Morphine causes an initial delay in gastric secretion of HCl which is later compensated by excessive secretion.

Absorption, Fate and Excretion

Although morphine is considered to one of the oldest and most efficacious drugs, pharmacokinetic information regarding its fate has not been clearly determined in animals or humans. One of the primary reasons for this has been lack of sensitive analytical method for detection of morphine and its various metabolites. Development of radioimmunoassay methodology has improved sensitivity for detection of compounds such as morphine over 100 fold.

Morphine is readily absorbed from the small intestine and some may be absorbed from stomach. It is absorbed promptly following SC injection but not absorbed from intact skin but scarified epithelium permits slow entrance to the circulation.

Biotransformation of morphine to morphine 3-0-glucuronide is the primary metabolite pathway for inactivation and eventual elimination of the drug. The principal catalyst in formation of morphine glucuronide is a hepatic microsomal uridine diaphosphate (UDP)-glucuronyl transferase which transfer a glucuronide acid moiety from UDP-glucuronic acid to morphine. With exception of the cat, approximately 50% of morphine administered to most of the mammals appears in urine as glucuronide forms. In the cat a deficiency in UDPGA and its associated glucuronide transferase enzyme does not favour glucurinidation of morphine. Increased toxicity of aspirin and salycylate drugs is linked to failure of cat to conjugate the compounds with glucuronic acid. The biologic half life of morphine would be expected to be longer in the cat because of its inability to form glucuronide. Surprisingly, the biologic half-life in plasma is only 3.05 hrs in the cat following SC injection of morphine (1 mg/kg). The biologic half-life of morphine in other species is probably shorter than in cat; these values were not located in literature.

Toxicity

Newborn animals are known to be more sensitive to morphine than adults. In morphine induced toxicity decreases with animals. The toxic dose of the morphine appears to be variable. Subcutaneous or intravenous fatal dose is 110 to 220 mg/kg. Convulsive seizure similar to strychnine occur in most species following administration of higher dose of morphine. Naloxone (Saloon) reverses these toxicity.

Addiction

Addiction is a rare problem encountered in animals because narcotics are not administered for long period. Cessation of morphine medication after repeated administration in animals leads to behavioural syndrome (abstinence). This is characterized by irritability or explosive motor, behaviour, wet-dog shakes, teeth chattering, increase hypermotility of G I tract, weight loss and ear blanching.

Dogs

Morphine is important in canine surgery to relieve pain, facilitates handling the patient for local or general anaesthesia, and decrease the amount of CNS depressants necessary to produce surgical anaesthesia. The peak effect of morphine following SC injection is between 30–45 mins. The analgesic effect last for 1–2 hrs. The SC dose of morphine for premedication vary from 0.1–2 mg /kg. Onset of action after IM or SC injection within a few mins. Atropine (0.045 mg/kg) is routinely administered subcutaneously or intramuscularly at the same time as morphine to prevent salivation and bronchial secretion. Very young, aged, and debilated dogs are more susceptible to morphine than normal, middle aged, vigorous ones. Emetic action of morphine may cause great inconvenience if it is not anticipated. It is a definite advantage to have stomach empty. The effect of morphine in event of fasting was sufficient prior to anaesthesia and surgery.

The premedication with sufficient morphine will decrease the total amount of general anaesthetic requirement to half or even one third. This support concept of balanced anaesthesia increase the safety of anaesthetic procedures.

Traditionally, morphine has been used cautiously in cesarean section of dogs because of its fetal respiratory depression. It now appears that fetal respiratory movement are not abolished by doses of morphine that depress maternal respiration and however they may be depressed by large dose. A large dose also interferes with uterine contraction and parturition.

Contraindication
Should be used with care in acutely uraemic and toxaemic dogs.

Cats
An effective analgesic dose of morphine subcutaneously in cat is 0.1 mg/kg. Other studies have shown SC administration of morphine (0.1 mg/kg) produces effective analgesia in cat. Phenothiazine tranquilizer (e.g. chlorpromazine, promazine) blocks central dopaminergic receptor, this probably explains satisfactory effects of this drugs in combination with morphine as observed in cat.

Guinea Pigs and Rats
Morphine may be used subcutaneously or intramuscularly as a preanaesthetic agent in guinea pigs and rats in the dose of 2–5 mg\kg. The usual analgesic dose of morphine exerts effect within 15 mins of SC administration.

Rabbits
The IM use of morphine (8 mg/kg) is advocated within 30 mins prior to IV thiamylal (20 mg/kg). Atropine (0.2 mg/kg) is also simultaneously administered with morphine.

Swine
Morphine has more CNS stimulant than depressant effect in pigs. However, it is used successfully for analgesic effect in pigs prior to chloralose and barbiturates. The recommended IM dose is 0.2–0.9 mg/kg.

Subhuman Primates
Comparatively large dose (1–3 mg/kg) of morphine are necessary for chemical restrain and sedation of chimpanzee.

Horse

Morphine and other opiates are used for relief of acute spasmodic colic. Morphine (0.22 mg/kg) is administered slowly by IV or IM route. The preanaesthetic dose of morphine is 0.12 mg/kg IV. Some horses show undesirable central stimulation and excitation. Loss of coordination in between 20–100 mins after IV administration of 2.4 mg/kg of morphine and last for 7 hours. Morphine has been satisfactorily used for sedation and analgesia.

CODEINE PHOSPHATE

Occurs in opium to extent of around 0.5%. Most of it is produced semi synthetically from morphine. The phosphate salts are more widely used than codeine sulphate. Codeine is metabolized rapidly by tissues of humans, dogs and rats. Metabolic alteration followed rapid urinary excretion begins a few mins after IM in injection and after a slight delay following oral administration. About one-half an ordinary dose is eliminated within 6 hrs and all within 24 hrs in dog. About 50% of dose is excreted in urine in conjugated form. Interestingly codeine is one-tenth as potent as morphine in intact animals and one-hundredth in isolated guinea pig ileum.

Codeine is widely used to depress cough centre. The dose of codeine should be increased proportionately over that of morphine to produce desired depression of cough reflex with less undesirable side effects. Codeine has some constipating action as that of morphine. Since the analgesic action of codeine is less than morphine, codeine is not commonly used in animals for analgesia. Addiction to codeine is uncommon.

Codeine is used as an expectorant in cough syrup mixture at 1.1–2.2 mg/kg to allay irritating coughs in dogs; this is administered orally 3–4 times daily.

Hydromorphone Hydrochloride

It is 5 times more potent as an analgesic than morphine. In the dog it produces less nausea and emesis and GI disturbances than morphine. It is soluble in three parts of water. The SC dose for dog is 1.1–2.2 mg/kg.

Oxymorphone Hydrochloride

It is approximately 2.5 times as potent as hydromorphone and about 10 times more potent than morphine on an mg/mg basis.

In the cat, a combination of oxymorphone (0.165 mg/kg) and triflupromazine (1.1 mg/kg) proved to be satisfactory. This neurolepsia analgesic mixture is followed by IV examination (1.1–2.2 mg/kg). The combination of oxymorphone and triflupromazine can be administered SC, IM or IV route. Examination not be administered until after oxymorphone and triflupromazine have taken effect because simultaneous administration of all three drugs induces prolonged apnea resembling the "locked chest" syndrome described in-humans.

When used alone, preanaesthetic effectiveness of oxymorphone is limited in the dog and cat because its CNS depressant effects are slight. It produces a mild ataxia and hyperesthesia in cat when used by itself. In combining the narcotic analgesic with a neurolepsia drug such as triflupromazine, a greater degree of neurolepsia or tranquilization is achieved.

Pethidine Hydrochloride

It was synthesized in Germany during a search for atropine like drug having spasmolytic activity. Meperidine is not only spasmolytic but also analgesic and sedative. The hydrochloride salt is used in medicine. It is a colourless crystalline powder with neutral reaction, a slight bitter taste.

Administration

Pethidine is best administered intramuscularly in animal. The SC route is not preferred because local irritation and pain may be produced. Oral administration is not advisable because of cost. IV injection must be made slowly to avoid drug shock and prostration.

Metabolism and Fate

Pethidine is absorbed rapidly following SC, IM or oral administration. The drug is largely inactivated in the liver. A small amount is excreted unchanged in urine, the major part of given dose is demethylated (normepridine) and hydrolyzed before being excreted. Both normepridine and parahydroxymepridine have analgesic activity.

Thermoregulatory effect: In the cat following SC injection of large doses (30–50 mg/kg) of mepridine, a marked rise to 40.5–41.6 C occurs in rectal temperature, is related to dose dependant phenomenon.

Cardiopulmonary effect: Following IM dose of 10 mg/kg, reduction in heart rate and drop in systemic arterial pressure in dogs. Generally, the fall in blood pressure is moderate, and occurs 10–20 mins after IM injection, with return to control level in 30 mins. The decline in systemic arterial pressure is probably the result of peripheral vasodilation following the release of histamine.

A significant degree of bronchoconstriction occurs in the dogs following an IV dose of 0.5 mg/kg. Also meperidine administered at 2.5 mg/kg IV produces 22% decrease in lung capacity.

Analgesic Action

The analgesic effect of meperidine is intermediate between codeine and morphine. In dogs meperidine (4.4 mg/kg) administered IM every 3–6 hrs has been used to depress the cough reflex and in treatment of cardiac asthma. In horse, mepridine produces analgesia within few mins following IV administration and 15–25 mins after an IM injection.

Spasmolytic Action

The spasmolytic activity of meperidine is significant but considerably less than morphine and methadone. Meperidine will relax the intestine, bronchi, ureter and to some degree uterus. Mepridine has an advantages of 75 to 1 over morphine when an analgesic drug is needed that does not depresses intestinal motility. Meperidine poses marked advantages over morphine for relief of postoperative pain.

DIPHENOXYLATE HYDROCHLORIDE

A derivative of meperidine combined with atropine in management of severe diarrhea in humans. Toxicity induced by the drug preparation in cats results in extreme excitement, restlessness and marked mydriasis with visual impairment. In the dog an oral dose of diaphenoxylate (2.5–5 mg) is used every 6 or 8 hours for antidiarrheal purposes. Nalaxone reverse the action of diphenoxylate.

Fetus

Meperidine is distributed widely throughout the body including placental and fetal tissue. It is used to allay parturition pains because it does not depress fetal respiration.

Toxicity

SC doses in excess of 20–30 mg/kg can produce excitement and clonic convulsion in cats. Convulsion can be controlled by pentobarbital. Saloon (naloxone) is an antagonist of respiratory depressant and toxic effect of mepridine.

Clinical Use

In dogs and cats meperidine given preanaesthetically eliminate the period of excitement and reduces the amount of anaesthetic needed.

Dogs and Cats

In the dog meperidine is used IM for preanaesthetic medication varying from 2.5–6.6 mg/kg. The postanalgesic dose is 5–10 mg/kg imp. Duration is approx. 45 mins. In the cat IM dose of meperidine is 2.2–4.4 mg/kg for preanaesthetic medication.

Methadone

Methadone is useful in human medicine for relief of postoperative pain and pain from several other causes. The analgesic effects of methadone are decreased intensity and duration by therapeutics doses of atropine or scopolamine. Narcotics action of methadone is antagonized by saloon.

Pentazocin Lactate

Chemically pentazocin is 2'hydroxy 5,9 diamethyl 2(3,3 diamethylalyl) 6,7 benzomorphone. Each ml of commercially available preparation contains 30 mg pentazocin. FDA has approved its use only in horse.

Pharmacologic Consideration

The principal effects of the analgesic agent are upon CNS and smooth muscle. The analgesic potency is one half that of morphine and 5 times than meperidine. The most significant response of pentazocin in dog is decrease in systemic arterial pressure by 25%. Blood pressure drop is only transient and returns to original in less than one min. Decrease in arterial pressure by meperidine returns to control after 5 min due to initial release of histamine.

Metabolism and Fate

The kinetics of disappearance of pentazocin from plasma following an IM in of 3 mg/kg have been determined in goats, swine, dogs and cats. After IV in pentazocin is distributed widely in the horse and binds extensively to plasma protein. Following an IM in of 0.66 mg/kg peak plasma level are attained in about 30 mins. The plasma half life of pentazocin and duration of action in humans are longer than in domestic animals. Pentazocin crosses the placenta less readily than meperidine. Fetal blood concentration are attained in humans at 60% of those observed in maternal blood.

Clinical Use

Pentazocin has been restricted primarily to preanaesthetic medication because of its lack of profound sedation in animals. Intramuscular dose in dog is 1.5–3 mg/kg. In the horse total IV doses 200–400 mg. Doses of 6–10 mg/kg in dog produced tremors and convulsions. Side effects in pony when 2.2–4.4 mg/kg was given IV or IM are in coordination tremors, hypertonicity and hypersensitivity. Pentazocin is used for control of pain caused by colic in horses. Dose is 0.33 mg/kg IV or IM. Pentazocin has also been used for treatment of wounds in horses. For preanaesthetic use in horses, an IV dose of 0.9 mg/kg is recommended.

Diethyl Thiambutine Hydrochloride

It is recommended for use only in dog because it has analgesic and pharmacologic properties similar to morphine. It produces tetanic muscle spasm, tremors and excitation. Thiopental sodium has been used to control spasm.

ANALGESIC ANTAGONIST

Narcotic antagonist of current importance in veterinary medicine are saloon hydrochloride and diprenorphine hydrochloride. Nalorphine and levallorphan tartate are only occasionally used in clinical practice. Saloon should be the drug of choice because it is virtually free of agonist activity. Other narcotic antagonist under study are nalbuphine hydrochloride and nalmexone hydrochloride.

Naloxone Hydrochloride

Chemically naloxone is 17-allyl-4,5α-epoxy-3,14-dihydroxymorphinan-6-one hydrochloride. It has a potency 10–30 times that of nalorphine. Unlike nalorphine it lacks agonist effect. It is regarded as virtually pure competitive antagonist. Consequently, it does not produce respiratory depression.

Action

In the dog and cat one part of saloon will antagonize respiratory depression produced by 15–20 parts of oxymorphine. Effects of morphine and meperidine are reversed by saloon to a lesser degree than oxymorphine. Saloon does not antagonize halothane barbiturates and procaine in the dog. Saloon will reverse the fentanyl component of droperidol. Saloon can alter expression of oestrogen induced daily surge in ovary ectomized rats.

Administration and Doses

Naloxone can be administered by all parenteral routes but IV route is preferable. In large wild species one mg injected iv is sufficient to antagonize one mg etotorhine or 10 mg fentanyl. Naloxone compares favourably with diprenorphine. Respiratory depressant effect of oxymorphine in dogs and cats can be reversed with a ratio of 0.1 mg saloon to 1.5 mg oxymorphone. The parenteral dose of saloon for dog is 0.04 mg/kg. Since naloxone also blocks α-endorphine, it is used in dog for reversal of hypovolemic shock. An IV bolus of 2 mg/kg and an infusion at 2 mg/kg/hr increases arterial pressure, left ventricular contractility and cardiac output. In canine endotoxic shock saloon also improve survival and cardiac performance.

Diprenorphine Hydrochloride

Most consistent results are obtained when an etorphine to diprenorphine ratio of 1:2 is used. Reversal of narcotics effect of etorphine is obtained by IV diprenorphine or saloon. Residual narcosis after diprenorphine is less than nalorphine. Diprenorphine is also recommended IV for reversal of effects of etorphine when employed in combination with acepromazine for immobilization of horse.

Nalorphine Hydrochloride

Chemically it is N-allylnormorphine, nalline, lethidrone. It is a morphine derivative in which an N-methyl group has been replaced with an N-allyl group. Although nalorphine is a partial agonist, it antagonizes many of the reaction of morphine.

Absorption and Fate

Nalorphine is relatively ineffective after oral administration but is promptly absorbed after SC or IM injection.

Action

Nalorphine usually acts as narcotics antagonist during the effect of narcotics. However in their absence, nalorphine acts like a narcotic and may produce CNS depression and analgesia as a result of its partial agonist activity.

The most prominent antagonist action of nalorphine is in preventing or relieving typical respiratory depressant activity of morphine and all its derivatives.

Dosage

One mg of nalorphine is recommended for every 10 mg of morphine or 20 mg of meperidine for reversal of narcotics effects. For the reversal of the effect of etorphine, a ratio of 10–20 mg nalorphine to 1 mg etorphine is required.

Toxicity

It has the same toxicity as morphine but provides less relief from pain. If the first dose fails to produce an effect on the depression, additional doses are contraindicated. In the event of an overdosage of nalorphine, respiratory supportive measures must be instituted.

Levallorphan Tartrate

It acts as an antagonist during CNS action of opiate and related analgesic. If it is administered in the absence of opiate derivative, it usually induces respiratory depression. Consequently partial agonist activity is seen.

Neurolept Analgesics and Narcotic Antagonist 61

It is ineffective in antagonizing respiratory depressant action of anaesthetic, barbiturates or non narcotics drugs. IV administration of levallorphane (0.022 mg/kg) has been used to relieve or prevent the excitable effects of morphine in the horse.

Bibliography

1. Clifford, D in L R Soma ed. Textbook *of Veterinary Anaesthesia,* p. 385. 1971.
2. Harthoorn, A. M. Application of pharmacological and physiological principals in restraint of wild animals, p 40. 1965.
3. Moller, A W in R W Kirk ed. Current veterinary therapy. Vol 3, Small Animal Practice p.421, 1968.
4. Muir, WW Scarda, R T and Sheehan Equine Pharmacology p.173, 1987.
5. Simon, E J in J R Smythies and R J Bradley ed. Receptor in Pharmacology p.257. 1977.
6. Soma L R , *Textbook of Veterinary Anaesthesia,* p.121–621. 1971.
7. Kumar P., *Textbook of Pain,* 1st ed. New Delhi Modern Publishers 2005.
8. Kumar P., *Textbook of Anaesthesiology,* 1st ed. Hyderabad, Paras Med. Pub. 2008.

7

Nonsteroidal Anti-inflammatory Drugs

CLASSIFICATION

a. Nonselective COX inhibitors
  - *Salicylates:* Aspirin, diflunisal
  - *Pyrazolone derivatives:* Phenylbutazone, oxyphenbutazone
  - *Indole derivatives:* Indomethacin, sulindac
  - *Propionic acid derivatives:* Ibuprofen, naproxen, ketoprofen, flurbiprofen
  - *Anthranilic acid derivatives:* Mephenamic acid
  - *Aryl-acetic acid derivatives:* Diclofenac
  - *Oxicam derivatives:* Piroxicam, tenoxicam
  - *Pyrrolo-pyrrole derivative:* Ketorolac

b. Preferential COX-2 inhibitors
  Nimesulide, meloxicam, nabumetone

c. Selective COX-2 inhibitors
    Celecoxib, rofecoxib, valdecoxib

d. Analgesic-antipyretic with poor anti-inflammatory action
  - *Paraaminophenol derivative:* Paracetamol
  - *Pyrazolone derivative:* Metamizol, propiphenazone
  - *Benzoxazocine derivative:* Nefopam.

SALICYLATE ANALGESIC

Salicylate analgesics were first introduced into clinical medicine in the late 19th century. Sodium salicylate was introduced in 1875 by Buss and acetylsalicyclic acid (aspirin) in 1889 by Dresser.

It relieves pain without causing unconsiousness as the general anaesthetic do. They are of value in relief of mild to moderate pain such as cephalgia, myalgia, athralgia and others pain from integumental structers rather than viscera. They also have an antipyretic action. Antipyretic drugs impair ability of pyrogens to "raise the set point".

Aspirin

Generically known as acetylsalicylic acid. It is a most commonly used anti-inflammatory agent because of its efficacy, low toxicity and low cost.

Pharmacological Consideration

It is potent inhibitor of prostaglandin synthatase. So prevents biosynthesis of PGs. It uncouples oxidative phosphorylation. It also inhibits other chemical mediators of inflammation, e.g. inhibits contraction of bronchial smooth muscle induced by SRS-A and bradykynin. It inhibits release of PGE_2, $PGF_{2\alpha}$ from thrombin stimulated platelets so platelet aggregation is inhibited. It has long been known by clinicians that bleeding time is prolonged following long term administration of aspirin, acetaminophen and sodium salicylate. It has a depressant action on pain by inhibiting local release of bradykinin regardless of type of stimuli. It favors production of PGI_2, inhibits platelet aggregation, and by inhibiting thromboxanes prevents plaque formation.

Toxicosis and Treatment

Aspirin is a phenol derivative, toxic to cats. Daily doses causes intoxication and pathological changes and low doses induce toxic hepatitis in 50% of animal. Signs are depression, poor appetite, vomiting, weight loss, death.

Given in suspension form, it produces severe gastric hemorrhage in dog, but not in solution form or intravenous form. Buffered form cause more severe lesion.

Given in high doses, it causes stillbirth, resorption, cleft palate in mice and rats. Low doses in rhesus monkey from day 25 to term doses not induce any anomaly in offspring. In rabbit inseminated doses given seven doses of aspirin prior to implantation reduce fertility and causes abnormal organogenesis and gestation. Aspirin antagonize therapeutic effect of several anti-inflammatory agents used in rheumatoid arthritis. Antagonism of GI effects of indomethacine following aspirin due to competitive antagonism so clinical use of aspirin in combination with other NSAIDs should be avoided. In sheep aspirin given IV to increase lung vascular permeability to fluid and protein and causing pulmonary edema.

Treatment of aspirin toxicity is removal of drug from body by gastric lavage or oral administration of activated charcoal. Elevating urine pH with IV $NaHCO_3$ and diuresis with mannitol. Peritoneal dialysis is effective in removal of aspirin from plasma.

Clinical Uses

Aspirin is used for relief of minor pain of musculoskeletal origin and for arthritic disease. Therapeutic dose is 10 mg/kg orally at 48 hour interval for cat and dog. And for horse 30–47.5 mg/kg 12 hourly. In cattle oral dose of 100 mg/kg 12 hourly is therapeutically effective. In swine 10 mg/kg orally 6 hourly is recommended.

SODIUM SALICYLATE

Pharmacological Consideration

Mechanism of action and primary action are similar to that of other salicylates. Plasma half lives of IV injection of it are 1,5.9, 0.78, 8.6, and 37.6 hours in pony, pig, goat, dog and cat respectively.

As adult cat is deficient in enzyme glucuronyl transferase, as neonates of any species are, so it may be a useful model for studying drug metabolism typical of newborn animal.

Suggested IV Doses

Horse: 35 mg/kg/6 hrs

Dog : 10 mg/kg/12 hrs

Salicylic Acid

It is used as external application because it is extremely irritating to gastrointestinal (GI) mucosa. In cattle used as antifermentative agent in dose of 16–24 g.

Salicylic acid and benzoic acid are used in combination as ointment such as Whitfield's ointment and alcoholic solution for antifungal action in treatment of dermatomycotic infection. This ointment contains salicylic acid 3 g, benzoic acid 6 g.

Paraaminophenol-derivatives

It includes acetanilide, acitophenetidin and acetaminophen.

Acetamenophen

In cat it is used at any doses in experimental studies, it causes marked cyanosis at 350 mg causing hemolysis of RBCs causing anaemia and hemoglobinuria. It covalently binds with macromolecules of tissue proteins causing analgesic induced renal disease, e.g. renal cell cancer.

Acetylcystein

It is used for treatment acetaminophen toxicity at dose of 140 mg/kg orally 8 hrly.

Pyrazolone Derivatives

It includes phenylbutazone and dipyrone as analgesic and antipyretic.

Phenylbutazone

It is used in treatment of painful arthritis and skeletomuscular diseases, e.g. Tendonitis, capsulitis and bursitis.

It is approved by US FDA. Prolonged administration of it causes necrotizing phlebitis of portal vein. Induction or stimulation of hepatic microsomal enzymes activity results in progressively lower plasma level. Therapeutic dose is 99% plasma protein bound.

Toxicity: Idiosyncrasy, hemorrhage, biliary stasis, renal tubular degeneration.

Clinical uses: Used as a anti-inflammatory, analgesic for laminitis in horse and osteoarthritis.

Dipyrone

It is used as a antipyretic and analgesic, injected slow IV, SC, IM in a dose of 10–20 ml (5–10g) 8 hrly. Dipyrone causing agranulocytosis, leucopenia.

PREFERENTIAL COX-2 INHIBITORS

Nimesulide

It is a relatively weak inhibitor of PG synthesis. It acts by mechanisms like reduced generation of superoxide, inhibition of PAF synthesis and TNFα release, free radical scavenging, etc.

Uses: Short lasting painful conditions like sports injuries, sinusitis, dental surgeries, bursitis, postop pain, fever, etc.

Side effects: Nausea, loose motion, rashes pruritus, dizziness.

Meloxicam

These newer congener of piroxicam has a COX-2:COX-1 selectivity ratio of 10:14. Gastric side effects are milder but ulcer complications are reported on long term use.

Nebumetone

It is a recently developed prodrug. It has a lower incidence of gastric erosion, ulcer and bleeding.

SELECTIVE COX-2 INHIBITORS

Celecoxib

It exerts anti-inflammatory, analgesic and antipyretic action with low ulcerogenic potential. Abdominal pain, dyspepsia and mild diarrhea are common side effects. It is used in osteo and rheumatoid arthritis in dose of 100–200 mg BD.

Rofecoxib

It is the most selective COX2 inhibitor. Dose is 12.5–25mg OD.

Side effects are headache, dizziness, pedal edema and rise in BP.

Valdecoxib

It has similar efficacy as rofecoxib. Dose is 10 mg OD to 20 mg BD.

OTHER SALICYLATE LIKE ANALGESICS

Meclofenamic Acid

It is NSAIDs with pharmacological similarity with aspirin. Mechanism of action antagonize CVS and respiratory effects of histamine, bradykinin, PGE_1, PGE_2.

Onset of action is slow, take 36–96 hours and peaks within 1–4 hours. Oral dose is 1 g/450 kg. Its adverse effects are buccal erosion, anorexia and GI discomfort.

It is used in treatment of osteoarthritis in horse and laminitis at oral dose of 2.2 mg/kg/day for 5–7 days.

Indomethcin

It inhibits biosynthesis of PGs. It is used for treatment of arthritic conditions and gout, not approved by FDA for animals.

Naproxen

It is propionic acid derivative with D isomer of naphthalinic acetic acid and approved by FDA for use in horse.

Mechanism of action: It inhibits PG biosynthesis. It is absorbed 50% orally and plasma half life after IV or oral route is 4 hours.

Toxicity: Gastric erosion and GI discomfort.

Clinical uses: For treatment of pain and lameness in tying-up syndrome (myositis) in horse.

Dose: Oral —10 mg/kg/12 hours. IV —5 mg/kg/12 hourly for 14 days.

OTHER NON NARCOTIC ANALGESICS

Flunixin Meglumine

It is NSAID with analgesic and antipyretic effects. Chemically it is pyridine carboxylic acid.

Clinically it is used for treatment of inflammation and pain, musculoskeletal disorders and for GI colic.

Dose: 1.1 mg/kg/day IV or IM for 5 days. Peak effect seen within 12 to 16 hours and duration of action is 24–36 hours. It is available as a 5% solution with 50 mg/ml.

Xylazine

Chemically it is dimethylphenylaminothiazine and pharmacologically analgesic and sedative but not neuroleptic or anaesthetic agent.

Mechanism of action: It is sympathomimetic agent with potent antinociceptive and analgesic action in rodents.

It produce muscle relaxation by inhibition of intraneuronal transmission of impulses at central level of CNS.

Toxicity: Arterial hypotension, cardiac depression, ventricular arrhythmias, sensitize heart to epinephrine. Bradycardia and 2nd degree AV block due to marked depressive effects of thiopentone and halothane.

Dose: Cattle –0.03–0.1 mg/kg IV and 0.1–0.2 mg/kg IM. Sheep: 0.05–0.1 mg/kg IV and 0.1–0.3mg/kg IM. goat : 0.01–0.5 mg/kg IV and 0.05–0.5 mg/kg IM.

Clinical uses: Dog and cats —used as a sedative and analgesic with IV barbiturate and inhalational anaesthetics. Smooth and rapid induction of anaesthesia with uneven recovery. Depth of analgesia insufficient for ET tube insertion. Ketamine along with xylazine for CS in dog. Also used as a premedication in cats during ketamine anaesthesia.

Horse: Provide satisfactory analgesia and sedation in standing horse. It is useful for suturing wounds and external surgical procedure.

Bibliography

1. Da Visle I. M., Zaslow, ed., *Veterinary Trauma and Critical Care;* Philadelphia, 1982.
2. Killian J. G., Jones E.W., Hamm D., et al., *Textbook of Veterinary Anaesthesia,* 1974.
3. Kumar P. *Textbook of Pain,* 1st ed., Modern Publication, New Delhi, 2005.
4. McCashin F.B., and Gabel A.A. *Textbook of Veterinary Anaesthesia,* p.111, 1971.
5. Riley W.F., Romane W.M., Ellis D.J., et al. *Textbook of Veterinary Anaesthesia,* p.115, 1971.

8

Local Anaesthetics

The first clinically used was cocaine hydrochloride. It is an alkaloid and first obtained from the leaves of *Erythroxylon coca,* a tree indigenous to Chile, Peru and Bolivia. The native runners of this area chewed coca leaves to allay hunger and fatigue and produce psychic stimulation while they carried messages through the forest.

TYPES OF LOCAL ANAESTHESIA

Local anaesthesia is produced in several ways. Topical and surface anaesthesia results when drug is applied to skin or mucous membrane. They are ineffectively used on broken skin.

Infiltration anaesthesia consists of making numerous SC injection into the tissue. Large amounts of dilute solution are often infiltrated.

Conduction or nerve block anaesthesia is produced by injecting local anaesthetic into vicinity of nerve. The drug anaesthetizes the area innervated by preventing any further conduction of impulses along the nerve. A small amount of local anaesthetic solution of relatively high concentration is used.

Epidural or extradural anaesthesia is produced by injecting local anaesthetic solution into epidural space of spinal canal at the level of lumbosacral space, or first or second intercoccygeal space. The anaesthetic acts upon the posterior spinal nerves before they leave the vertebral column.

Paravertebral anaesthesia is a special form of conduction anaesthesia, wherein local anaesthetic is applied to spinal nerves as they emerge from intervertebral foramen. This method is used for rumenotomies. Landmarks for blockade of the spinal nerve can be located relatively easily in dairy cows. In beef cattle, landmarks for injection of local anaesthetic is difficult to locate because of obscuring fat deposits.

Spinal anaesthesia is seldom used to induce local anaesthesia in animals. Intrathecal anaesthesia has been accomplished in sheep by injecting the drug into spinal fluid. Frequently, intrathecal or spinal anaesthesia is confused with epidural or extradural anaesthesia or vice versa.

Regional anaesthesia is a term used rather loose to refer anaesthesia of large region. It may be produced by several methods, epidural, intrathecal, paravertebral, or conduction anaesthesia. The procedure of inducing surgical anaesthesia by intravenous injection of local anaesthetic into a limb, with circulation briefly occluded by a tourniquet has been employed in animals and humans. This form is referred to as IV or retrograde regional anaesthesia.

REQUIREMENTS OF AN IDEAL LOCAL ANAESTHETIC

Ideal local anaesthetic should produce reversible paralysis of sensory nerves but not other tissues, have nonaddictive properties, readily soluble and stable in water, possess a neutral pH, and be nonirritating to tissue. It should possess minimum local toxicity, absorbed slowly to minimize danger of systemic toxicity and prolong the effect at local site. After systemic absorption, compound should be readily and rapidly detoxified. It should be compatible with epinephrine to prolong its action. There should be no hyperesthesia following recovery of sensation by tissue. The local anaesthetic should withstand heat sterilization and be relatively inexpensive.

Mode of Action

Local anaesthetics are generally water soluble acid salts. When these salts are injected into tissues that are normally slightly alkaline, acid salts form of local anaesthetic is neutralized. This release free amine or alkaloid base through hydrolysis, which is necessary to penetrate liquid membrane of cell membrane to produce anaesthesia. After alkalinisation, the solution becomes turbid and the free base precipitate out. Local anaesthetic decrease the cell membrane permeability. The amino group of classic local anaesthetic drugs such as procaine and others, interacts with polar groups of cell membrane to decrease permeability of the nerve cells and stabilize the membrane. As a result, diffusion of potassium and sodium ion cannot occur and the changes which give rise to nerve impulse are blocked. When the cell membrane stabilize in a resting state, generation and transmission cannot occur.

Another mechanism, along with stabilization of cell membrane and lack of sodium and potassium ion diffusion, and involves the influence of local anaesthetic upon membrane calcium. Many authoritative sources indicate that both calcium and local anaesthetics have a stabilization effect upon excitable membranes; e.g. the threshold of electrical stimulation of the membrane is elevated by calcium and local anaesthetics. Consequently, there is a blockade in transmission or conduction of nerve impulse with no change in resting membrane potential. It has been suspected that calcium is crucial in genesis of nerve impulse. It is displacement or removal of calcium ions from nerve membrane sites by depolarization that result in transient increase in permeability of the cell membrane to sodium ions during action potential. Calcium ions and local anaesthetics act upon the same mechanism that is necessary for conveyance of sodium through the nerve cell membrane. Local anaesthetics produce deformation or expansion of cell membrane that result in anaesthesia. Alternation in the membrane Ca^{++} may responsible for this.

Although expansion in membrane volume occurs by at least 4–6% and with increase in fluidity of membrane. However, it is believed that binding of local anaesthetic molecules to hydrophobic regions of cell membrane and expansion of some critical regions in the membrane could also prevent an increase in sodium ion permeability.

According to Lee, the cell membrane slit of the sodium channel is surrounded by a ring like structure, which is composed of lipid molecules and exists in crystalline or gel state. In the presence of a local anaesthetics, rigidity of this structure is believed to reduced from solid to a crystalline state.

Fate

The principal metabolic pathway of local anaesthetic with ester or amide linkages is enzymatic hydrolysis. Derivative of 4-amino-benzoic acid are primarily hydrolyzed in the plasma and liver by nonspecific pseudocholinesterases. Products of hydrolysis either directly excreted or more commonly undergo metabolic transformation. Procaine complexed with penicillin at one time was believed to be protected against action of plasma esterase. The complexed procaine-penicillin molecule escaped hydrolysis.

Hydrolysis of local anaesthetic with amide bonds generally proceeds less rapidly or not at all. Another common pathway in biotransformation of local anaesthetic is dealkylation. Dealkylation probably occurs within the hepatic microenzymes. As most LA contain alkaline amino radicals, excretion in an acid is greater because of increased ionization. In alkaline urine, renal elimination of LA is delayed because the drugs remains principally in the nonionized form.

Toxicity

The symptoms arise primarily from stimulation of the CNS and consist chiefly of restlessness and muscular tremors that progress into clonic convulsion. Death usually result from respiratory failure. Susceptibility to convulsion is related to the degree of development of the CNS; primates are more susceptible than other species.

An elevated ambient temperature may influence toxicity of drugs, e.g. analgesic dose of procaine may produce seizures in puppies during hot weather. In domestic animal death caused by local anaesthetic are uncommon.

Prevention of Toxicity and Treatment

Resuscitatory measures include barbiturates IV to control CNS stimulation. Diazepam IV is drug of choice in treatment of acute local anaesthetic toxicity. Sodium thiopental is also used. Atropine is given IV if there is decrease in heart rate and ephedrine is given IV to restore arterial pressure.

Effects of Epinephrine and Hyluronidase

Addition of epinephrine will prolong the action of local anaesthetic. The concentration of 1 part of epinephrine in 50000 parts of LA should not be exceeded and 1:100000 is preferred. It also decreases toxicity of LA.

LOCAL ANAESTHETIC AGENTS

Procaine Hydrochloride

It is white crystalline powder relatively stable while exposed to air. It is nonirritant and promptly effective when injected SC.

Metabolism and Excretion

It is hydrolyzed in liver and blood plasma by nonspecific pseudocholinesterases. Half life is 25 mins.

Toxicity

Cocaine is slowly metabolized while procaine is rapidly detoxified by liver. Its toxicity is same as other LA.

Contraindication

It is contraindicated in epidural anaesthesia in dog and cat where shock may be a major factor during or following surgery.

Clinical Use

It is used for relief of pain routinely. It was used in veterinary medicine for infiltration, conduction and epidural anaesthesia. It is rarely used for surface anaesthesia. It is also used to induce analgesia for tail docking in lamb or dog, nerve block in bovine foot and enucleation of eye in cattle (Table 8.1).

Table 8.1: Average LD50 of procaine (g/kg)

Species	Route	
	SC	IV
Guinea pig	0.43	0.05
Rabbit	0.46	0.055
Cat	0.45	0.045
Dog	0.25	

Hexylcaine Hydrochloride

It is a long lasting anaesthetic for epidural anaesthesia in cattle, horses and dog. It is soluble in water to a conc of 12%. It is clear and colorless. It can be stored for 3 months at room temperature. It is 4–8 times active than procaine. Injected IV it causes lethal toxicity. Subconvulsion doses cause ataxia, salivation and vomiting.

Lignocaine Hydrochloride

It (α-diethylaminoaceto 2,6-xylidide) is a white slightly yellow powder with a characteristics odour relatively stable but insoluble in water.

Metabolism and Fate

It is metabolized in liver and excreted in urine. A large amount is conjugated with sulphate and excreted in this form. It rapidly crosses placenta.

Action

It is used for infiltration, nerve conduction, epidural and topical anaesthesia. Onset occurs in 5 mins and effects last for 30 mins. It is effective at half concentration of procaine.

Toxicity

Overdoses will cause muscular twitching, hypotension, nausea and vomiting. Local irritation is rare.

CLINICAL USE

Dogs and Cats

Epidural use of lignocaine will block cranially to L1 and 1 ml of 2% solution 3.4 mg/kg will block to T5 in average dog and cat. It has been recommended as a topical anaesthetic for endotracheal intubation in cat.

Swine Goat and Sheep

Doses is determined by length of animal from external occipital protuberance to 1st coccygeal vertebra. The dose of 2% lignocaine upto 40 cm length is 1 ml, then 1.5 ml is added for every 10 cm increase. Lignocaine is used for corneal nerve block of goat and epidural anaesthesia in sheep.

Cattle

It is preferred for a no of surgical procedures. A dose of 4 ml of 2% solution is used for low epidural and 60 ml for high epidural analgesia.

Horses

It is used for nerve block in the horse.

Tetracaine hydrochloride: It is a white crystalline powder soluble in water. It is used for surface conduction and infiltration anaesthesia. A few drops of 0.5 to1% solution on the eye of rabbit will produce excellent anaesthesia.

Piperocaine hydrochloride: It is a white crystalline powder soluble in water. It is used for surface infiltration and conduction anaesthesia. It is 3 times toxic tan procaine.

Proparacaine hydrochloride: It is comparable to tetracaine. It is used for cauterization of corneal ulcers, removal of foreign bodies from eye and ear, tonometry, minor surgery and catheterization.

Prilocaine hydrochloride: It is similar to lignocaine chemically and pharmacologically, however, onset and duration of action are longer. An unusual side effect is methhaemoglobinaemia.

Mipivacaine hydrochloride: It is 2 times potent than procaine. It is used in horse only.

Bupivacaine hydrochloride: It is an amide type local anaesthetic chemically related to mepivacaine. It is used for epidural anaesthesia in cat and spinal anaesthesia in sheep.

Benoxinate hydrochloride: It has antibacterial and antifungal property. It is benzoic acid ester chemically related to procaine.

Cocaine hydrochloride: It is a white crystalline substance readily soluble in water.

Administration: It will anaesthesize if there is abrasion, desquamation or hyperemia. It is not effective on intact skin.

Action: Sensory nerve endings are completely and reversibly paralysed. It block uptake of catecholamines at adrenergic nerve endings. Local vasoconstriction also occur.

Use: It is used only for topical anaesthesia. In concentration of 5–10% it is applied on mucous membrane of nose larynx and buccal cavity.

Toxicity: Acute toxicity can occur from overdoses rapid absorption or improper administration. The range of safety is 300–420 mg when used on mucous membrane of horse.

Dibucaine hydrochloride: It is most toxic and potent. It is used for relief of insect bite, minor burns, cuts and itching of skin.

Ethyl chloride: In addition to local anaesthetic it is occasionally used as general anaesthetic. Its spray is used for repeated blood sampling from marginal ear vein of rabbits.

Bibliography

1. Gellatt, K.N., *Veterinary, Opthalamic Pharmacologic and Therapeutics,* 2nd ed., p.23, 1978.
2. Goodman and Gilman, *The Pharmacological Basis of Therapeutics* 2nd ed., 1955.
3. Heinze C. D., *Bovine Medicine and Surgery and Herd Health Management,* p.795., 1970.
4. Ritche J. M. and Green N. M., *The Pharmacological Basis of Therapeutics,* 6th ed., p.300, 1980.
5. Kumar P. *Textbook of Anaesthesiology* 1st ed., Paras Med. Publishers, Hyderabad, 2008.

Section 2

Techniques
of Anaesthesia

9

Intrathecal and Epidural Anaesthesia

INTRATHECAL ANAESTHESIA

Accomplished by introduction of a local anaesthetic solution into the spinal fluid, the drug temporarily paralyzes the spinal nerve routes in the subarachnoid space. Spinal anaesthesia was first performed with cocaine by Corning in 1885 in a dog.

The technique has never become popular because of the difficulties and dangers associated with it. The vertebra in animals are more compressed, so the spinal column can not be flexed as readily as in humans. The risk of trauma to spinal cord is increased.

Experimentally spinal anaesthesia has been most satisfactorily performed in sheep. Bupivacaine has been successfully evaluated in sheep following intrathecal administration. In cattle the technique of administering a local anaesthetic (5% procaine) intrathecally via a Tuohy needle and catheter at the thoracolumbar interspace has been reported. After injection of 1.5–2 ml procaine, segmental analgesia occur within 7–10 mins.

EPIDURAL ANAESTHESIA

Epidural anaesthesia is attained by injecting local anaesthetic solution into the epidural space. This method of inducing local anaesthesia is much safer than using the intrathecal technique.

Application of epidural anaesthesia in veterinary medicine is most important in large animal practice. By using this technique in cattle, sensory anaesthesia can be produced as far forward as the flank and abdominal wall without affecting respiration and circulation. Epidural pressure appear to exert an effect on distribution and possibly vascular uptake of local anaesthetic in the space.

An improvement in the technique of epidural injection has been introduced through adaptation of epidural anaesthesia to so called caudal anaesthesia.

Mechanism of Action

The site of action of epidural anaesthesia has been a matter of considerable study. It appears that nerve tracts are not blocked at one specific site but at several. Three possible mechanism of action are: 1. Nerve are blocked distal to the dural sheaths after leaving the intervertebral foramina, producing a multiple paravertebral block, 2. Local anaesthetic directly act on dura covered nerve roots and dorsal root ganglia in the epidural space, 3. Diffusion across the durometer into the subarachnoid space and spinal fluid, resulting in a true but slow onset form of spinal anaesthesia.

In the dog one 10th of epidural anaesthetic can be detected from CSF in first 2 hours following injection and about 25% of an epidural anaesthetic enter azygous venous system within 40 mins following injection. The amount of local anaesthetic in circulation is reduced by one half by addition of 1:2,00,000 epinephrine hydrochloride to anaesthetic solution. Large dose of local anaesthetic may result in hypotension and seizures.

Sensory nerves in spinal nerves trunks are paralysed more rapidly than motor ones. Sensory nerves are smaller in cross section and greater surface exposure in proportion to volume contained in nerves fibres.

Onset and Duration

The onset of epidural anaesthesia is between 5–20 mins. Rapidity of onset varies with age as well as species. Epidural anaesthesia is most rapid in sheep and calf followed by ox, pig and horse. It is less rapid in dog and cat and slower in horse.

Metabolism

Procaine injected epidurally is probably absorbed by blood and lymph vessels of epidural space and then metabolized.

Drugs

For successful epidural anaesthesia the drug should have following characteristics: 1. Low absolute and relative toxicity, 2. High degree of potency, 3. Short latent period, 4. Prolonged duration and 5. High degree of diffusibility.

Phenothiazine is contraindicated in epidural anaesthesia because of hypotension. Drugs such as diazepam, xylaine hydrochloride, ketamine, morphine or meperidine may be used for restraint depending upon the species involved.

Cattles

Epidural anaesthesia is divided into two types: 1. Anterior, 2. Posterior.

It is advisable to leave the needle in epidural space (between 1st and 2nd coccygeal vertebrae). This permit local anaesthetic to be given in low or large volume over 5–10 mins. Local anaesthetic commonly used for epidural anaesthesia in cattle are procaine and lidocaine.

Posterior Plane

Posterior epidural anaesthesia provide sensory anaesthesia for skin areas of tail and croup. As far as midsacral region and posterior aspect of thighs. Motor control of hind legs are unaffected, although there may be paralysis of anal sphincter. If motor paralysis of adductor muscles of hind leg does appear, the cow lies down and shows no excitement, defecation is inhibited. The posterior rectum tends to balloon. Stretching of vulva has no response, and the vagina dilates. Parturient cow stopped straining but uterine contraction is unaffected.

Lignocaine 2% in a dose of 5–10 ml is used in cattle to induce posterior epidural anaesthesia for repair of vaginal prolapse for about 1 hour.

Anterior Plane

Anterior epidural anaesthesia result in loss of sensation spreading from the croup between hind limb to inguinal region, prepuce, scrotum and mammary glands, and over the hind legs, and finally, the flanks and abdominal areas forward to the region of umbilicus. Motor paralysis of hind limb varies from partial to complete: (a) If partial some moderate restraint may be necessary, (b) If complete animal should be kept on its sternum for 10–15 mins to provide bilateral anaesthesia. If unilateral anaesthesia is necessary the animals should be restraint with the side which is to be anaesthetised downward. After the spinal nerves on one side are anaesthetized, the animal may be turned to expose the operative areas.

A dose of 120 ml of 1% of LA injected between 1st and 2nd coccyx for reduction of prolapse of inner integument of penile sheath in bull of weight 495 kg. One day after epidural anaesthesia the animal was unsteady.

Lumbar Plane

Epidural anaesthesia is for anaesthetizing last thoracic and first two lumbar nerves for rumenotomies. This is advantageous over past earlier methods in which one injection site is necessary for anaesthetizing left flanks. Above 10 ml of 4% procaine in 1st lumbar space anaesthetizes entire left flank in dairy cattle.

Bilateral anaesthesia is attained by inserting the spinal needle close to midline. Anaesthesia and analgesia last longer in cattle blocked unilaterally (87±14.8 mins) than following bilateral block (70.3 ± 4.3 mins). Pelvic limbs weakness is seen in 85% cows in which analgesia of udder exist, all animals are unable to stand.

Horses

Epidural anaesthesia in the horse has not been as successful as in the cow. Epidural anaesthesia has been employed for numerous operation in horses including tail setting, perineal operation and numerous other kind of surgery on the rear part of animal. Regional anaesthesia of rear part of the animal can be induced by single injection of 2% lignocaine (6–10 ml) at level of 1st and 2nd coccyx. The injection needle is inserted at 45 degree with horizontal; this technique permits injection of local anaesthetic dorsal to 1st coccyx.

Sheep and Goat

Epidural anaesthesia has been used for tail amputation or docking in 2–6 months old lamb. The injection site is about 0.5 cm in diameter in either sacrococcygeal or first intercoccygeal space. Procaine (5% with epinephrine) is injected in a volume of 2 ml; analgesia or anaesthesia occurs within 5 mins. Ataxia results upto 30 mins after administration of the local anaesthetic. Recovery appears to complete in 6–15 hrs.

The above dose of Bupivacaine used in adult sheep (40–60 kg). Lignocaine (2%) in a dose 8–12 ml is used in adult sheep weighing 30.2–36 kg. Anaesthesia occur on in average of 4.6 mins. Anaesthesia is preceded by a brief period of muscular twitching, followed by excellent relaxation. Surgical procedure up to 80 mins duration can be performed.

Swine

Neuroleptanalgesia is sometimes necessary prior to giving an epidural injection in swine. Droperidol-fentanyl citrate administered IM (1 ml/30–50 kg) upto no more than 4 ml is recommended; atropinization is also necessary. The site of injection into epidural space on midline between most of cranial prominence of the wing of ileum on either side

1% lignocaine with 1:2,00,000 epinephrine has been used epidurally in pigs upto 50 kgs for surgical repair of rectal prolapse and scrotal hernia. Epidural anaesthesia can be successfully umbilical hernia, inguinal hernia, castration, scirrhous cord operation and prolapse of uterus.

Dog and Cat

The procedures consist of use of a 7.6 cm, 17 G Touhy needle. A catheter is passed through the needle and into the epidural space. The catheter provides a means for continuous epidural anaesthesia. The Touhy needle is cautiously removed by "feeding" the catheter as needle is withdrawn. A blunt 23 G needle is connected to the catheter so that a local anaesthetic solution (2% lignocaine with 1:2,00,000 epinephrine) can be injected. It is recommended that the local anaesthetic used for epidural anaesthesia be in single-use preservative ampules.

Epidural anaesthesia develops rapidly in 3–12 min after 2% lignocaine with 1:200000 epinephrine is injected. Duration of anaesthesia is 45 to 90 min. An advantage in use of lignocaine over other local anaesthetic is that it induces considerable sedation of the animal.

Lignocaine (2%) for epidural anaesthesia in the dog is estimated at 1 ml per 4.5 kg, this results in sensory blockade cranially upto L1. Dose of 2% lignocaine will induce blockade cranially to T5. Lignocaine (2%) with 1:100000 epinephrine has been used in dog for epidural anaesthesia. Prior to epidural injection all animals received 1.2 mg/kg morphine and 0.47 mg/kg atropine sulphate. A test dose of 0.5–1 ml 2% lignocaine is injected to determine if the epidural space has been penetrated.

A dose of 1 ml/2.3 kg 2% lignocaine with 1;100000 epinephrine is used for dogs undergoing cesarean delivery. Normally pregnant bitches require only 1 ml/4.5–5.4 kg. Onset of anaesthesia is rapid and lasts for 2–2.5 hrs. Some workers have used procaine 2% in a dose of 8.8 mg/kg for dogs upto 9 kg.

In Sweden mepivcaine or lignocaine is most often used for epidural analgesia. Mepivacaine (1%) in 1,200000 epinephrine is preferred for epidural blockade in dogs over other concentration. The local anaesthetic preparation is injected at a dose of 0.5 ml every 30 seconds until disappearance of rear limb toe reflex. Duration of motor blockade for 1% mepivacaine in 1,200000 epinephrine is 149±13 min.

Epidural Morphine

Preservative free morphine is injected epidurally relives pain cancer patients with in 5 min after administration. Epidural mepridine (100 mg) provided pain relief in labour upto

150 min in humans, while 25 mg provided duration of action of 55 min. Arterial pressure remains constant and nerve motor blockade after this dose.

Epidural Fentanyl

Fentanyl citrate given epidurally in human patients after cesarean section elicit analgesia upto 4 hours.

Bibliography

1. Lumb W. V. and Jones E.W., *Veterinary Anaesthesia,* p.416. Philadelphia, Lea & Febiger, 1973.
2. Wright J.G., *Veterinary Anaesethesia,* 2nd ed., Vailliere, Tindall & Cox, London, 1947.
3. Wright J.G. and Hall. L.W., *Veterinary Anaesthesia.* 5th ed., Baltimore: Williams & Wilkins, 1961.
4. Kumar P., *Textbook of Anaesthesiology,* 1st ed., Hyderabad, Paras Med. Publishers, 2008.

10

Fluid Therapy

The purpose of fluid and electrolyte therapy is to correct dehydration or overhydration and/or electrolyte imbalance. These state may occur as a result of gastrointestinal (GI), renal, cardiac, or hepatic disease, trauma; or a host of other conditions. Fluid therapy may be indicated to correct a condition of acidosis or alkalosis, treat shock, give parenteral nourishment, or even stimulate organ function (i.e. the kidneys).

INVESTIGATIONS

History Taking and Examination

Includes duration and frequency of diarrhoea and vomiting, consistency of stool, skin turgor, colour of mucus membrane and sclera, weight loss or gain.

Urinalysis

Includes tests for specific gravity, glucose, acetone, pH, albumin and microscopic sediments examination.

Causes of fluid, electrolyte, and/or protein loss include situations wherein substances are not available because of lack of supply or condition of the animal, e.g. an animal with a fractured mandible may be unable to eat or drink because of the primary disease state, other causes of fluid, electrolyte, and/or protein imbalances may involve excessive elimination.

Vomiting and diarrhea result in loss of specific electrolytes and resulting homeostatic mechanisms cause apparently paradoxical changes in plasma electrolytes. Persistent and severe vomiting causes loss of H^+ and Cl^- in the vomitus. To compensate for the proton loss the animal preferentially exchanges K^+ for Na^+ in the gastric mucosa, renal tubular cells, and other tissues. Production of more H^+ to replace losses is dependent upon formation of carbonic acid (H_2CO_3) from carbon dioxide (CO_2) and water. Clinically, the animal shows a metabolic alkalosis, with plasma bicarbonate levels usually higher than normal. Diarrhea causes large amount of loss of K^+, Na^+, H^+, Cl^- and HCO_3^-. Excessive salivation as well as kidney disease may cause imbalances; either condition may be responsible for marked fluid and electrolyte changes. Specific disease such as diabetes insipidus and mellitus may also cause excessive fluid loss. Excessive panting, hyperventilation, pulmonary disease, and inhalational anaesthesia may all cause dramatic changes in acid-base balance and, via compensatory mechanism, other electrolyte shifts. Great imbalances may result from abnormalities of skin and cutaneous glands and losses from body exudates and wounds.

1. A lack of water will cause the osmolarity and Na^+ concentration of the blood to increase, and the urine will be highly concentrated if the kidneys are functional. The animal will have oliguria, fever, circulatory collapse, dry mucous membranes, lack of skin pliability, constipation, weight loss, and sunken eyes. Muscular twitching may appear towards the terminal phase and the animal may lapse into coma and finally die.

2. Too much water causing reverse osmolarity and sodium decrease leads to polyurea and intracranial hypertension and mental confusion, pulmonary edema as well as nausea, vomiting, weakness, coma, convulsion and death.

3. Lack of adequate sodium with decrease in ECF volume, hemoconcentration, uremia and circulatory collapse.

4. Hypocalamia result in muscular weakness, ECG changes, metabolic alkalosis, paralytic ileus, impaired glucose tolerance hypercalamia charecterised by ECG changes, muscular weakness and cardiac arrest.

5. Hyperphosphatemia with hypocalcemia and tetany.

6. Hypocalcemia result in tetany, circulatory failure, abnormal muscular contraction, hypercalcemia result in calcium deposits in body and cardiac arrest.

7. Carbohydrate depletion increase catabolism of protein, water and electrolyte loss and ketosis, carbohydrate overintake result in hyperglycemia, glucosurea, obesity and hepatic failure.

8. Hypoproteinemia result in weakness, ascitis, hydrothorex, delayed wound healing.

Laboratory Examination

Laboratory examination of blood includes hematocrit, plasma CO_2, serum calcium, serum sodium, B.urea, N and creatinine determination.

Fluids to be used: Acid base changes include metabolic acidosis —excess of H^+ and deficit of HCO_3 in ECF. Keton and excess Cl^- tends to replace HCO_3. The compensatory mechanism for metabolic acidosis include hyperactive aspiration to remove H_2CO_3.

Treatment for this includes H_2CO_3 2.2 mEq/kg/15 mins, ringer lactate solution and sodium gluconate.

Metabolic Alkalosis

Excess of HCO_3 caused by deficit of H^+ in ECF. The compensatory mechanism require kidney to excrete HCO_3 and retain H^+. Treatment of this is by acidifying solution which includes NaCl, NH_4Cl.

Respiratory Acidosis

Retention of CO_2 as a consequence of alveolar hypoventilation. The fall in pH predictable from Henderson-Hasselbalch equation. Clinical signs includes respiratory distress, CNS depression with progressive disorientation, weakness and CO_2 narcosis. Treatment for this involves proper ventilation and use of alkalinizing solution.

Respiratory Alkalosis

Deficiency of H_2CO_3 thereby H^+ causes are fever, hypoxia, heat prostration, hysteria.

Clinical signs include hyperapnea, hyperactive tendon reflex, CNS stimulation with or without convulsion. Treatment of this include acidifying solution.

It has purposely dealt with single etiologic processes in the genesis of acid-base abnormalities in the pure sense. Such states rarely exist in real life. Mixed disturbances occur much more frequently, and treatment will often convert one type of acid-base disturbance into another. With careful appraisal of repeated laboratory determinations and close observation of the clinical situation, these mixed disturbances can be identified, evaluated, and managed successfully.

The most conservative fluid therapy consists of using a balanced electrolyte solution. This fluid should be incapable of inducing abnormalities in the patient and should be isotonic. Since bicarbonate cannot be autoclaved, most commercial solutions do not contain this substance. Lactate or acetate ions are metabolized by the liver or bicarbonate and these substances are usually incorporated commercially. If substantial liver disease exists, these compounds are not easily converted and their beneficial effects are not realized. The conservative approach is indicated when there are no particular electrolyte disturbances or there is no way to determine which if any electrolyte imbalance exists. Use of such a balanced solution is not an effective means of correcting severe acidosis, alkalosis, hyponatremia, or hypokalemia.

When metabolic acidosis is present, an unphysiologically high concentration of bicarbonate must be given. When additional sodium is also required, a very useful solution is obtained by adding 3–5 g $NaHCO_3$ to each liter of lactated ringer's solution. Nearly pure $NaHCO_3$ can be purchased in bulk from a laboratory supply house. The powder can then be measured into 3 g and 5 g individual packets, which can be gas sterilized. The packets can then be stored until needed. If Na^+ are not abnormally low, fluid given should be high in bicarbonate but not abnormally high in Na^+. In this case, a slightly, hypertonic solution of $NaHCO_3$ (approximately 300 m Osm) can be made by adding sterile distilled water (q.s. to 1L) to 13 g sterile $NaHCO_3$ powder. If it is impossible to monitor the patient, a crude estimate of the amount of bicarbonate needed can be made. An animal in severe acidosis will usually have bicarbonate levels of 10–15 mEq/L. Normal bicarbonate levels for most species vary between 20 and 30 mEq/L. Therefore, animals in acidosis will have deficits of about 10–15 mEq/L ECF. Since the ECF is about 20% of body weight, it is impossible to calculate the volume of ECF for each other. The number of mEq of bicarbonate needed is calculated by multiplying the bicarbonate deficit by the ECF volume.

Example A: A 450 kg horse with estimated bicarbonate deficit of 10 mEq/L ECF; 450 kg × 20% × 10 mEq/L = 900 mEq needed.

Example B: A 20 kg dog with estimated bicarbonate deficit of 10 mEq/L ECF; 20 kg × 20 % × 10 mEq/L = 40 mEq needed.

In cases of severe acidosis associated with anesthesia, surgery, and/or shock, it may be desirable to administer a bolus of $NaHCO_3$. Commercial solutions containing this concentration can be made by mixing 84 g gas-sterilized $NaHCO_3$ q.s to 1000 ml with sterile water. This solution should be given at the rate of 2.2 mEq/kg every 15 minutes as needed. The solution should be injected intravenously at the rate of approximately 10 ml/min. Horses present some special problems in acid-base management. In cases of severe diarrhea, shock, and intestinal obstruction, the horse seems predisposed to rather severe metabolic acidosis. Respiratory acidosis is a very common sequel to closed-circuit inhalation anesthesia in the horse. An abnormally low concentration of Na^+ is also common problem in dehydrated horse. Dangerous hyperkalemia , with blood levels >6–7 mEq/L, may be associated with acidosis in foals. Prompt correction of the acidosis will usually correct the hyperkalemia.

Ruminants also present special fluid and electrolyte management problems. Grain overloading will result in severe dehydration and metabolic acidosis. Calf diarrhea also results in severe dehydration and metabolic acidosis. If hyperkalemia exists, one should guard against administration of even more K^+.

When dealing with herbivors, it is important to remember that normal feed contains high levels of K^+. When these animals are anorexic, they frequently become depleted in K^+. The best way to replace K^+ deficits is by consumption of hay of grass, but K^+ must be added parenterally when the situation dictates.

Special problems in fluid and electrolyte management for all species are presented by heat exhaustion, and burns. Heat exhaustion is due to excessive loss of Na^+. Renal excretion of Na^+ ceases but water excretion continues. Conversely, heat prostration involves loss of both Na^+ and Cl^-. With burns more electrolyte than water is lost. The end result is a hypotonic dehydration of ECF. With loss of ECF electrolyte, fluid moves into cells, causing swelling and edema. The latest forms of therapy involve use of hypertonic electrolytes that replace Na^+. The goal of this therapy is a gradual restoration of ECF volume.

Calculating fluid requirement: Calculation of how much fluid to use must be based on a total of the normal turnover of water plus replacement of the abnormal losses, for practical purposes, 65 ml/kg/24 hr average water turnover for mature animals and 130 ml/kg/24 hr for immature animals of all species. From these assumptions, an average, 1 mature dog weighing 20 kg requires about 1300 ml for a daily maintenance supply of water. A horse weighing 445 kg would require about 29 L/day.

Replacement of abnormal losses must be in addition to maintenance requirements. To calculate this quantity, one must estimate the degree of dehydration present. This is accomplished by application of the following guidelines.

An animal with 4% dehydration (mild or no evidence of clinical dehydration) will have a history of fluid loss (vomiting, diarrhea), the skin will be slightly leathery, the mucous membranes will still be moist, and there will be evidence of a history of thirst. These signs dictate replacement of water to 4% of body weight (i.e. a 20 kg dog –800 ml).

With a 6% dehydration (moderate), the animal's skin will be leathery, when the skin is lifted, it will peak but will return to normal slowly; the hair coat will be dull and the mucous membranes dry, but the tongue will still be moist. In this case, replace fluids to 6% of body weight (20 kg dog –1.2 L).

Animals with severe dehydration (i.e. 8%) will show a lack of skin pliability and elasticity. When picked up, the skin will peak and stay, both the mucous membranes and tongue will be dry, and the eyeballs will be soft and sunken. These animals require replacement of water to 8% of their body weight (20 kg dog –1.6 L).

Circulatory insufficiency is the severe extension of the dehydration syndrome. All the classic signs of a circulatory collapse are evidenced. Water is replaced up to 12% of body weight (20 kg dog –2.4 L). In classic signs of acute shock, water is replaced up to 15% of body weight (20 kg dog –3 L).

Example A: A 2 month old, 20 kg dog 6% dehydrated clinically is losing approximately 120ml water/day while undergoing treatment for a Orather severe diarrhea. This animal needs: (1) Maintenance –130 mi/kg × 20 kg –2600 ml, (2) Replacement –0.06 × 20 kg –1.2 L or 1200 ml, (3) Continuing loss = 120 ml, (4) Total fluid required a, over the first 24 hours –3920 ml.

Example B. A mature 450 kg horse with severe obstructive colic and 8% dehydration clinically is presented. This animal needs: (1) Maintenance –65ml/kg × 450 kg = 29,250 ml, (2) Replacement 0.08 × 450 kg = 36 L or 36,000 ml, (3) Total during the first 24 hours = 62,250 ml.

Additional circumstances that must be considered are:

1. Dehydration affects young animals much faster than adults.
2. Old animals with chronic diseases (especially impaired renal function) require more water than other animals.
3. Animals need more fluids if they are very active or if the weather is hot and/or humid.
4. Drugs such as corticosteroids and diuretics will alter fluid and electrolyte requirements.
5. Animals that have been under various forms of anesthesia may require additional water for a few days.

Rate of Administration: The rate of fluid and/ or electrolyte replacement should parallel the severity of dehydration. Fluids should be administered rapidly at first and then at decreasing rates until the condition is corrected. Most workers have felt that rates of about 15 ml/kg/hour were reasonable.

Conservative and reasonable practice would dictate infusion rates of about 50 ml/kg/hour in severely dehydrated cases. Less severe cases should tolerate rates of 15–30 ml/kg/hour. In all cases the rate of infusion should be slowed after the first hour of administration and should be slowed considerably if no urine flow is established. After 4 or more hours of fluid administration without urine flow, rate of administration should be 2 ml/kg/hr or less. Every attempt must be made to establish renal function if no urine flow is detected after 2 hours of fluid administration. In administration of fluids, common sense and clinical judgement must be exercised. If an animal is severely dehydrated and in shock, it is almost impossible to administer fluids too fast. If, however, an animal is almost normally hydrated and the aim is, only to maintain hydration, the rate should be slowed considerably. The importance of renal function has been repeatedly emphasized. A commonly used method of determining if the kidneys are capable of functioning is to inject a small bolus (1–25 ml, depending on size of the animal) of 50%

glucose. The urine is then checked every 5 minutes for the presence of glucose which indicates glomerular filtration is occurring.

Route of Administration: The route of fluid administration depends on the type of illness being dealt with and the severity of the condition, degree of dehydration, condition of the patient, type of electrolyte imbalance, organic functions of the patient, and time and equipment available.

Probably the earliest, most physiologic, and most overlooked route of administration of fluid and electrolytes is oral or nasogastric. The oral route is least dangerous, since the solution can be administered without strict attention to tonicity, volume, and asepsis. Replacement of electrolytes by using combination of electrolyte salts, glycine, and dextrose has been especially successful.

The most commonly used and perhaps most practical routes of fluid and electrolyte administration are parenteral routes: intravenous (IV), subcutaneous (SC) or intraperitoneal (IP).

Evaluation: The only effective method for evaluation of the success of fluid therapy is the application of clinical judgment and experience. One must observe a return to normal of the clinical signs presented by the patient as well as of the various physiologic parameters being monitored.

Bibliography

1. Kirk R. W., *Current Veterinary Therapy,* Vol. 3, *Small Animal Practice,* Philadelphia W. .B Saunders, 421, 1968.

11

Transfusion

Transfusion: Use of whole blood, blood plasma, and blood serum occupies an important place in veterinary therapy. Major indications for whole blood therapy include hemorrhage or shock, anemia, coagulation abnormalities, and provision of specific and nonspecific antibodies. Whole blood is also known to supply substances of metabolic benefit.

Donor selection: Although five isoantibodies have been demonstrated in blood serums of transfused dogs the only known blood factor causing transfusion reactions of clinical significance is the A factor. Approximately 63% of all dogs seem to be positive for factor A and 37% are negative. Unless the practitioner is able to type each donor and recipient before transfusion, it is desirable to maintain A-negative donor dogs (universal donors) that have never received a transfusion. Blood from these animals can be given safely to any other dog, whereas A-positive blood can be given only to A-positive recipients.

Although A-negative donors are the most desirable, finding them is difficult. Interpretation of blood types requires a technician with training and experience. The inexperienced clinician is not likely, to be able to make the necessary readings. In addition, serum for typing dogs for the A factor is almost impossible to obtain. The best sources are large research facilities or institutional hospitals with well-managed laboratory animal facilities. Serum for typing human blood is not adequate for dogs.

CROSS MATCHING

It is of limited value in dogs. Since an incompatible recipient will not be detected unless it or the donor has previously had a transfusion with incompatible blood. Confusing results are often obtained with cross matching, since blood factors other than A cause production of antibodies easily detected with this technique. The other factors are apparently not important in transfusion incompatibilities. From a practical standpoint, however, cross matching will prevent use of incompatible types and is essential when repeated transfusions from unknown donors are used.

Dangers in using A-positive blood for an A negative recipient are delayed destruction of the transfused cells 7–10 days following the first transfusion, sensitization of the animal to subsequent transfusions of A-positive blood, immediate transfusion reaction if the recipient has been previously sensitized, and hemolytic disease in A-positive pups from an A-positive sire and A-negative bitch transfused with A-positive blood. This can be avoided if pups are not allowed to suckle during the first 24 hours of life.

There is little information on blood typing in cats. It appears that most cats have the same blood type, but complications after single or repeated transfusions have been experienced by many clinicians. For practical purposes, blood normally will be used in emergency situations only and rarely more than once. The likelihood of experiencing a transfusion reaction under these circumstances is greatly reduced. Cross matching should be used if repeated transfusions are indicated.

Cross matching techniques: Blood samples are collected from both recipient and donor and allowed to clot. The serum is removed from each tube and labelled. A suspension of erythrocyte from each animal is made by resuspending cells from the clot in several ml of saline. The cell suspension should be the consistency of thin tomato juice. One drop of donor cell suspension is mixed with two drops of recipient serum (major test). One drop of recipient cell suspension is mixed with two drops of donor serum (minor test). The tubes are incubated 5–8 minutes at 37 °C in a water bath or for 30 minutes at room temperature. The tubes are then centrifugated at 1000 rpm for one minute. The cells are then resuspended by jarring the tubes sharply against the hand or flipping with a finger. A strong agglutination can be detected macroscopically. A drop of the contents is placed on a microscope slide without a cover slip and examined at a magnification of 100, results are reported as strong, weak or negative agglutination. If there is a doubt that agglutination has occurred the slide is rotated from side to side for a few minutes. If agglutination is occurring it will become stronger. If not any clumps that have formed will break up.

Blood collection: Direct transfusions are usually unsatisfactory in veterinary medicine for two reasons. Lack of patient cooperation and clotting in collection and / or administration apparatus. The general technique of collection is the same whether the blood is to be stored or used directly. Commercially available collection equipment with disposable evacuated bottles containing acid citrate dextrose solution is available and practical for small animal use. In cats blood may be drawn directly into a syringe with heparin and injected into the recipient after cross matching. Blood with heparin cannot be stored for more than a few hours. Collection bottle should be stored in the refrigerator before collection to reduce initial haemolysis and they must be rotated gently during the entire collection period for all species, blood should be collected under sterile condition. For large animals 3.8 L containers can be autoclaved and partially filled with 400 ml 4% solution of sodium citrate. Blood can be collected by gravity flow from the jugular vein through a 10 G needle in larger species or the collection can be speeded with use of a suction device.

Collected blood should be stored in the refrigerator at a temperature of 5.6–6.7 C. Dog blood can be stored safely for 21 days. However it is best to remove the plasma for future use after 16 days. Cat blood is usually collected only as needed as are horse and cattle blood.

Plasma can be aspirated from the top of a stored container of blood after atleast 12 hrs in the refrigerator to allow for separation. It can then be stored in the refrigerator for several months or frozen and kept for as long as two years. All containers should be adequately identified.

Administration and dosage: Inexpensive, sterile, disposable equipment with built in filters is commercially available in a variety of designs. Speed of administration best controlled by the gauge of the needle or the catheter. Venous cut down and insertion of large bore cannula is a much preferred method if a more rapid injection rate is indicated.

Rate of administration is determined by severity of signs and the calculated dose. A large animal may be able to handle rates of 40–60 ml/kg/hr or more in a case of severe shock whereas a 10 kg dog or a 5 kg cat might not tolerate a rate much about 5–10 ml/kg/hr. The usual recommended dose of blood or plasma is 10–20 ml/kg depending on the severity of the condition.

Interspecies transfusions: It is known that 50 % of transfused canine red blood cells are destroyed in the cat within 6 hrs after injection. Hemolysed cells are not beneficial to the animal and cause additional problem in excretion of breakdown products by already stressed liver and kidneys. More than one transfusion of blood from one species into another may cause severe anaphylactic reaction and death.[1]

Washed red blood cells: In most instances the only reason for use of blood is to provide oxygen carrying capacity. It is not necessary to use whole blood for volume expansion. If the need is for oxygen carrying capacity the incidence of transfusion can be reduced significantly by use of washed red blood cells. The donor and the recipient should still be cross matched. To each 500 ml collected blood, 500 ml an isotonic electrolyte solution is added. The mixture is agitated gently and centrifuged at 1000 rpm or allowed to settle. Then, the supernatant is removed and the process is repeated atleast three times. Sterile procedure must be maintained throughout.

Plasma volume expanders: It has been assumed that plasma itself is an ideal expander of blood volume in shock therapy because it is well retained in the vascular space. Incomplete retention is frequently accompanied by urticaria which may be prevented by use of anti histamines or coticosteroids.

Artificial plasma volume expanders are generally considered to be somewhat inferior to plasma itself. The two most commonly used agents in veterinary medicine are dextran and gelatin.

Dextran is a polysaccharide obtained by bacterial fermentation of sucrose. It is administered intravenously as a 6% solution in physiological saline. Approximately 50% is excreted by the kidney within first 24 hrs. The remainder traverse the capillary wall very slowly and is oxidized within few weeks. Dextran appears to have no significant deleterious effects on renal, hepatic or other vital functions. But does have some antigenic action that may result in pruritis, urticaria, joint pain and other minor side effects.[2]

Sterile gelatine solution are also available for use as infusion colloids. These agents are excreted rapidly by the kidneys and may produce extra stress for that organ. Use of this agent is not recommended for animals with renal disease. Gelatine is antigenic and minor allergic type reactions occur following its use in some animals.

Parenteral alimentation: The first continuous intravenous delivery technique for long term administration of nutrients was employed in dogs. The technique is specially useful in inflammatory lesion of the bowel requiring healing time that can be guided only by placing the gut completely at rest. Hypermetabolic states associated with extensive burns, severe infections or multiple injuries all respond to this therapy.

Meticulous care of an indwelling central venous catheter is essential to safe long term parenteral feeding. The catheter tip must extend into the anterior vena cava or even the right atrium. The size of the catheter will depend on the size and dose requirement of the animal to be maintained. In very small animal jugular vein cut down will be necessary and the catheter should be exteriorized through a subcutaneous tunnel to a point on the dorsal aspect of the neck or between the scapula. Catheter placement must be done under aseptic condition. Withdrawal or administration of blood through the catheter should be avoided since blood in the lumen is more likely to increase the possibility of contamination slugging or clotting.

Alimentation solution cannot be autoclaved because of caramilisation at elevated temperatures. However most large hospitals, pharmacies are equipped to prepare this solution using a laminar flow filtered air hood for mixing and a small micropore membrane filter for sterilization.

Bibliography

1. Kumar Pramod, *Textbook of Anaesthesiology,* 1st ed., Hyderabad, Paras Med. Publishers, 2008.
2. Thornton G.W., In Robert W. Kirk ed., *Current Veterenary Therapy,* 5th ed., page 47, Philedelphia, W.B. Saunders, 1974.

12

Diuretics

In general, diuretics are not as effective as other available agents. Their continued use often leads to loss of effectiveness and gastric irritation may become a problem.

Aldosterone antagonists: Spironolactone is an oral preparation often marketed in combination with thiazide diuretic. This combination is rational, since the potassium excretion encountered with thiazide diuretics is mainly the result of exchange of sodium.

For potassium in the distal tubule, an exchange that is almost entirely under the control of aldosterone, this combination of agent enhance diuretic action and controls the side effects of thiazide agents.

Spironolactone is a true competitive antagonist of aldosterone which enhances direct resorption of sodium in more proximal area of the distal tubule of the nephrons. The more distal area of the distal tubular network, aldosterone promotes sodium resorption by enhancement of exchange mechanisms with either potassium or hydrogen ions. Spironolactone blocks both these actions of aldosterone.

Spironolactone may exert some oestrogen like activity but is not diabetogenic. The usual dose is 0.5–1.5 mg/kg alone or in combination with a thiazide or other diuretics. No parenteral form is available. In patients with diminished renal function, i.e. high BUN >50 mg%, these agents should be used with care. During the withdrawal period, it may be necessary to continue use of thiazide or other diuretic for 48–72 hrs to promote potassium excretion.

Heparin prevents release of aldosterone by the adrenal gland. When indicated for therapy of other conditions, one may take advantage of this diuretic action as well.

POTASSIUM RETAINING AGENTS

Triemterene: It is acting directly on tubular transport of sodium. This effect appears to be independent of the plasma level of aldosterone. The incidence of hyperkalemia with prolonged administration is greater. The reduced rate of potassium excretion associated with use of this compound has been attributed to inhibition of potassium secretion in the distal tubular network. The usual oral dose is 0.5–3 mg/kg. onset of action is usually within 2–3 hrs and may last 6–8 hrs. with three times a day administration, the action of the drug seems to become more pronounced on the 2nd and 3rd day of treatment. No parenteral form is available.

Amiloride: 1 mg/kg IV in an anesthetized sheep; urine potassium decrease to one third of the baseline and sodium excretion increased 6–180 fold. Clinical doses in animal has not been established.

Loop of henle diuretics: It acts by affecting resorption of sodium in the ascending limb of loop of henle. These drugs are the only diuretic agents that have a significant effect on patient with impaired renal function. The diuretic response to these agents is not significantly altered by changes in the acid base balance of the patient. The ability of the kidney to regulate bicarbonate resorption is apparently not altered.

Furosemide: It is an orthochlorosulfonamide compound but it has an additional carboxyl group that differentiate it from thiazides. Furosemide is available in 12.5 mg and 50 mg tablets for oral administration and 50 mg/ml injectable form is available for parenteral use.

The dose of furosemide for dogs and cats is approximately 5 mg/kg. following oral administration response is often seen within 30 min. The effective dose for horses is 1.5 mg/kg the drug is not approved by FDA. It has been used for udder edema in dairy cattle. It is also used at race tracks in horses as prophylaxis therapy for epistaxis.

Ethacrynic acid: It is apparently very similar to furosemide, its chemical structure is quite different. Mechanism of elimination and side effects are similar to furosemide. High dose may produce hypokalemia. It is available for both oral and parenteral form. For dog and cats dose is 5 mg/kg.

Bibliography

1. Grant C. L., *Rational Drug Therapy,* Vol. 6., W.B. Saunders, Philadelphia:, 1972.
2. Goth A., *Medical Pharmacology,* p.458. St. Louis, C. V. Mosby, 1972.

13

Shock

Circulatory shock has been defined as an acute circulatory insufficiency in which cardiac output is not adequate to provide for normal perfusion to tissues. Metabolic and cellular changes are sequential and their severity varies with time as well as the degree of initial disturbance. Once shock is evoked the progression of events is largely dependent of the initiating mechanism.

Circulatory insufficiency is common to all form of shock. Diminished blood flow results in insufficient tissue oxygenation. Treatment of shock centers on prevention and correction of cellular hypoxia.

Commonly observed signs include tachycardia; weak, thready or nonpalpable arterial pulse; collapse of peripheral veins; cold, pale mucous membranes; prolonged capillary refilling time; dry shriveled tongue; mental depression or unconsciousness; subnormal temperature and lack of surface warmth; and oliguria or anuria. Digital pressure applied to gingival membranes is followed by an extended capillary refilling time.

Aetiology and types: Circulatory shock may be classed as three major types according to primary etiology. This basic classification includes hypovolemic shock, vasculogenic shock, and cardiogenic shock. The scheme of classification is as follows:

A. Reduction in blood volume (hypovolemic shock):
1. Loss of whole blood —external hemorrhage, internal hemorrhage
2. Loss of plasma —surface exudation due to thermal or chemical burns, exudation into body cavities —inflammatory process
3. Loss of water and electrolytes —acute water deprivation, excessive sweating, vomiting, diarrhea and fluid loss in acute intestinal obstruction.

B. Primary changes in venous capacitance or peripheral resistance (vasculogenic shock)
1. Endotoxin
2. Anaphylaxis or acute hypersensitivity
3. Vasomotor paralysis from central nervous system trauma or depression.

C. Acute changes in cardiac pumping effectiveness (cardiogenic shock)
1. Interference with cardiac filling

a. Cardiac tamponade
b. Positive pressure ventilation.
2. Improper ventricular emptying
   a. Acute pulmonary heart disease
   b. Abrupt increase in systemic vascular resistance
   c. Rupture of chordae tendinae
   d. Severe toxic myocardial depression
   e. Significant cardiac dysarrhthmias.

REDUCTION IN BLOOD VOLUME (HYPOVOLEMIC SHOCK)

Hypovolemic shock is due to volume loss from the circulation. In a healthy animal rapid loss of 30% or more of normal blood volume induces signs of circulatory loss. Plasma loss occurs when increased pulmonary vascularity develops over a large area such as superficial burns or acute intestinal perforation. Significant depletion in plasma volume also occurs in rapid dehydration from excessive sweating, prolonged diuresis or persistent vomiting and diarrhea.

Changes in venous capacitance or peripheral resistance (vasogenic shock): Severe bacterial infection are a significant cause of shock due to bacterial toxins. Endotoxins are capable of inducing shock. Septicemia caused by organism such as *E.Coli*, Proteus species and Klebsiella species. Endotoxins cause increase portal vein pressure because of hepatic vein constriction and an increase in pulmonary artery pressure because of pulmonary constriction. Cardiac output falls and large quantity of blood are sequestered in hepato portal system.

Acute changes in cardiac pumping effectiveness (cardiogenic shock): In animal it may result from the heart failing to fill properly or empty properly. Incomplete emptying may be due to rupture of chordae tendinae, severe depression of myocardial contractility or onset of arrythmias. It is characterised by low cardiac output, hypotension, increased systemic resistance and elevated CVP. In this case auscultation or ECG examination is performed.

Pathophysiology: In response to hypoxia and hypotension reflex neuroendocrine stimulation occurs. Intense sympathetic activity occurs. Catecholamine is released at neuro effector endings and from the medulla. Pituitary release ADH. Rennin angiotensin aldosterone mechanism is also activated. Sympathetic cardiac stimulation cause in increased heart rate and contractility.

Reduced renal blood flow results in decreased GFR and leads to oliguria and anuria. Prolonged renal ischemia may lead to tubular necrosis due to hemoglobinemia or myoglobinemia in case of trauma. Renal shutdown is marked by azotemia, hyperkalemia and metabolic acidosis.

With lack of adequate tissue perfusion, decreased aerobic oxidation and increased anerobic glycolysis that leads to increased circulating pyruvate and lactate levels. So metabolic acidosis occurs.

In acidotic state and limited cerebral blood flow may cause cerebral depression. In circulatory shock progressive myocardial depression, microcirculatory slugging of blood and development of DIC may occur.

Therapy: Early correction of shock is mandatory. The need for fluid and blood administration to the hypovolemic patient is urgent. Volume expansion is standard therapy in hypovolemic shock and is also useful in septic and cardiogenic shock. The red cell mass is usually adequate to support life if the effective circulating volume can be restored. Requirement for large quantities of replacement fluids center around the following considerations. Certain losses may be hidden or inapparent, especially in traumatic shock, loss of vascular tone, necessitate a greater than normal filling volume, loss of capillary volume integrity and moderate overfilling of vascular system resulting in enhancement of cardiac output.

Blood: Whole blood is indicated in significant hemorrhage or hemolysis. Blood should be administered at the rate of 20–40 ml/kg, except where blood loss is continuing. Administration of blood should be accompanied by balanced electrolyte solutions in a ratio of 1 part blood to between 2 and 6 parts fluid.

PLASMA AND PLASMA EXPANDERS

Plasma, serum, and fractionated protein solution should be considered to expand blood volume without additional cells. 2–5 ml/kg plasma may be given intravenously rapidly, then slowly to a total quantity of 5–20 ml/kg. Limitation of use of plasma is cost and availability. Canine plasma albumin solutions are commercially available. Several type of plasma expander like dextran solution and low molecular weight dextran solution are available. The initial IV dose of Dextran 40 is 10–15 ml/kg and total dose should not exceed 20 ml/kg over a 24 hour.

Electrolyte solutions: Initial administration of sufficient amount of fluid is ·most vital measure in shock therapy. Treatment should be based on achieving volume expansion sufficient to effect satisfactory arterial pressure, adequate urine output, and good peripheral perfusion without excessive elevation of CVP or severe reduction in plasma oncotic pressure.

Administration of various type of electrolyte solutions has been advocated, particularly isotonic saline and ringer lactate.

The most danger of use of fluids is pulmonary oedema and congestive heart failure. CVP provides a reliable information for additional volume load. Food administration should be stopped when the auscultatory and clinical signs of pulmonary oedema develop.

Oxygen and ventilatory assistance: In patients suffering from lack of adequate ventilation or in which there is interference with diffusion of gases across the respiratory oepithelium, oxygen is administered by inhalation of 40–100% atmosphere by mask or ET tubes. In the majority of patients suffering from shock, limitation in tissue oxygenation result primarily from reduced cardiac output and AV shunting in poorly ventilated pulmonary capillaries. This condition is corrected more successfully by improved alveolar ventilation that is provided by patent airway and ventilatory assistance.

CARDIOSTIMULATORY AND VASOACTIVE DRUGS

Sympathetic Agonists

Norepinephrine, epinephrine and isoproterenol have been used in treating shock, particularly when other measures fail to raise arterial pressure. Norepinephrine is most valuable as a pressor agent . When diluted to a concentration of 8 mcg/ml in 5% dextrose, it may be given as a continuous IV drip at a rate of 0.5 ml/min for average size dog. Epinephrine 0.1–0.5 ml 1:1000 dilution may be given iv to average size dog for cardiac stimulation and vasomotor effects. Isoproterenol is effective in improving cardiac output and lowering CVP via cardiac stimulation. Its beta adrenergic action has a marked ionotropic effect greatly accelerate heart rate and causes vasodilatation particularly in skeletal muscle. It should be diluted to a concentration of 10 mcg/ml in 5% dextrose and given continuous IV drip at a rate of 5–10 mcg/min. Dopamine —a precursor of norepinephrine and epinephrine, possesses beta-adrenergic and only minor alfa-adrenergic effect. It is useful in treatment of cardiogenic shock.

Potentially harmful effects of catecholamines include intensification of tissue ischemia, reduction in plasma volume because of increased capillary filtration, increase in oxygen requirement resulting from the direct calorigenic effect and induction of tachyarrythmia and ventricular fibrillation.

Sympathetic Antagonist

Phenoxybenzamine and phentolamine are beneficial in sustained, deep shock.

Steroids: Administration of massive dose of corticosteroids has a become a principle step in shock therapy. Some controversy still exist regarding the benefits of steroids administration in routine regime of shock. Steroids in very large doses affect microcirculation, producing sustained vasodilatation and significantly improve tissue perfusion and cardiac output.

Steroids may be considered in the treatment of shock as the most nearly ideal vasodilator available to the practitioner. Other effects of steroids which are beneficial in shock therapy include protection of capillary endothelial integrity during hypoxia, stabilization of lysozomal membranes and reduction in sensitivity to endotoxins.

An optimal dose for use in shock is 4–6 mg/kg dexamethasone, or equivalent doses of methylprednisolone, (25–30 mg/kg), prednisolone. (35–40 mg/kg), or other glucocorticoid. Following adequate fluid volume replacement, steroids should be given as a single IV injection (bolus) over a 1–3 minute period. The more soluble succinate and phosphate salts of steroids are purported to have a more rapid onset of action. Improvement in circulation may be noted in some patients within 5–10 minutes and may persist for as long as 4 hours. If arterial pressure is not reestablished following volume replacement and vasodilator therapy, positive inotropic agents such as norepinephrine, epinephrine, or isoproterenol may be used more effectively and at lower dosage than when not preceded by steroid-induced vasodilation.

OTHER THERAPEUTIC MEASURES

Antibiotics: Use of broad-spectrum antibiotics is specifically indicated whenever shock is the result of sepsis or trauma. Antibiotics are important for prophylactic management of shock from other causes as well. It is advisable to consider possible adverse effects, including moderate circulatory depression, that are attributed to certain antibiotics, especially the aminoglycosides.

Heparin: Administration of heparin sodium, USP, should be restricted to patients in which DIC has been demonstrated. DIC is the syndrome of widespread thromboses in microcirculatory vessels because of combined effects of capillary stagnation and stimulation of the coagulation process. The latter may occur from acidosis, hemolysis, bacterial toxins, or presence of tissue damage and necrosis. DIC may be ameliorated by correction of the acidosis, volume expansion, vasodilator therapy, or administration of heparin. Heparin is administered intravenously at a dose of 250 units/kg and may be repeated every 4 hours. It is not indicated in the latter stages of DIC.

Hypothermia: Hypothermia as an adjunct in treatment of shock is of uncertain benefit. While it has been a long-accepted procedure to maintain or restore normal body temperature, evidence suggests that a moderate hypothermia (33°C) may be effective in increasing survival rate in both hemorrhagic, and endotoxic shock. In any event, one should attempt rapid restoration of body temperature in a shock patient by devices or, procedures supplying large quantities of heat to the body surface. Rapid surface warming results in diversion of blood flow to the skin from more critical areas.

Other cardiotonics: Cardiotonic agents, other than the sympathomemitics described above, may be of use in strengthening cardiac contractility. Calcium salts are capable of increasing circulatory performance through their positive inotropic effects, particularly when hyperkalemia exists. Calcium gluconate is safer than the more highly ionized calcium salts. Intravenously, the dose of calcium gluconate is 10–20 mg/kg administered slowly.

Glucagon, is a polypeptide hormone with significant cardiostimulatory activity. It produces a moderately sustained inotropy and chronotropy and has been reported to be of value in treatment of experimental cardiogenic shock in dogs. Because of marked action in stimulating cardiac output and absence of arrhythmogenic effects, glucagon is potentially a useful drug in management of circulatory shock. It may be administered at a dose of 50 ug/kg intravenously and may be repeated at 30-minutes intervals.

Rapid-acting digitalis glycosides such as deslanoside, or digoxin may be employed.

Mannitol: Urine output tends to be clearly reduced at arterial pressures of less than 80 mm Hg and generally ceases at arterial pressures below 50 mm Hg. In shock, following restoration of effective circulatory volume and the normalization of arterial pressure, renal function may not necessarily recover promptly or adequately. Mannitol effects a return of urine flow by further increasing intravascular volume, promoting increased renal blood flow, retaining glomerular filtrate within renal tubules, and reducing cellular edema in the renal tubular epithelium. Doses of 1–3 g/kg enhance urine flow in oliguric or anuric animals that have received adequate fluid replacement. An inotropic effect of mannitol results from a slight increase in plasma extracellular osmolarity.

SPECIAL CONSIDERATIONS

Acute Adrenocortical Insufficiency: An acute shock like state occurs in animals that develop sudden loss of adrenocortical function. The disease complex is marked by weakness, prostration, hypovolemia, and electrolyte imbalances. There is hyperkalemia usually hyponatremia, along with an absolute sodium deficit. ECG changes include P-wave suppression, widening of the QRS interval, and increased amplitude of T waves. Because acute adrenal crisis represents a medical emergency, IV fluids and corticosteroids must be administered immediately. Fluids containing potassium should be avoided. Use of 5% dextrose in normal saline may be used for volume expansion and correction of sodium deficit.

Hydrocortisone hemisuccinate, (cortisol hemisuccinate), preparations administered intravenously are ideal for rapid supplementation of glucocorticoids. In addition, mineralocorticoids such as deoxycorticosterone acetate, USP (percorten, descotone, DOCA acetate), are required. Extended therapy includes mineralocorticoids and increased dietary salt intake.

Anaphylactic shock: Anaphylaxis is an acute systemic reaction that occurs upon administration of an antigen to any suitable sensitized subject and is mediated by pharmacologically active substances. Anaphylactic reactions are the result of the interaction of antigen and IgE antibody and the subsequent release of mediators from mast cells and basophils. These pharmacologically active substances are principally histamine, serotonin, and slow-reacting substance of anaphylaxis, in addition to plasma kinins. These agents, through their own effects and by initiating certain physiologic reflexes, cause anaphylaxis.

The most important step in treatment of anaphylaxis is the prompt administration of epinephrine. Epinephrine, with its α-and α-adrenergic effects; is clearly the treatment of choice. Intramuscular administration of 0.1 ml 1 : 1000 epinephrine is used in dogs of average size. Hypotension, bronchospasm, pruritus, and urticaria are commonly relieved if epinephrine is employed early. If the clinical signs persist, epinephrine may be repeated at 15–20 minute intervals.

Diphenhydramine hydrochloride (benadryl), administered intravenously at a dose of 2 mg/kg is suggested when the symptoms of anaphylaxis are severe or when the response to epinephrine is not satisfactory. In mild reactions, antihistamines may be given orally. Specific antagonists of mediators other than histamine are recognized and may become useful in treatment of anaphylaxis in which histamine is not the primary mediating substance. Aminophylline, 10 mg/kg intravenously is indicated when bronchospasm persists. Corticosteroids should not be considered as primary therapy in anaphylaxis but employed as adjunctive therapy where shock persists.

If anaphylaxis proceeds to a state of circulatory collapse and shock, the measures described above for the management of shock are indicated. These include volume expansion, massive quantities of corticoids and the vasoactive and inotropic agents.

Acute colitis syndrome in horses: A particularly malignant form of circulatory shock is observed in horses afflicted with the acute colitis (colitis X) syndrome. The disease onset is extremely rapid. Its specific etiology is uncertain but its development may relate to exhaustion and other forms of physical and physiologic stresses. There is early elevation of body temperature, which later falls to normal or below. A profuse diarrhea develops, but at times death occurs so quickly that the diarrhea is not observed. There are dark, congested mucous membranes; focal areas of sweating; shallow, rapid respiration; and, commonly, outward signs of colic.

Hemoconcentration is marked by a rise in PCV. In more advanced stages, the animals exhibit signs of extreme distress, central nervous depression, and mania. The survival rate is low and clinical management must begin early and be pursued vigorously.

The principal consideration in treating acute colitis is in maintaining an adequate circulatory fluid volume. Balanced electrolyte solutions in quantities as great as 12 L/hr (1 L/5 min) may be required for expansion and maintenance of adequate circulatory volume. Metabolic acidosis is best corrected by first measuring the negative base excess (base deficit) and administering sodium bicarbonate in appropriate amounts. Alternatively, in presumed severe acidosis, the base deficit may be estimated to be 0–15 mEq/L.

As in other forms of shock, a comprehensive regimen also requires use of steroids, antibiotics, vasoactive drugs where indicated, and other forms of supportive therapy as discussed above.

Bibliography

1. Goth A., *Medical Pharmacology*, p. 458., St. Louis, C. V. Mosby, 1972.
2. Grant C. L., *Rational Drug Therapy*, Vol. 6., Philadelphia, W.B. Saunders, 1972.

14

General Consideration in Anaesthesiology

The anaesthetist aims to prevent awareness of pain, provide immobility and, whenever this is needed, relaxation of the skeletal muscles. These aims must be achieved in such a way that the safety of the patient is not jeopardized during the preanaesthetic period.

Many animals fear and resist the restraint necessary for the administration of anaesthetics thereby increasing not only the technical difficulties of administration but also the dangers inseparable from their use. A fully conscious animal forced to breathe a strange and possibly pungent vapour struggles to escape and the sympathoadrenal stimulation produced greatly increases the risks associated with the induction of anaesthesia. For this reason, veterinary anaesthetists often employ sedative drugs to facilitate the completion of general anaesthesia as well as to overcome the natural fear of restraint inherent in animals and control any tendency to move suddenly during operations under local analgesia. In addition, the anaesthetist must recognize that not only does the response of each species of animal to the various anaesthetics differ due to anatomical and physiological differences, but that there is often a marked variation in response between breeds within each particular species. Another factor which must be considered is that many veterinarians have to carry out tasks without highly skilled assistance and, when employing general anaesthesia, after inducing it themselves, have to depute its maintenance to a nurse or even a lay attendant. For all these reasons the continued development in recent years of safe, simple, easily applied techniques of general anaesthesia and regional analgesia is particularly welcome.[1]

TYPES OF ANAESTHESIA

Broadly speaking, two distinct types of substances are used in anaesthesia. The first have selective, transient paralytic actions on sensory nerves and nerve endrings. They are applied in aqueous or oily solution by topical application to mucous or abraded surfaces; by intradermal, subdermal or submucous infiltration; and by peripheral, paravertebral or spinal perineural injection. The anaesthesia, or analgesia as it is better described (for unconsciousness is not featured), is classified as local or regional. In veterinary practice lignocaine hydrochloride is probably the drug most often used for these purposes.

The second type of substance has a depressant, and ultimately paralytic, action on the central nervous system, producing progressive loss of consciousness and voluntary motor function. In the main these substances fall into two distinct groups: volatile or gaseous agents, typified by enflurance, halothane, isoflurane and nitrous oxide, which are given by inhalation; and non-volatile agents such as propofol, etomidate, metomidate and the barbiturates, which are usually administered by intravenous injection.[2]

Thus, the subdivisions of the subject of anaesthesia are:

1. *Local analgesia*
   (a) by surface application
   (b) by intra and subdermal infiltration
   (c) field analgesia — the blocking of an area by linear infiltration of its margins
2. *Regional analgesia*
   (a) by perineural injection
   (b) spinal block
        (i) by epidural injection
        (ii) by intrathecal injection
3. *Sedation*
   (a) in combination with local analgesia
   (b) as an adjunct to general anaesthesia
4. *General anaesthesia*
   (a) by inhalation
   (b) by the intravenous administration of non volatile or non-gaseous anaesthetics (some may be given by intraperitoneal, intramuscular or other routes)
   (c) by a combination of the above two with or without premedication.

ANAESTHETIC RISK

Anaesthesia is not a naturally occurring state and its induction with drugs which are never completely devoid of toxicity must constitute a threat to the life of the patient. This can be a major or trivial threat depending on the circumstances, but no owner must ever be told that anaesthesia does not constitute such a risk. When the owner raises the question of the risk involved the veterinarian, before replying, needs to consider:

1. *The state of health of the animal:* Animals presented for anaesthesia may be fit and healthy or suffering from disease; they may be presented for 'cold' surgery or as emergency cases needing immediate attention for obstetrical crises, intractable haemorrhage or thoracic injuries. In the USA the American Society of Anesthesiologists has adopted a classification of physical status into categories, an 'E' being added after the number when the case is an emergency:

   Category 1 — normal healthy patient with no detectable disease.

   Category 2 — slight or moderate systemic disease causing no obvious incapacity.

   Category 3 — slight to moderate systemic disease causing mild symptoms (e.g. moderate pyrexia, anaemia or hypovolaemia).

Category 4 — extreme systemic disease constituting a threat to life (e.g. toxaemia, uraemia, severe hypovolaemia, cardiac failure).

Category 5 — moribund or dying patients. This is a useful classification but it is most important to appreciate that it refers only to the physical status of the patient and is *not necessarily a classification of risk* because additional factors such as its species, breed and temperament contribute to the risk involved for any particular animal.[3]

2. *The influence of the surgeon:* Inexperienced surgeons may take much longer to perform an operation and by rough technique produce intense and extensive trauma to tissues thereby causing a greater metabolic disturbance. Increased danger can also arise when the surgeon is working in the mouth or pharynx in such a way as to make the maintenance of a clear airway difficult, or is working on structures such as the eye or larynx and provoking autonomic reflexes.

3. *The influence of available facilities:* Crises rising during anaesthesia are usually more easily over come in a well-equipped veterinary hospital than under the primitive conditions which may be encountered on farms.

4. *The influence of the anaesthetist:* The competence, experience and judgement of the anaesthetist have a profound bearing on the degree of risk to which the patient is exposed. Familiarity with anaesthetic techniques leads to greater efficiency and the art of anaesthetic administration is developed only with experience.

GENERAL CONSIDERATIONS IN THE SELECTION OF THE ANAESTHETIC METHOD

The first, consideration will be the nature of the operation to be performed; its magnitude, site and duration. In general the use of local infiltration analgesia will suffice for simple operations such as the incision of superficial abscesses, the excision of small neoplasms and the castration of immature animals. Nevertheless, what seems to be a simple interference may have special anaesthetic requirements. The equine capped elbow is an example, for with this lesion the degree of subdermal fibrosis is often such as to make local infiltration impossible to effect. Again, the site of operation, consequent on the complexity of the structures in its vicinity, may render operation under local analgesia dangerous because of possible movement by the conscious animal, e.g. operations in the vicinity of the eyes.[4]

When adopting general anaesthesia the likely duration of the procedure to be carried out will influence the selection of the anaesthetic. Minor, short procedures may be performed quite satisfactorily after the intravenous injection of a small dose of an agent such as propofol or thiopentone sodium. For longer operations, a longer-acting agent supplemented by local analgesia may be chosen, or it may be decided to induce general anaesthesia with an ultrashort acting agent and maintain it with an inhalation anaesthetic with or without tracheal intubation. For most major operations under general anaesthesia, preanaesthetic medication ('premedication') will need to be considered, particularly when they are of long duration and the animal must remain quiet for several hours after the procedure. Undesirable effects of certain anaesthetics such as the provocation of salivation may also be controlled by suitable premedication. Although sedative premedication may significantly reduce the amount of general anaesthetic required it may also increase the duration of recovery from anaesthesia. Premedication may be omitted for out-patients when a rapid return to full awareness is desirable.[5]

The species of animal involved is, of course, a pre-eminent consideration in the selection of the anaesthetic method. The anaesthetist will be influenced not only by size and temperament but also by any anatomical and physiological features peculiar to a particular species or breed. In general it may be taken that the larger an animal is, the greater are the difficulties and dangers associated with the induction and continuation of general anaesthesia. Methods which are safe and satisfactory for the dog and cat may be quite unsuitable for the horse or the ox. In heavy and vigorous creatures like horses the mere upset of locomotor coordination may entail risks, as also may prolong recumbency.

The Horse

In horses, the need for adequate restraint, even for quite simple operations, may necessitate recumbency of the animal to ensure the safety of the surgeon and of the patient. The old-fashioned process of casting the fully conscious animal with ropes and tackle is not only frightening to the animal but exposes it to injury unless the assistance of an experienced casting team is available. Such assistance is most unlikely to be generally available today but, by way of compensation, we now have very effective sedatives available to facilitate horse management. It was sometimes claimed that the use of muscle-paralysing drugs as the means of casting the conscious animal entailed less risk, was more convenient and no more distressing to the animal than forcible casting with ropes and tackle. However, most veterinarians (including the authors) reject this view and consider that the use of muscle-paralysing drugs for this purpose is both more dangerous for the animal and inhumane. The recent introduction of drugs which induce very transient periods of unconsciousness enable this problem to be resolved in a way which cannot be challenged on either of these grounds. The facility with which certain of the peripheral sensory nerves can be 'blocked' in horses should always be borne in mind.

An important consideration when selecting a general anaesthetic for the horse, particularly when it is proposed to use one of the intravenous agents to be administered in the standing position, is that induction shall be unassociated with excitement. Moreover, when using agents from which recovery is relatively slow it is important that this period too shall be free from excitement and that the horse shall be able to rise to its feet relatively soon after the completion of the operation. When it does so, locomotor power and coordination must have been regained to a degree whereby the animal is able to retain the standing position without floundering or falling. These requirements preclude the use of some intravenous anaesthetics and sedatives.

Cattle, Sheep and Goats

Cattle, sheep and goats are unsuitable subjects for inhalation anaesthesia unless endotracheal intubation is practised. For work in the field, general anaesthesia by intravenous injection without abortion of the swallowing and belching reflexes gives satisfactory results, especially if combined with some form of local analgesia. It is in these animals that regional analgesia has attained its greatest development. For major abdominal operations, paravertebral or lumbar epidural injections are most satisfactory; for obstetrics, caudal epidural block is extensively employed; for dehorning, perineural block is suitable; for surgery on digits, intravenous regional analgesia (IVRA) can be ideal.

Pigs

The continuous squealing and struggling provoked by restraint makes most veterinarians disposed to adopt general anaesthesia for all but the most rapidly performed operations. Fortunately the pig is a good subject for general anaesthesia provided its airway can be kept patent by maintaining its head normally flexed on the neck with the lower jaw pushed forward. Where this is not possible endotracheal intubation is mandatory and the pig is probably the most difficult of the domestic animals to intubate. In the little pig most operations can be satisfactorily carried out under heavy sedation combined with local infiltration analgesia and some of the recently introduced sedative drugs now enable this to be done with the minimum of trouble.

Dogs

In dogs anaesthetic methods have now attained a degree of perfection so that general anaesthesia is used not only for practically all surgical operations but in many instances for examination procedures also. It must be borne in mind that breeds having a markedly brachycephalic type of skull with depression of the nasal bones, the bulldog, the Pekingese, etc. are bad subjects for general anaesthesia without endotracheal intubation because relaxation of the jaw muscles may cause obstruction of the airway and particular care will always be required when using agents which give rise to a slow recovery from anaesthesia. Some of the more recently introduced sedative and opioid drugs can be combined to produce profound sedation and in a busy practice there is the temptation to use them to control dogs undergoing procedures such as radiography when a veterinarian is not present. While this may be safe in healthy, fit young animals, older dogs with cardiopulmonary disorders are likely to be far safer when general anaesthesia with a guaranteed clear airway and oxygen administration is employed.

Cats

The cat is often a difficult subject to anaesthetize quietly and smoothly, for restraint may provoke violent struggling and sometimes frenzy. Cats should always be handled gently, using the minimum of restraint, and when this is done the most satisfactory method of inducing general anaesthesia is by intravenous injection. For young cats, inhalation anaesthesia without the use of an intravenous induction agent, but with forcible restraint, was often used in the past and although it proved to be quite safe it cannot be denied that it was very distressing for the animal. Today, there are agents which can be given by intramuscular injection to produce a quiet, trouble-free onset of unconsciousness and there is little excuse for subjecting a fully conscious cat to the unpleasant experience of induction with an inhalation anaesthetic.

The variable reaction of the different species of animals, and of individuals, to the various anaesthetic agents will also influence the choice of anaesthetic.

Sometimes the barbiturates, when used in subaneasthetic doses in an attempt to sedate horses, provoked marked excitement, whilst a cat under the influence of large doses of opioids may become maniacal stimulated. Factors causing increased susceptibility to the toxic actions of anaesthetic agents must also be borne in mind. These include:

1. *Prolonged fasting:* This, by depleting the glycogen reserves of the liver, greatly reduces its detoxicating power and, when using parenterally administered agents in computed doses, allowance must be made for an increased susceptibility to them.

2. *Diseased conditions:* Toxaemia causes degeneration changes in parenchymatous organs, paretic the liver and heart, and great care must be taken in giving computed doses of agents to toxaemic subjects. Quite often it is found that a toxaemia animal requires very much less than the 'normal' dose. Toxaemia may also be associated with a slowing of the circulation and unless this is recognized it may lead to gross overdosing of intravenous anaesthetics. In those diseases associated with wasting there is often tachycardia and a soft, friable myocardium; animals suffering from such diseases are, in consequence, liable to develop cardiac failure when subjected to the stress of anaesthesia. It is most important that the presence of a diseased condition is detected before anaesthesia is induced.[6]

EXAMINATION OF THE PATIENT BEFORE ANAESTHESIA

It is probable that most veterinary operations are performed on normal, healthy animals. The subjects are generally young and represent good 'anaesthetic risks'. Nevertheless, enquiry should be made to ensure that they are normal—bright, vigorous and of hearty appetite. Should there be any doubt, operation is best delayed until there is assurance on this point. Many a reputation has been damaged by performing operations such as castration or spaying on young animals which are in the early stages of some acute infectious disease.

When an operation is to be performed for the relief of disease, considerable care must be exercised in assessing the factors which may influence the choice or course of the anaesthetic. Once these are recognized the appropriate type of anaesthesia can be chosen and other measures enforced preoperatively and postoperatively to diminish or, where possible, prevent complications. The commonest conditions affecting the course of anaesthesia are those involving the cardiovascular and respiratory systems, but the state of the liver and kidneys cannot be ignored.

History

The owner or attendant should always be asked whether the animal has a cough. A soft, moist cough is associated with the presence of airway secretions and these may give rise to respiratory obstruction and lung collapse when the cough reflex is suppressed by anaesthesia. Severe cardiovascular disease may be totally asymptomatic and the object of taking the history is to gauge the level of functional incapacity and to indicate the underlying pathophysiology. Enquiry should be made to determine whether the animal suffers from undue breathlessness (respiratory distress) after exertion, or indeed appears unwilling to take exercise, since these signs may precede other signs of cardiac and respiratory failure by many months or even years. Dyspnoea on exercise is generally the first sign of left ventriculi failure.

A history of excessive thirst may indicate the existence of advanced renal disease, diabetes mellitus or diabetes insipidus.

Examination

The actual examination may be restricted to one which is informative yet will not consume too much 'time nor unduly disturb the animal. While a more complete examination may sometimes be necessary, attention should always be paid to the pulse, the position of the apex beat, the presence of cardiac thrills, the heart sounds, the jugular venous pressure and any signs arising from the respiratory system. Examination of urine for the presence of albumin and reducing substances is also valuable.

Tachycardia is to be expected in all febrile and in many wasting diseases and under these circumstances is indicative of some degree of myocardial weakness. It can, however, also be due to nervousness and where this is so it is often associated with rather cold ears and/or feet. Bradycardia may be physiological or it may indicate complete atrioventricular block. In horses, atrioventricular block that disappears with exercise is probably of no significance. Careful inspection of the external jugular vein is a most helpful guide towards making the diagnosis. If the head is lowered to a position where jugular vein pulsation can be seen, it will be observed that, whilst with physiological bradycardia the usual three waves appear in a regular sequence (Fig. 14.1), in cases of complete atrioventricular block two kinds of waves occur. The first is the largest and obvious pulsation caused by:

1. The distension of the atrioventricular valves as they close producing a shock wave back in the jugular veins.
2. The pulse in the underlying carotid artery.

The second kind of wave occurs at a regular but different rhythm and is due to atria. In small animal patients, or where the jugular vein pulsation cannot be seen, an electrocardiogram may be the only way of determining whether bradycardia is physiological or is due to heart block. The jugular venous pressure is also important. When the animal is standing and the head is held up so that the neck is at an angle of about 45° to the horizontal, distension of the jugular veins should, in normal animals, be just visible

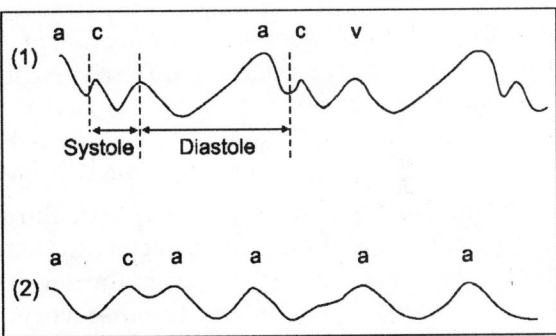

Fig 14.1: Pressure tracings of (1) the normal jugular venous pulse and (2) of the jugular pulse in a horse suffering from complete atrioventricular block: a = atrial contraction preceding the carotid pulse, v = rise in atrial pressure due to continuous venous filling whilst the tricuspid valve is closed c = inconstant wave due to arterial pulsation and/or deformation of the atrium with bulging of the tricuspid valve during early systole

at the base of the neck. When the venous distension rises above this level, even in the absence of other signs, it indicates an obstruction to the anterior vena cava or a rise in the right atrial or ventricular pressures. The commonest cause of a rise in pressure in these two chambers of the heart is probably right ventricular hypertrophy associated with chronic lung disease although congenital conditions such as atrial septal defects may also be indicated by this sign and it should be remembered that cattle suffering from constrictive pericarditis, or bacterial endocarditis, may have a marked increase in venous pressure.

The presence of a thrill over the region of the heart is always a sign of cardiovascular disease and suggests an increased risk of complications arising during anaesthesia. More detailed cardiological examination is warranted when a cardiac thrill is detected during the preoperative examination.

Auscultation of the heart should never be omitted but the findings are perhaps of only limited interest to the anaesthetist. The timing of any murmurs should be ascertained by palpation of the pulse while listening to the murmur. Diastolic murmurs are always indicative of heart disease and, while they may be of little importance in relation to cardiac function during anaesthesia, it is unwise to come to this conclusion unless other signs such as displacement of the apex beat are absent. Systolic murmurs may or may not indicate the presence of heart disease, but if other signs are absent they are probably of no significance. Accurate location of the apex beat is possibly the most important single observation in assessing the state of the cardiovascular and respiratory systems. It is displaced in most abnormal conditions affecting the lungs (e.g. pleural effusion, pneumothorax, lung collapse) and in the presence of enlargement of the left ventricle. In the absence of any pulmonary disorder a displaced apex beat indicates cardiac hypertrophy or dilatation.

Oedema in cardiac failure has multiple causes which are not fully understood but include a failing right ventricle and an impaired renal blood flow that gives rise to secondary aldosteronism and excessive reabsorption of salt and water by the renal tubules. The tissue fluid appears to accumulate in different regions in different species; in horses in the limbs and along the ventral body surface, in cattle it is seen in the brisket region and in dogs and cats the fluid tends to accumulate in the abdominal cavity. The differential diagnosis of peripheral oedema includes renal disease, liver disease and impaired lymphatic drainage.

Pulmonary disorders provide particular hazards for an animal undergoing operation or anaesthesia and any examination, no matter how brief, must be designed to disclose their presence or absence. On auscultation, attention should be directed towards the length of the expiratory sounds and the discovery of any rhonchi or crepitations. If rhonchi or crepitations are heard, excessive sputum is present, and the animal is either suffering from, or has recently suffered, a pulmonary infection. Prolongation of the expiratory sounds, especially when accompanied by high-pitched rhonchi, indicates the existence of narrowed airways or bronchospasm. Respiratory sounds may be absent in animals with pneumothorax, extensive lung consolidation, or severe emphysema; they are usually faint in moribund animals. Uneven movement between the two sides of the chest is a reliable sign of pulmonary disease and one which is easily and quickly observed. The animal should be positioned squarely while the examiner stands first directly in front of it and then directly behind it. In small animals uneven movement of the two sides of the chest is often better appreciated by palpation rather than by inspection.

The mouth should be examined for evidence of anaemia denoted by paleness of the mucous membranes, and the presence of loose teeth which might become dislodged during anaesthesia and inhaled into the tracheobronchial tree.

Urine testing is particularly important in dogs, for in these animals renal disease is common. In dogs suffering from chronic nephritis, curtailment of water intake associated with general anaesthesia and operation may provoke a uraemic crisis. Urine testing may also uncover previously undiagnosed diabetes mellitus.

Haematological examinations and scanning of biochemical data may be of value in some cases but their routine use is debatable, for in the vast majority of cases they constitute an unnecessary expense.

Provided a brief examination such as that described is carried out thoroughly, and that the examiner has sufficient skill to realize the significance or lack of significance of the findings, most of the conditions which have a bearing on the well-being of an animal during and after anaesthesia will be brought to light so that appropriate measures can be taken to protect it from harm.

SIGNIFICANCE OF CONDITIONS FOUND BY PREANAESTHETIC EXAMINATION

During the course of even a brief examination the examiner will form some opinion of the animal's temperament. Animals which are unduly nervous or aggressive need special care in the immediate preoperative period and many of them may be difficult to handle or nurse postoperatively. The appropriate choice of sedative and analgesic medication can do much to facilitate the handling of such subjects. An impression of the 'real' age of an animal as opposed to its chronological age will also have been gained. This is most valuable for the young animal which looks, for example, several years older than its chronological age is liable under stress to behave as an older animal might be expected to.

Heart Disease

A knowledge of the exact nature of the cardiac lesion is less important in anaesthesia than a knowledge of the effective function of the heart. A broad division into congenital and acquired heart disease is, however, of some value. In animals, acquired disease is more commonly encountered than is congenital disease, for animals suffering from congenital disease usually die or are killed in early life. Acquired disease is of more serious import since, unlike congenital disease, it tends to affect both the myocardium and the valves so that even in its earliest stages the heart muscle is weakened. Fitness for anaesthesia must be assessed from a knowledge of what the heart can do both at rest and at exercise set against such factors as the importance and urgency of operation coupled with experience of how animals similarly affected have behaved in like circumstances. It is rarely possible to state that an animal will not tolerate anaesthesia because of heart disease. Of course, major operations on large animals suffering from heart disease can seldom be justified on economic grounds, but in small animal practice such considerations may not apply. Provided that the anaesthetist is aware of the existence of a heart lesion and exercises care in the administration of the anaesthetic, these small animal patients will usually tolerate anaesthesia and the operation well.

A feature of complete atrioventricular block is the occurrence of syncope due to ventricular asystole, the so called "Stokes-Adams attack'. In these attacks the animal loses consciousness, lies limp, still and pulse-less, with fixed dilated pupils; breathing, however, continues. As a rule, ventricular contractions are resumed and recovery occurs quite spontaneously, but sometimes ventricular fibrillation supervenes.

Episodes may occur under anaesthesia and may not be noticed unless an electrocardiogram is being recorded or a very careful watch is being kept on the pulse. Sudden asystole is also a feature of aortic stenosis and in this condition it may occur at any time, even when the animal is apparently at rest. It is uncertain whether such animals are more liable to sudden death when under anaesthesia than they are at any other time, but many have survived carefully administered anaesthetics without incidence. In these cases survival depends on the force of ventricular contraction and agents such as thiopentone sodium, which is known to decrease this, must be used with caution. Physiological bradycardia is associated with a marked ability to increase the cardiac output to meet extra demands but, except in horses, where it is physiological at rest, the presence of heart block implies

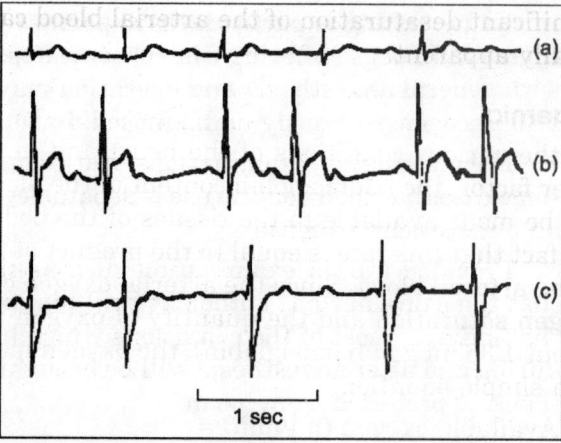

Fig. 14.2: Electrocardiogram (ECG) tracings from dogs showing first-degree heart block, (a) second-degree block, (b) and complete block, (c) In (a) there is an increased P-R interval, in (b) some impulses are transmitted whilst others arc not and in (c) none of the P waves are transmitted to the ventricles. If the P-R interval lengthens progressively until a P wave occurs without a QRS complex this is known as a Mobitz type-I block and is benign. Sudden failure of atrioventricular conduction without previous lengthening of the P-R interval is known as a Mobitz type-II block; this has a very different connotation because sudden asystole is a very real hazard and the majority of cases have widespread fibrosis of the conducting tissues

an inability to produce more than a fractional increase in output. Thus, whereas animals with physiological bradycardia are well able to withstand the stresses of anaesthesia, animals (other than horses) with heart block are liable to develop circulatory failure when exposed to such strains as the vasodilatation induced by anaesthetic agents and hypovolaemia due to haemorrhage (Fig. 14.2). Except in emergencies drugs have no place in the modern management of bradyarrhythmias.

Other important, common causes of fixed low cardiac output are constrictive pericarditis and mitral stenosis.

Respiratory Disease

Hypoxaemia results from many pulmonary conditions. Horses afflicted with the syndrome which is commonly referred to as 'broken wind' where there is marked hypoxaemia, hypercapnia and polycythaemia and other animals suffering from conditions such as chronic bronchiolitis, asthma and alveolar emphysema may be difficult to keep well oxygenated during anaesthesia unless high concentrations of oxygen are administered. Pneumonitis, or lung collapse such as may occur with space-occupying lesions of the thorax or ruptures of the diaphragm, disturbs the ventilation-perfusion relationships within the lungs, and alveoli which are perfused with blood but not ventilated act as venous-arterial shunts.

Significant desaturation of the arterial blood can result from this, even if cyanosis is not readily apparent.

Anaemia

All the various conditions of the heart and lungs which have been mentioned, and one other factor, the haemoglobin content of the blood, clearly affect the rate at which oxygen can be made available to the tissues of the body. Nunn and Freeman[7] drew attention to the fact that this rate is equal to the product of the cardiac output and the oxygen content of the arterial blood. Since the arterial oxygen content approximates to the product of the oxygen saturation and the quantity of oxygen which can be carried by the haemoglobin (about 1.36 ml/g of haemoglobin), the oxygen made available to the body can be expressed by a simple equation:

Available oxygen (ml/min) =

Cardiac output (ml/min) × Arterial saturation (%) × Haemoglobin (g/ml) × 1.36

This equation, of course, makes no allowance for the small quantity of oxygen which is carried in physical solution in the plasma, but it serves to illustrate the way in which the three variables combine to produce an effect which is often greater than is commonly supposed.

If any one of the three determining variables on the right-hand side of the equation is changed, the rate at which oxygen is made available to the tissues of the body is altered proportionately. Thus, if the cardiac output is halved, the available oxygen is also halved. If two determinants are lowered simultaneously while the third remains constant, the effect of the available oxygen is the product of the individual changes. For example, if the cardiac output and the haemoglobin concentration are both halved while the arterial oxygen saturation remains at about the normal 95%, only one-quarter of the normal amount of oxygen is made available to the body tissues. If all three variables are reduced the effect is, of course, even more dramatic.

The full significance of these facts can, perhaps, be best illustrated by considering a hypothetical case. If a 500 kg horse has a cardiac output of 30 l/min, a haemoglobin level of 15 g/dl of blood, and the arterial blood is 95% saturated, then the oxygen made available to the tissues of the animal is equal to

$$30,000 \times \frac{95}{100} \times \frac{15}{100} \times 1.36 \text{ ml/min}, \text{ i.e. approximately 5700 ml/min.}$$

Thus, the oxygen made available to the horse would be adequate for its needs, since at rest its oxygen consumption is of the order of 1400 ml/min, corresponding to an arteriovenous oxygen difference of 5 ml/dl of blood, and a mixed venous blood saturation of about 75%. (because different organs extract widely differing amounts of oxygen from the blood, a mixed venous saturation of about 20% is the minimum that can be tolerated by the body: some organs and especially the heart already extract most of the oxygen from their arterial supply).

If this hypothetical horse is now assumed to become anaemic so that its haemoglobin concentration falls by one-third to 10 g/dl of blood, and is anaesthetized by an agent which reduces the cardiac output by one-third to 20 l/min, and the arterial oxygen saturation decreases to 64%, then the oxygen made available to the tissue equals

$$20\ 000 \times \frac{64}{100} \times \frac{10}{100} \times 1.36\ ml/min$$

That is approximately 1700 ml/min. Since the oxygen consumption is unchanged, making oxygen available at this rate would lead to the haemoglobin in the mixed venous blood being almost completely desaturated — a condition which is incompatible with life. It is important to note that none of the values substituted on the right-hand side of the equation would, individually, cause alarm. A reduction of one-third in the cardiac output is often encountered in anaesthesia, oxygen saturation of 64% may occur without obvious cyanosis and haemoglobin levels of 10 g/dl are common place. Nevertheless, these three apparently mild departures from normal can, in combination, be lethal.

In most cases, especially when it is limited by disease, little can be done to increase the cardiac output, and this is the factor which determines the lowest permissible levels of the other two variables. The haemoglobin level, however, is capable of being raised and in a critical situation every effort must be made to do this. The concentration is often low preoperatively and may be further reduced by transfusion of plasma or plasma volume expanders. Pulmonary conditions which are likely to interfere with blood oxygenation should, if possible, be treated before anaesthesia to reduce the severity of their effect. When this cannot be done the administration of high concentrations of oxygen during anaesthesia may be life saving.

Hypoproteinaemia

Most drugs are carried in the bloodstream partly bound, usually by electrostatic bonds, to the proteins of the plasma, albumin being by far the most important for the majority of agents. Light or moderate protein binding has relatively little effect on drug pharmacokinetics and pharmacodynamics. Heavy protein binding with drugs such as thiopentone results in a low free-plasma concentration of the drug which may become progressively augmented as the available binding sites become saturated. The bound drug is, of course, in dynamic equilibrium with free (active) drug in the plasma water.[8]

Anaemia is often associated with hypoproteinaemia and this can have marked effects in anaesthesia. In conditions where there is anaemia and hypoalbuminaemia, a greater fraction of a given dose of a drug will be unbound and this will be even greater if other bound drugs have already occupied many of the binding sites. This can result in an increased peak activity of the drug. Liver disease giving rise to hypoalbuminaemia can result in reduced binding of drugs such as morphine so that smaller than normal doses of this analgesic will be effective when pain relief is needed. A rapid intravenous injection of an albumin-bound drug may also lead to increased pharmacological activity because the binding capacity of the albumin in the limited volume of blood with which the drug initially mixes is exceeded and more free (active) drug is presented to the receptor sites. Plasma protein binding enhances alimentary absorption of drugs by lowering the free plasma concentration and thereby increasing the concentration gradient for diffusion from the gut lumen.

An apparent exception to the increased activity of drugs in hypoproteinaemic animals is the resistance to tubocurarine seen in cases of liver disease. This is explained by the fact that tubocurarine binds to γ-globulin rather than albumin);[8] dose requirements are related to globulin and reversed albumin/globulin ratios are common in hepatic diseases.[9,10]

Renal Disease

Chronic renal disease is common in dogs, and affected animals cannot produce concentrated urine. Dehydration from any cause deprives the kidneys of sufficient water for excretory purposes, so that urea and other waste products are retained, giving rise to uraemia. Curtailment of water intake for a day when a general anaesthetic is administered may easily be responsible for uraemia in dogs suffering from chronic nephritis. Uraemia precipitates a vicious circle as it causes malaise and vomiting which not only themselves limit the water intake, but also produce further water depletion (Fig. 14.3). To guarantee that these animals receive an adequate fluid intake it may be necessary to administer fluid by intravenous infusion if the length of anaesthesia and/or the recovery period is prolonged. A uraemic circle can also be set up in animals suffering from chronic renal disease if the arterial blood pressure falls as a result of anaesthetic overdose or haemorrhage and renal ischaemia ensues (Fig. 14.4). The replacement of blood as it is shed is very important in these animals.[11]

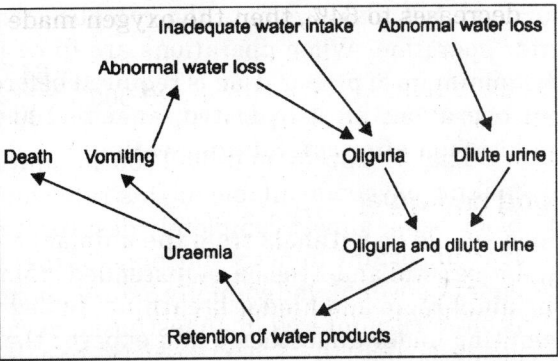

Fig. 14.3: Illustration of how curtailment of water intake may give rise to uraemia in dogs suffering from chronic nephritis

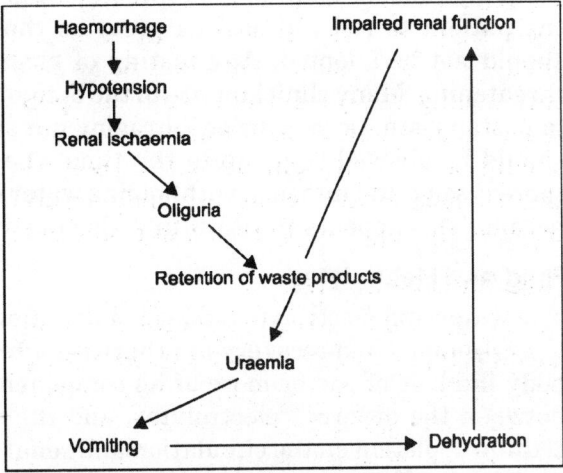

Fig. 14.4: Illustration of the development of uraemia when an animal suffering from chronic nephritis is subjected to haemorrhage

PREPARATION OF THE PATIENT

Certain operations are performed in emergency when it is imperative that there shall be no delay, and little preparation of the patient is possible. Among these operations are those for repair of thoracic injuries, the control of severe, persistent haemorrhage, and certain obstetrical interferences where the delivery of a live baby animal is of paramount importance. For all other operations, time and care spent in preoperative preparation are well worthwhile since proper preparation not only improves the patient's chances of survival, but also prevents the complications which might otherwise occur during and after operation. When operations are to be performed on normal, healthy animals, only the minimum of preparation is required before the administration of a general anaesthetic, but operations on dehydrated, anaemic, hypovolaemic or toxic patients should only be undertaken after careful preparation.[12]

Food and Water

Food should be withheld from the animal on the day it is to undergo an elective operation under general anaesthesia. A distended stomach may interfere with the free movement of the diaphragm and hinder breathing. In dogs, cats and pigs, a full stomach predisposes to vomiting under anaesthesia and exposes the animal to the danger of inhaling vomitus. A full or distended stomach may rupture when a horse is forcibly cast or falls to the ground as unconsciousness is induced. In ruminants, a few hours of starvation will not result in any appreciable reduction in the volume of the fluid content of the rumen, but it seems to reduce the rate of fermentation within this organ, thus delaying the development of tympany when eructation is suppressed by general anaesthesia. Excessive fasting exposes the patient to risks almost as great as those associated with lack of preparation and should not be adopted. Any fasting of birds and many small mammals is actually life threatening. Many clinicians are of the opinion that prolonged fasting in horses predisposes to postanaesthetic colic by encouraging gut stasis. In non-ruminants, free access to water should be allowed right up to the time when premedication is given, but in ruminants there is some advantage in withholding water for about 6 hours before abdominal operations because this appears to result in a slowing of fermentation in the rumen.

Fluid and Electrolytes

The water and electrolyte balance of an animal is a most important factor in determining the uncomplicated recovery or otherwise after operation. The repair of existing deficits of body fluid, or of one or more of its components, is complex because of the inter-relations between the different electrolytes, and the difficulties imposed by the effects of severe sodium depletion on the circulation and renal function. Fortunately, the majority of animal patients suffer only minor and recent upsets of fluid balance so that treatment by intravenous infusion with isotonic saline, Hartmann's solution or 5% dextrose, depending on whether sodium depletion or water depletion is the more predominant, is all that is required. An anaesthetic should not be administered to an animal which has a decreased circulating blood volume, for the vasodilatation caused by anaesthetic agents may lead to acute circulatory failure, and every effort should be made to repair this deficit by the infusion of blood, plasma or plasma volume expander before anaesthesia is induced. In many instances, anaesthesia and operation may be safely postponed until the total fluid deficit is made good and an adequate renal output is achieved but, in cases of intestinal obstruction, operation should be carried out as soon as the blood volume has been restored. Attempts to restore all the extracellular deficit before the intestinal obstruction is relieved result in further loss of fluid into the lumen of the obstructed bowel and make subsequent operation more difficult, especially in horses. When in doubt about the nature and volume of fluid to be administered, it is as well to remember that, with the exception of toxaemic conditions and where severe hypotension due to hypovolaemia is present, an animal's condition should not deteriorate further if sufficient fluid is being given to cover current losses. These current losses include the inevitable loss of water through the skin and respiratory tract (approximately 20–60 ml/kg/day depending on age and species of animal), the urinary and faecal loss, and any abnormal loss such as vomit.[11]

Haemoglobin Level

As already mentioned, anaemia may be treated to raise the haemoglobin concentration to more reasonable levels before any major premeditated surgery is performed. When operation can be delayed for 2 or more weeks, the oral or parenteral administration of iron may raise the haemoglobin to a satisfactory concentration, but when such a delay is inadvisable the transfusion of red blood cells is indicated.[12]

Treatment of Diabetes Mellitus

It is sometimes necessary to anaesthetize a dog or cat suffering from diabetes mellitus and if the condition is already under control no serious problems are likely to be encountered. However, if the normal dose of insulin is given, starvation before surgery and inappetence afterwards may give rise to hypoglycaemia. There are over 30 commercially available preparations of insulin and they have different durations of action. Short-acting insulins (e.g. soluble insulin) have a peak effect at 2–4 hours and their effects last for 8–12 hours. Medium-acting insulins (e.g. semilente) have a peak effect at 6–10 hours and activity for up to 24 hours. Long-acting insulins (e.g. lente, protamine zinc) have a peak effect at 12–15 hours and one dose lasts for at least 36 hours. For this reason it is advisable to switch to purely short-acting insulin a few days prior to elective surgery. By doing this, there is effectively no active long-acting insulin preparation left on the day of operation and it becomes much easier to control the blood sugar around the preoperative period.

If an emergency operation has to be performed on an uncontrolled diabetic then the condition of the animal requires careful assessment and treatment. Ketonuria is an indication for treatment with glucose and soluble insulin, whilst overbreathing is a sign of severe metabolic acidosis. This must be treated by the infusion of sodium bicarbonate solution but the amount of bicarbonate needed in any particular case can only be calculated when the acid-base status is known from laboratory examination of an anaerobically drawn arterial blood sample. In veterinary general practice, facilities for such examination of arterial blood samples are unusual and metabolic acidosis has to be treated by infusing 2.5% sodium bicarbonate solution until the animal ceases to over-breathe. Because of the presence of an osmotic diuresis, many uncontrolled diabetics also require treatment for dehydration. The object of management is not to try to correct all disturbances as quickly as possible so achieving in an hour or two what normally should take 2–3 days. Doing this can produce swings in serum osmolarity which may be responsible for the development of cerebral oedema. All that is necessary prior to emergency surgery is to correct any hypovolaemia and ensure that the blood glucose level is declining.

INFLUENCE OF PRE-EXISTING DRUG THERAPY

Modern therapeutic agents are often of considerable pharmacological potency and animals presented for anaesthesia may have been exposed to one or more of these. Some may have been given as part of the preoperative management of the animal but whatever the reason for their administration they may modify the animal's response to anaesthetic agents, to surgery and to drugs given during and following operation. In some cases drug interactions are predictable and these may form the basis of many of the combinations used in modern anaesthesia, but effects which are unexpected may be dangerous.

In an ideal situation a drug action would occur only at a desired site to produce the sought-after effect. In practice most drugs are much less selective and are prone to produce 'side-effects' which have to be anticipated and taken into account whenever the drug is administered. (A side-effect may be defined as a response not required clinically, but which occurs when a drug is used within its therapeutic range). Apart from these unavoidable side-effects which are inherent, adverse reactions to drugs may occur in many different ways which are of importance to the anaesthetist. These include:

1. *Overdosage:* For some drugs exact dosing may be difficult. Overdosage may be absolute, as when an amount greater than the intended dose is given in error, or because the nature of the preparation differs from one manufacturer to another (e.g. thyroxine) in spite of apparently strict pharmaceutical specifications, so that bioavailability is inconstant. Drugs may also be given by an inappropriate route, e.g. a normal intramuscular dose may constitute a gross overdose if given by accidental intravenous injection. Relative overdosage may be due to an abnormality of the animal; for example an abnormal sensitivity to digitalis is found in hypokalaemic animals, and newborn animals are sensitive to non-depolarizing relaxants. The use in dogs and cats of flea collars containing organophosphorus compounds may reduce the plasma cholinesterase to low levels and prolong the action of a normal dose of the relaxant drug suxamethonium.

Overdose manifestations vary from acute to chronic and may produce toxicity by a quantitatively enhanced action which can be an extension of the therapeutic action, e.g. neostigmine in excess in the antagonism of competitive neuromuscular block resulting in a depolarizing block. They may also be due to side-effects (e.g. morphine producing respiratory depression).

2. *Idiosyncrasy:* Some animals may have a genetically determined response to a drug which is qualitatively different to that of normal individuals, e.g. the porcine hyperpyrexia syndrome ('porcine malignant hyperthermia').

3. *Intolerance:* An intolerant animal exhibits a qualitatively normal response but to an abnormally low or high dose. This is usually simply explained by the Gaussian distribution of variation in response to drugs seen in any animal population. The normal distribution curve includes responses in individuals unusually sensitive to the drug as well as responses in resistant animals.

4. *Allergy:* Allergic responses are, in general, not dose related and the allergy may be due to the drug itself or to one of its metabolites or even the vehicle in which it is presented (e.g. cremophor in preparations of steroid anaesthetics). Most drugs which produce allergic responses do so because they are small molecules which act as haptens combining with a body protein to form the antigen against which immunological activity is directed and which in turn produces antibodies and/or antigen-reactive T

cells. These latter then react with any antigen remaining or subsequently formed (by further administration of the same or related compound) to elicit one of the characteristic allergic responses. The reaction may take a number of forms: anaphylactic shock, asthma or bronchospasm, hepatic congestion from hepatic vein constriction, blood disorders, rashes or pyrexia. Usually there is a history of previous exposure to the drug or to a related compound but there are exceptions to this general rule.

5. *Drug interactions:* Despite the importance of drug interactions there is little information in the veterinary literature on this subject and for this reason only the general principles can be reviewed here. Drug interactions can occur outside the body as when two drugs are mixed in a syringe before they are administered or inside the body after administration by the same or a different route. It is generally unwise to mix products or vehicles in the same syringe or to administer a drug into an intravenous infusion for this may result in the precipitation of one or both drugs or even possibly the formation of new potentially toxic or inactive compounds.

The result of the interaction between two drugs inside the body may be an increased or decreased action of one or both or even an effect completely different from the normal action of either drug. The result of interaction may be simply the sum of the actions of the two drugs (1 + 1 = 2), or greater (1 + 1 > 2) when it is known as 'synergism'. When one agent has no appreciable effect but exaggerates the response to the other (0 + 1 > 1) the term 'potentiation' is used to describe the action of the first on the effect of the second. An agent may also antagonize the effects of another and the antagonism may be 'chemical' if they form an inactive complex, 'physiological' if they have directly opposing actions though at different sites, or 'competitive' if they compete for the same receptors. Non-competitive antagonism may result from modification by one drug of the transport, biotransformation or excretion of the other. In the liver the non-specific process of oxidation and conjugation are implicated in the metabolic degradation of many drugs and many different agents have the ability to cause an increase in the activity of these systems, enzyme induction, whilst a few decrease the activity, enzyme inhibition. In experimental animals, enzyme induction has been reported to double the size of the liver but this does not seem to have been recorded in clinical cases. The barbiturates, some other anticonvulsants, chloral hydrate and analgesics such as phenyl-butazone cause enzyme induction and can produce a great increase in the rate of metabolism of substrates. For example, barbiturate treatment of epilepsy may almost halve the half-life of dexamethasone with a consequent marked deterioration in the therapeutic effect of this steroidal substance.

Most drugs are carried to their sites of action and elimination by the bloodstream and are present in the blood either in simple solution or partly bound to proteins of the erythrocytes or plasma. The degree of binding varies widely with different drugs and the veterinary anaesthetist needs to be aware that competition for binding sites and the displacement of one drug from the bound to the unbound (active) form may lead to increased toxicity. For example, warfarin (which is sometimes used in the management of navicular disease in horses) is displaced by several agents, including the analgesic drug phenylbutazone, with a resulting risk of haemorrhage.

USE AND ABUSE OF DRUGS IN ANAESTHESIA

While the rationale behind the concept of modern anaesthesia is undoubtedly sound, there has been a regrettable tendency towards ever-increasing complexity in the number of drugs given to anaesthetized animals. If potentiation can occur in respect to desirable drug actions it may, as already indicated, also occur in relation to toxic effects. It is, therefore, likely that some of the difficulties encountered in anaesthesia today are produced by the anaesthetist in the sense that they are aggravated, if not caused, by the misuse of sedative, anaesthetic and analgesic drugs and their pharmacological antidotes. In the hands of the inexperienced or careless anaesthetist the apparently rational use of a combination of drugs, each employed for a specific purpose, can easily degenerate into polypharmacy in which the advantages become lost by the development of complications, the origin of which is promptly made more obscure by the administration of antidotes that often introduce further complications. This is not to say, however, that anaesthetists should revert to deep general anaesthesia to produce satisfactory operating conditions, or avoid the use of muscle relaxants, for this would be a very retrograde step, but the number of agents used in any one case should be kept to a minimum. The skilled anaesthetist, keeping to this minimum, using each agent for a specific purpose and bearing in mind the pharmacokinetics of the agents used as well as their principal pharmacological actions, can easily demonstrate that the advantages can outweigh the alleged safety of the old, simple depression techniques.

References

1. Prys Roberts C., *British Journal of Anaesthesia,* 59, 1341, 1987.
2. Levinson B. W., *British Journal of Anaesthesia,* 37, 544, 1965.
3. Cherkin A. and Harroun P., *Anesthesiology,* 34, 469, 1971.
4. Eich E., Reeves J. L. and Katz R. L., *Anesthesia and Analgesia,* 64, 1143m 1985.
5. Gray T. C. and Rees C. J., *British Medical Journal* II, 891, 1952.
6. Dodson B A. and Miller K. W. *Aneasthiology,* 62, 615, 1985.
7. Nunn J. F. and Freeman J. *Anaesthesia,* 19, 120, 1964.
8. Stovner J., Thcodorsen L. and Birlke E., *British Journal of Anaesthesia,* 43, 385, 1971.
9. Sherlock S. *Diseases of the Liver and Biliary System,* 2nd edn., Blackwel Scientific, Oxford, 1958.
10. Ford E. J. H. and Ritchie H. E. *Journal of Comparative Pathology,* 78, 207, 1968.
11. Kumar P. *Textbook of Anaesthiology,* Ist ed. Hyderabad, Paras Med. Publishers, 2008.
12. Kumar Pramod, *Clinical Methods in Anaesthesia,* 1st ed. Mumbai, National Books, 2008.

15

Anaesthesia Apparatus

Apart from simple needles and syringes which can be disposable, there are various other instruments used in veterinary practice; the disposable catheter over the needle hubs which allow the operator to see the blood which runs back when the needle punctures the vein. Three important factors govern the choice of catheter. First, it should be no longer than strictly necessary. The length of most catheters (up to 7 cm) is always adequate and there is no need for the larger diameters to be longer.

The second important feature is the wall thickness. It is the external diameter which largely determines the size chosen in any given situation and catheters with thinner walls obviously permit more rapid infusions. The third factor is that the external shape should be as smooth as possible, for catheters with smooth contours are the easiest to insert (Fig.15.1).

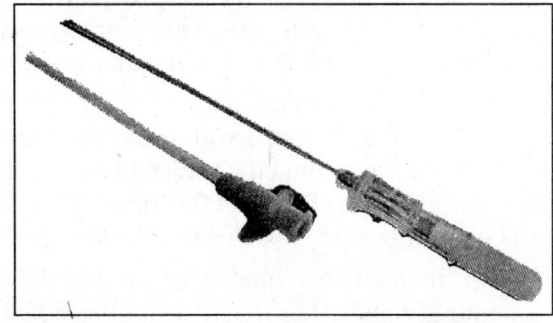

Fig. 15.1: Disposable plastic 'catheter over-needle'

Longer catheters are available for special purposes such as measurement of the central venous pressure. Although it is possible to obtain some sizes of the catheters described above up to 13.3 cm in length (which may be adequate for central venous pressure measurement in cats and small dogs), the longer catheters are generally not provided with introducing needles. These long catheters may be introduced into the vein through a large-bore needle but this method of placing a catheter can be dangerous, as the end of the catheter may be severed by the point of the needle. Such catheters should, therefore, be placed by cutting down surgically on to the vein or else passed through short, large-bore catheters previously introduced into the vessel for this purpose. Some long catheters are supplied with an additional short, wider-bore catheter of the 'over-needle pattern' that is introduced into the vein so that the longer one can be threaded through it.

A slightly different design of long catheter which is particularly easy to introduce is the E-Z Cath. A needle lies inside the tip of the catheter to assist introduction; it is attached to a wire which passes through the length of the catheter. A split inserting handle attached to a protective sleeve surrounds the catheter, and the catheter can be worked up the vein by advancing it with the inserter, using one hand, and holding it inside its protective sleeve with the other hand.

The tube should be as short, and the diameter as large as possible. It must be noted that a small change in diameter has a large effect on flow.

At very high flows it may be found that the resistance is disproportionately high. There is a critical flow velocity at which the flow changes from streamline to turbulent. During turbulence the driving pressure is largely used up in creating the kinetic energy of the turbulent eddies. The flow no longer depends on the viscosity of the fluid but on its density. However, the critical velocity at which turbulence occurs depends mainly on the viscosity and density of the fluid as well as the radius of the bore of the tube through which it is flowing. In an intravenous infusion system the critical velocity is likely to be exceeded at very high flow rates and also at local points in the apparatus at which, because of sudden change in internal configuration, the velocity of flow momentarily rises. Thus, at points at which the internal diameter changes suddenly, turbulence will occur.

The viscosity of blood is considerably greater than that of water, mainly because of the presence of erythrocytes. It increases with the haematocrit and above about 60% haematocrit blood hardly behaves as a fluid. Viscosity is also increased by a drop in temperature, and the viscosity of blood at 0°C is about 2.5 times as great as at 37°C. Blood-warming coils are, therefore, justified on grounds of increasing the speed of transfusion as well as of preventing the development of hypothermia in the recipient.

An alternative to a catheter for very small veins is a needle attached to a hub by a length of plastic tubing. There are at least nine types of 'small-vein' needles currently available (Fig. 15.2). Some have winged handles to aid insertion and subsequent fixation to the patient. The flow performance of most of the 'infant scalp-vein sets' or 'butterflies' is surprisingly poor, and it is usually best to choose one with the shortest length of tubing attached.

An infusion set' consists of an outlet tube which may or may not incorporate a filter depending on whether the set is for blood and blood products or crystalloid fluids alone, a drip chamber and a long length of plastic delivery tubing which can be occluded by some form of clamp. If it is intended for use with bottles of fluid an air inlet with a filter is incorporated. All plastic sets include a short piece of rubber tubing towards the needle mount end of the delivery tube so that injections can be made into the infusion fluid while administration proceeds. Injections are made through a fine-bore needle whilst the tubing is pinched between the finger and thumb on the drip chamber side of the injection site to prevent the pressure created by the injection from damming back fluid in the drip chamber. The flow rate is controlled by means of the clamp and can be estimated by counting the number of drops which pass through the drip chamber in 1 minute. For example, with most sets 40 drops/min means the administration of approximately 500 ml in 4 hours. Much more accurate control of infusion rate can be obtained by the use of drip rate controllers between the fluid container and the patient. These are electronic devices which monitor the drip rate with a sensor attached to the drip chamber and, by changing the effective cross-sectional area of a section of the standard administration set tubing, maintain a constant drip rate. The automatic control eliminates the need for frequent adjustment of the drip rate. However, drip rate controllers are expensive and cannot compensate for variations in drop size.

Drip rate pumps are similar in cost and appearance to drop rate controllers and most operate satisfactorily with standard administration sets. They generate a pressure by peristaltic fingers or rollers acting on deformable tubing to give a constant infusion rate. As with drip rate controllers the actual volumes delivered depend on drop size.

Volumetric pumps (Fig. 15.2) are designed to avoid problems associated with variations in drop size. Very good volumetric accuracy is obtained with either a reciprocating-piston-type pump or by peristaltic pumping on an accurately made tube which forms part of the administration set. With the piston-type pump no fluid is delivered to the patient during the refilling stage of the cycle so that at low flow rates significant fluctuations in delivery rate occur. The need for a dedicated infusion set adds to the cost of each infusion and the volume of fluid required to prime these sets can also be in the region of 20 ml which may give rise to significant wastage of expensive solutions. These pumps arc, however, particularly valuable for longer procedures where the solution can be withdrawn from a large container such as a 3 litre plastic bag.

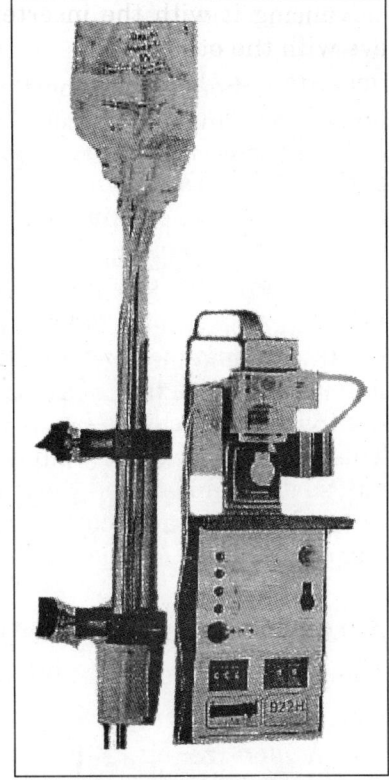

Fig. 15.2: Volumetric or constant-infusion pump. Types such as this drive a disposable pump unit and the need to refill the barrel of the pump means that the infusion rate is not actually constant

Electrically driven syringe drivers overcome many of the problems associated with the administration of relatively small volumes of fluid (e.g. to cats, or the continuous administration of drugs during anaesthesia). They are usually calibrated for a particular type and size of syringe. The delivery rate control alters the rate of plunger travel, and hence the cross-sectional area of the syringe barrel is critical in ensuring that the delivery rate is correct. The syringe can be filled from a large container of fluid and connected to the intravenous catheter with a simple administration extension set so that the priming volume is minimal. Syringe drivers are generally less expensive than volumetric pumps or drip rate pumps or controllers as well as being more portal. Further developments include the use of microprocessor control with an ability (if the pharmacokinetics of the infused substance are known) to deliver a changing infusion rate such that a steady state of blood concentrations can be achieved and maintained (Fig. 15.3).

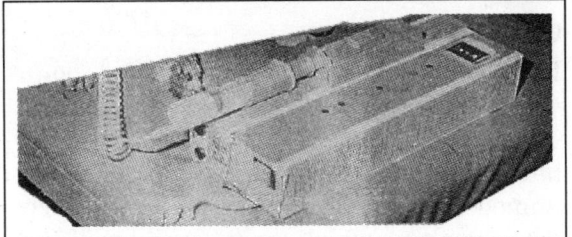

Fig. 15.3: Syringe driver. Many different types of electrically driven syringe drivers are available. Some must be used with one specified size of syringe, others can be used with a variety of syringes

When fluids are administered under the influence of gravity the speed of infusion depends more on the bore of the needle or catheter than on the pressure (i.e. the height above the needle or catheter at which the container is held). Doubling the diameter of the needle or catheter gives a 16-fold increase in the rate of flow, whereas a fourfold increase in the pressure is required to double the rate. In the case of the 'flutter-valve' apparatus, traditional and so popular in veterinary practice, the vertical distance between the needle and the air inlet opening determines the rate at which air enters the system; increasing this distance increases the rate of air entry and hence the speed of infusion. The 'flutter valve' is unreliable and there is no real justification for its continued use in veterinary practice.

In circumstances where the maximum size of the needle or catheter is limited, the maximum rate of flow of fluid can be increased by pressurizing the system. Where bottles are in use, they can be pressurized by pumping air under pressure through the air inlet. This procedure carries a high risk of producing air embolism if the supply of fluid runs out, so it should be used with caution and the infusion never left unattended. More safely, pressure can be applied to plastic bags of fluid by placing them in a second pressurized bag or container for there is then no danger of air embolism.

ADMINISTRATION OF INHALATION AGENTS

The administration of an inhalation anaesthetic requires:

1. A source of oxygen (which may be air)
2. A vaporizer or a source of anaesthetic gas
3. A 'patient' or 'breathing' circuit

In its simplest form modern anaesthetic apparatus consists of an oxygen cylinder, with a pressure gauge, pressure regulator and flowmeter delivering oxygen to a suitable patient breathing circuit. A vaporizer for an inhalation anaesthetic agent may be included inside or outside the patient breathing circuit. Such a simple apparatus is not as versatile as more elaborate equipment but is adequate for most veterinary purposes.

Oxygen Cylinders

For medical use, oxygen is obtained compressed at high pressure (2000 Ib/in^2) in metal cylinders or as liquid oxygen in special containers. For veterinary purposes cylinders are usually used; they are colour-coded black with a white top. When delivered, all cylinders have a plastic seal over their outlet to exclude dust and this seal should be removed only immediately before use. There are two types of cylinder outlet. Some cylinders fit into a yoke over pins which are indexed for different gases so as to make it impossible to attach an incorrect cylinder. A small washer termed a 'Bodcock seal' is needed around the inlet on the yoke of these pin-indexed fittings. Other cylinders utilize 'bull-nose' linings which screw into place and require no sealing washer.

Pressure Gauge

It is essential for the anaesthetist to know that there is an adequate supply of oxygen in the cylinder so when in use they are coupled to a pressure gauge to register the pressure inside and, therefore, the quantity of oxygen available. These gauges are most commonly of the Bourdon type (Fig. 15.4), consisting of a metal tube, the end of which is attached to a pointer. The application of pressure to the inside of the tube causes it to straighten and moves the pointer over a scale.

Reducing Valves or Regulators

A pressure reducing valve is necessary for three reasons:

1. Once the flow has been set for any particular level, frequent readjustment of the flowmeter control, which would be necessary as the pressure in the cylinder fell off, is obviated. Because the reducing valve exerts this automatic control it is often referred to as a 'regulator'.

2. By supplying a low gas pressure to the control valve spindle small variations in the gas flow can be made easily. When a high-pressure cylinder is controlled directly by a simple needle-type valve large changes in flow rate result from very small movements of the control valve spindle.

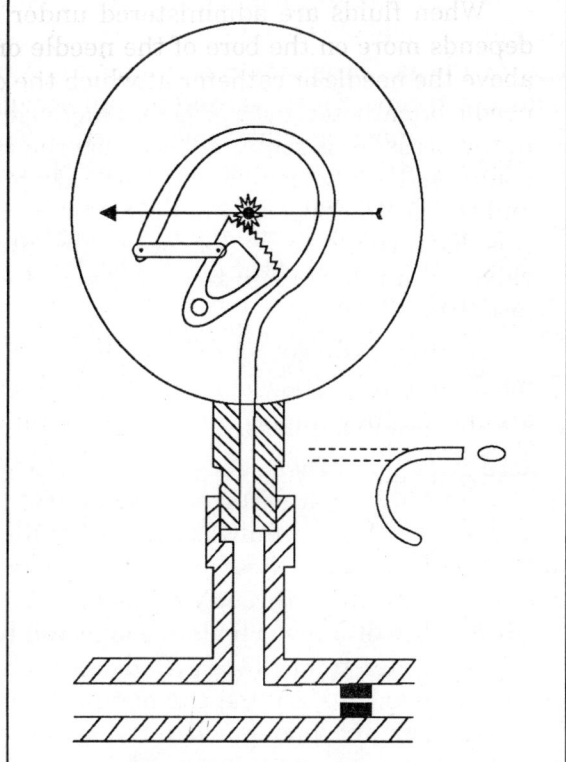

Fig. 15.4: Bourdon gauge. These are used for measuring gas pressure and, placed before an orifice, for gas flow measurement

3. The regulator limits the pressure within the connecting tubing to a low level and the likelihood of bursting the connecting tube when the flow is shut off by the flowmeter control is very much reduced.

The regulators in common use in anaesthesia usually reduce the pressure at which oxygen is delivered to below 13.8 atm (200 lb/in^2) and many modern anaesthetic machines incorporate the valve into the block featuring the cylinder pin index so that on superficial inspection of the machine they may be difficult to identify.

Flowmeters

Today most of the flowmeters used in anaesthesia in the UK are known as 'rotameters' (Fig.15.5). They make use of the interdependence of flow rate, size of orifice and pressure difference on either side of an orifice. The rotameter consists of a glass tube inside which a rotating bobbin is free to move. The bore of the tube gradually increases from below upwards. The bobbin floats up and down the tube, allowing gas to flow around it. The higher the bobbin in the tube the wider the annular space between the tube and bobbin (orifice) and the greater the flow rate through it. The bobbin, usually made of aluminium, has an upper rim which is of a diameter slightly greater than that of the body, and in which specially shaped channels are cut. As the gas enters the rotameter tube it impinges on the bobbin and causes it to rise and to spin because the rim with its set of channels acts like a set of vanes. The result is that the bobbin rides on a cushion of gas thereby eliminating errors due to friction between the tube and bobbin. The gas flow rate is read from the top of the bobbin against a scale etched on the outside of the glass tube. If the tube is mounted in a truly upright position these meters are capable, of readings of an accuracy of ± 2% but only for the gas for which they have been calibrated.

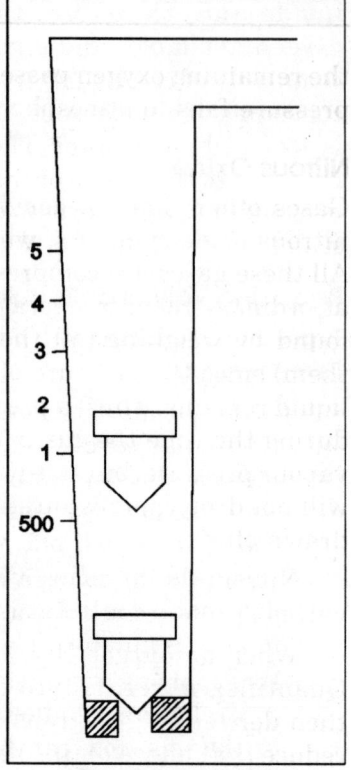

Fig. 15.5: Rotameter

Central Pipeline Systems

Where large quantities of oxygen (or other gases) are used, it is more convenient and more economical to utilize larger cylinders. As these are awkward to handle they are kept outside the operating theatre and the gas is supplied to the anaesthetic machine through a pipeline. The central depot has a number of large cylinders connected to a manifold so that gas is taken from all the cylinders in the bank. Warning devices are included so that the manifold can be changed to a second bank of cylinders when the supply pressure drops, or, with more complex apparatus where there are two or more manifolds the change to the bank of fresh cylinders takes place automatically. If extremely large quantities of oxygen are used daily the cylinder bank may be replaced by a liquid oxygen container but this is most unlikely to be necessary for veterinary practice.

The outlets from the pipelines in the theatre are colour coded and indexed so that, at least in theory, pipes from the anaesthetic machine cannot be connected to the wrong outlet. Oxygen is delivered at a low pressure to the anaesthetic machine and does not need a reducing valve or pressure regulator so the piped supply is fed directly to the flowmeter. However, most pipeline machines also carry a small oxygen cylinder and an associated pressure regulator for emergency use in the event of a failure in the pipeline supply.

Oxygen Failure Warning Devices

Devices which warn the anaesthetist that the pressure of the oxygen supply is low have been very neglected in veterinary anaesthesia, yet it is in this field, when often there is minimal assistance available to monitor the oxygen delivery, where they should be considered an essential feature of the anaesthetic machine. Some types depend on a second source of gas, usually nitrous oxide, for their operation. When the oxygen pressure falls a diaphragm moves to allow the second gas to pass through a whistle and an easily audible warning note is emitted. In other types a valve opens as the oxygen pressure drops and the remaining oxygen passes through the whistle; the whistling noise ceases as the oxygen pressure falls to atmospheric pressure.

Nitrous Oxide

Gases other than oxygen which are commonly found on anaesthetic machines include nitrous oxide cylinders, which are colour-coded blue and carbon dioxide (grey cylinder). All these gases are compressed into the cylinders under a pressure which liquefies them at ordinary room temperatures. The amount of gas present in the cylinder can only be found by weighing (all these cylinders have their full and empty weights stamped on them) since the pressure of gas above the liquid remains almost constant as long as any liquid remains. Thus, a pressure gauge at the cylinder outlet will register only a small fall during the time the gas is being drawn off due to cooling causing a fall in the saturated vapour pressure, but this will rise again as the cylinder warms and the pressure registered will not drop rapidly until all the liquid has been vaporized and the residual gas is being drawn off.

Nitrous oxide, oxygen and carbon dioxide cylinders need to be fitted with reducing valves ('pressure regulators'). However, the use of CO_2 gas has been stopped longback.

When an oxygen flow is being mixed with a nitrous oxide flow without the aid of a Quantiflex mixer, failure of the oxygen supply is disastrous because the machine will then deliver 100% nitrous oxide. Oxygen warning devices such as those described above reduce the chance of this happening without the knowledge of the anaesthetist, but many modern machines incorporate a cut-off device so that should the oxygen flow cease the nitrous oxide flow is also cut off. This cut-off device may prevent the machine from being fitted with some types of oxygen failure alarm.

Vaporizers

The ideal vaporizer is one that delivers a suitable and accurately known quantity of a volatile anaesthetic agent at all times and under all conditions of use.

Factors which have most influence on the vaporization of volatile anaesthetics include temperature, gas flow rate through the vaporizer, and back pressure transmitted during IPPV. A low resistance to gas flow may also be important if the vaporizer is to be used in the breathing circuit.

Uncalibrated Vaporizers

If a liquid anaesthetic is contained in a bottle it is possible to bubble gas from a cylinder through it or to allow the gas to flow over its surface. This arrangement is sometimes known as a 'plenum vaporizer' because gas is being forced into a chamber and a 'plenum' is a chamber or container inside which the pressure is greater than outside it.

In these the method of varying the concentration of anaesthetic vapour utilizes a permanent partition to prevent the direct passage of gases from the flowmeters to the patient. When the control lever is in the 'off position all gases are diverted around the partition but away from the bottle. With the tap in the 'on' position all gases pass through the bottle containing the liquid anaesthetic agent. The control tap can be placed in any intermediate position and this determines how much of the total gas flow passes through the bottle. A further means of controlling the vapour concentration is also provided. The gases are made to pass through a J-shaped tube before emerging into the space above the liquid anaesthetic in the bottle. The open end of the J-tube is covered by a metal hood which can be positioned as required by moving the rod attached to it up or down. As the hood is pushed downwards, the gas is deflected nearer and nearer to the surface of the liquid and finally, when the open end of the hood is pushed below the surface of the liquid, gases are made to bubble through the liquid anaesthetic. When the tap is in the 'on' position and the hood, or cowl, fully depressed, the whole of the gas flow is made to bubble through the liquid and the maximum concentration of the anaesthetic vapour is picked up. Boyle-pattern vaporizers for potent agents such as halothane have a single, straight inlet tube with a side port and no cowl arrangement.

When air or other gas flows over the surface of a liquid, the vapour of the liquid is carried away, and is replaced by fresh vapour. This continuous process of vaporization is accompanied by a corresponding loss of heat, the magnitude of which is determined by the rate at which the vapour is removed and by the latent heat of vaporization of the liquid. The loss of heat results in a fall in the temperature of the liquid unless heat is conducted to the liquid from some outside source. With a fall in the temperature of the liquid there is a corresponding decrease in the speed of vaporization and, if the gas flow remains constant, the concentration of anaesthetic vapour in the gas stream from a Boyle pattern vaporizer decreases with time until the heat loss due to vaporization is balanced by the conduction of heat through the glass of the bottle from the surrounding atmosphere to the liquid anaesthetic. The vaporizers, O_2, N_2O gases, circle absorbes are attached in a prototype Boyles apparatus (Fig. 15.6).

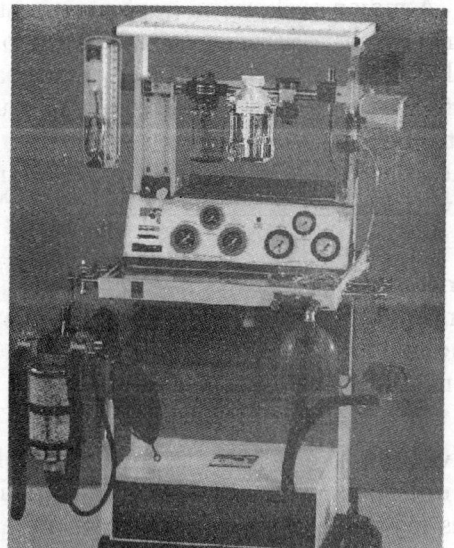

Fig. 15.6: Boyles anaesthesia apparatus

Calibrated Vaporizers

There are today many precision vaporizers on the market, all designed to deliver an accurately known concentration of volatile anaesthetic agents over a wide range of gas flow rates. Among the best known of these are the various 'tecs' (e.g. Fluotec, and the vapor (Drager). All these consist of a vaporizing chamber and a bypass. The fresh gas stream flowing into the vaporizer is divided into two portions, the larger of which passes straight through the bypass. The smaller portion is ducted through the vaporizing chamber, where it becomes saturated with the vapour, and this ensures that:

1. There is no sudden burst of high vapour concentration when the vaporizer is first switched on.
2. The output of the vaporizer is unaffected by shaking.

As already pointed out, the vaporization of the liquid anaesthetic results in the removal of heat from a liquid with a resultant fall in its temperature. If this fall is not checked the rate of vaporization will fail and the output concentration of the vaporizer decreases with time. In various 'tecs' (e.g. Fluotec for halothane) temperature compensation is achieved by means of a bimetallic strip valve. This valve is arranged to act as a control of the volume of gas passing through the vaporizing chamber. As the temperature of the liquid falls, the bimetallic strip opens the valve further, allowing more gas to pass through the chamber. In the vapor, the vaporizer is constructed from a large mass of copper. The high thermal conductivity of this metal allows heat to pass into the liquid from the room and this, together with the high thermal capacity of its mass, supplies the necessary heat for vaporization, holding the liquid temperature constant. In the 'tec' and vapor vaporizers temperature compensation is automatic and the only control to set is the output concentration.

A major problem in vaporizer design lies in the design of the splitting valves. In the earlier 'tec' vaporizers it proved impossible to ensure that the flow division ratio of this valve remained constant over a wide range of flow rates, and the vaporizers were supplied with graphs which needed to be consulted when the vaporizers were used with gas flow rates below 4 1/min. In current models (e.g. Mark Fluotec) this problem has been overcome and it is claimed that they are accurate at flow rates, above 500 ml/m with various advantages (Fig. 15.6).

Pressure fluctuations produced by IPPV may have a considerable effect on the output concentration of vaporizers. This 'pumping effect' can result in doubling the output concentration at low fresh gas ' flow rates and modern vaporizers incorporate a nonreturn valve to overcome this.'

All the vaporizers described so far have a high resistance to gas flow, which is unimportant when the carrier gas is pushed through them by the power of the compressed gases in their cylinders. If the vaporizer is to be used in the breathing circuit, where the gas flow is powered by the respiratory efforts of the animal, then a low-resistance vaporizer is essential.

Low-resistance vaporizers: Vaporizers offering a low resistance to gas flow are usually of a simple type with wide-bore entry and exit ports and no wicks to impede the flow of gases. A simple low efficiency vaporizer of this type often used in dental surgery is the Goldman vaporizer (Fig. 15.7).

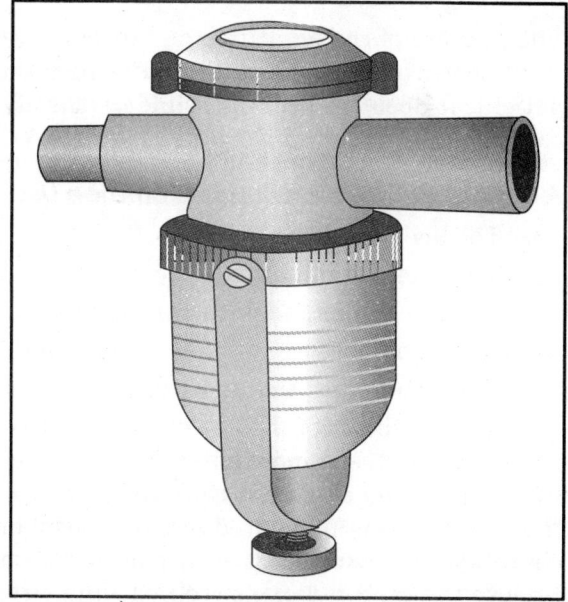

Fig 15.7: Goldman vaporizer for halothane. This is a simple low- resistance vaporizer which may be placed in the inspiratory limb of circle breathing systems

The EMO vaporizer (Epstein-Macintosh-Oxford) (Fig. 15.8) was specifically designed for the use of ether and is generally recognized as the best of this type of vaporizer. It is portable, has a temperature-compensating device and is employed in a non-rebreathing system. Its place in small animal anaesthesia was assessed by ether/air anaesthesia administered from it met criteria for acceptability in general practice where the veterinarian may be assisted in the operating theatre by a nurse or may be entirely alone.

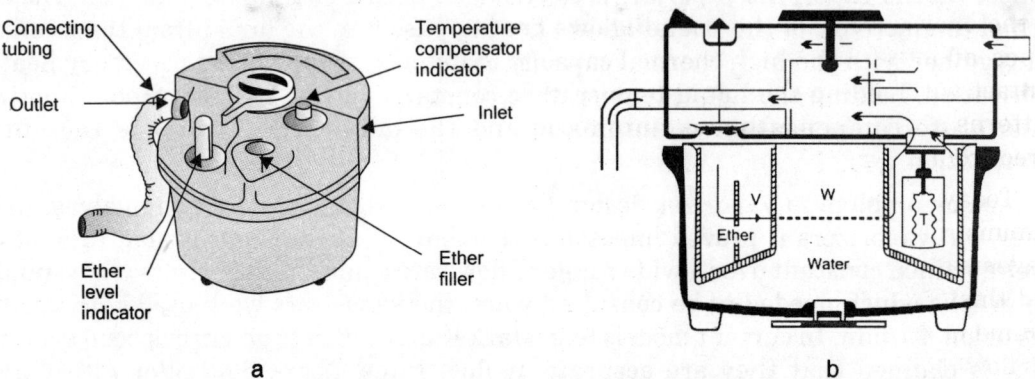

Figs 15.8: (a and b): The EMO vaporizer for ether. This draw-over, temperature-compensated unit may be used in situations where supplies of oxygen are not readily available

Breathing Circuits

The purpose of the breathing circuit of an anaesthetic apparatus is to convey oxygen and anaesthetic to the patient, and to ensure the removal of carbon dioxide produced by the patient. It does not seem possible to classify all the ways in which this can be done in a completely logical manner and as yet there is no universally agreed system.

A System of Classification in Common Use

a. The open method
b. The semi-open method
c. The closed method with carbon dioxide absorption
d. The semi-closed method with carbon dioxide absorption
e. The semi/closed method without carbon dioxide absorption

This classification has been criticized on the grounds that it is impractical and does not lit all systems. A more clinically useful definition of circuits is based on the two methods by which carbon dioxide is removed from the circuit. Either the circuit is designed so that the expired gases are vented to the atmosphere and cannot be rebreathed (non-rebreathing circuits) or the expired gases are passed through an absorber which contains soda lime to remove the carbon dioxide (rebreathing circuits).

The open and semi-open methods were used to volatilize agents such as chloroform and ether. The methods are often referred to as 'rag and bottle anaesthesia' and they survived through over a 100 years of anaesthetic history. In the semi-open or 'perhalation' method all the inspired air was made to pass through a mask on which the vaporization of the agent occurred. In horses and cattle, special masks (Fig. 15.9) were often used for the semi-open administration of chloroform. These masks were cylinders of leather and canvas applied over either the upper or both jaws. Chloroform was applied to a sponge inserted in the open end of the cylinder. In the cruder types of mask the sponge was actually in contact with the nostrils, but in more refined patterns a wire mesh partition prevented this direct contact.

Today, the open and semi-open methods of administration are seldom used. The anaesthetic agents are diluted to an unknown extent by air and this dilution is greatest when the minute volume of breathing is large so the inspiratory gas flow rate is high. The greater the ventilation (and, hence, the dilution of the anaesthetic inhaled), the closer the alveolar concentration of the anaesthetic will approach zero, and anaesthesia lightens as ventilation increases. On the other hand, depression of breathing decreases the

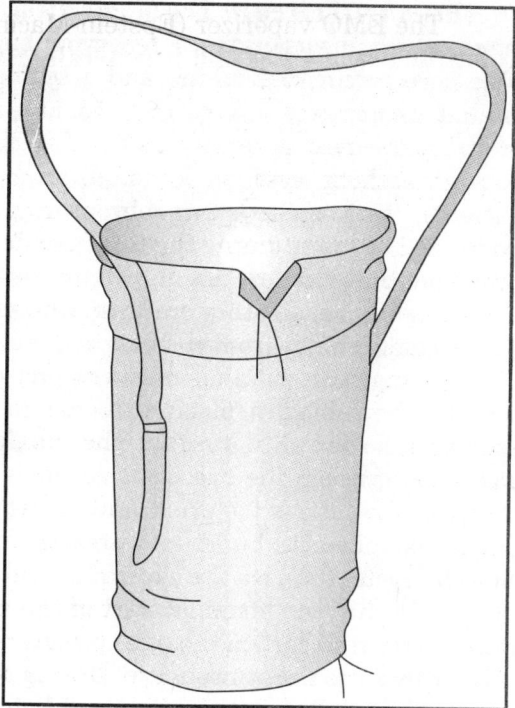

Fig. 15.9: Face-mask used for the administration of chloroform to horses and cattles

air dilution and thereby increases the concentration of anaesthetic inspired. Under these circumstances, unless there is an increase in the uptake of the anaesthetic by the body, the alveolar concentration of the anaesthetic must rise. A rise in the alveolar concentration produces deeper unconsciousness and further respiratory depression. In addition, deepening anaesthesia reduces the cardiac output and hence the uptake of anaesthetic by the body, thus adding still further to the rise in the alveolar concentration. If this process is allowed to proceed unchecked, unconsciousness deepens until the ventilation becomes inadequate. In other words, with the open and semi-open methods of administration, animals which become more lightly anaesthetized tend to continue awakening and animals which become more deeply anaesthetized tend to continue becoming more depressed and nearer to death.

Non-rebreathing Circuits

The general principle behind non-rebreathing circuits is that fresh gases flow from the anaesthetic machine into a reservoir from which the patient inhales and the exhaled gases are spilled, usually through an expiratory valve, to the atmosphere. Carbon dioxide removal depends on the fresh gas flow rate, and on the minute and tidal volumes of respiration of the patient. Many circuits have been devised but in general, they are all variations of those classified by Mapleson (Fig. 15.10). In veterinary anaesthesia the most commonly used semi-closed non-rebreathing circuits are the Magill circuit (Mapleson A), the T-piece (Mapleson E) and coaxial circuits (variations of Mapleson A and D).

The magill circuit: The Magill attachment, which incorporates a reservoir bag, wide-bore corrugated tubing and a spring-loaded expiratory valve (Fig. 15.11), is probably the most generally useful of all the non-rebreathing systems for small animal patients. With this system rebreathing is prevented by maintaining the total gas flow rate from the cylinders slightly in excess of the patient's respiratory minute volume. The animal inhales from the bag and wide-bore tubing; the exhaled mixture passes back up the tubing displacing the gas in it back into the bag until it is full. The exhaled gases never reach the bag because the capacity of the tube is too great and once the bag is distended the build upto pressure inside the system causes the expiratory valve to open so that the terminal part of the expiration (rich in carbon dioxide) passes out of the valve into the atmosphere. During the pause which follows expiration and before the next inspiration fresh gas from the anaesthetic apparatus sweeps the first part of the exhaled gases from the corrugated tube out through the expiratory valve.

To ensure minimal rebreathing of the expired gases the fresh gas flow rate should be equal to, or greater than, the minute volume of respiration of the patient.

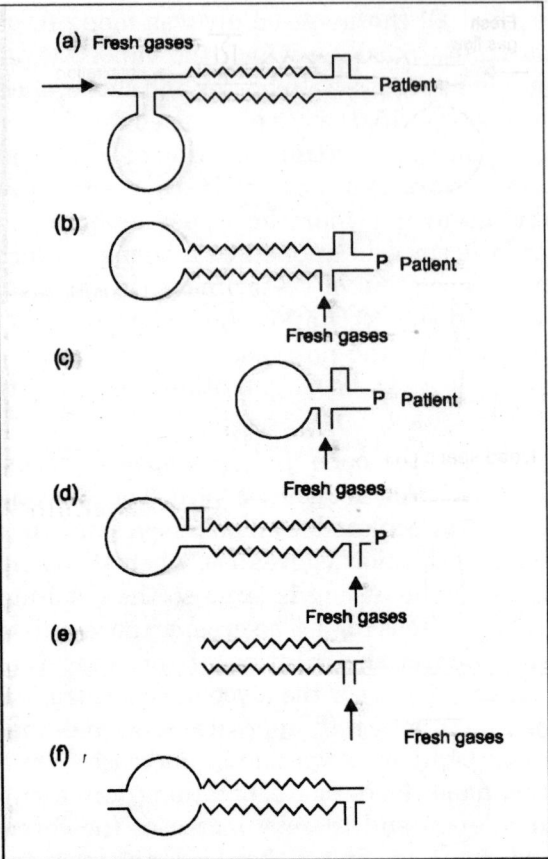

Fig. 15.10: The Mapleson classification of patient breathing circuits. This is a most comprehensive classification, system (a) = Magill and Lack circuits; (e) = T-piece circuit

However, as the system leads to the preferential removal of alveolar gas, a lower fresh gas flow rate (equal to the alveolar ventilation) may be adequate and, in spontaneously breathing patients significant rebreathing does not occur until the fresh gas flow rate falls below 70% of the patient's minute volume. If, however, IPPV is applied by compression of the reservoir bag, then very much higher fresh gas flow rates are needed to prevent rebreathing because under these circumstances the fresh gas is spilled through the expiratory valve at the end of inspiration. Various non-return valves Ruben's and, in veterinary anaesthesia, Weaver's valve, have been incorporated in the Magill system in place of the simple spring-loaded expiratory valve. These valves prevent any rebreathing of the exhaled gases other than those contained in the 'dead-space' of the valve itself and its connections. Where they are used the gas flow rates from the apparatus require frequent adjustment, for any alteration in the rate or depth of the patient's breathing affects the degree of distension of the reservoir bag. If the gas flow rate is constant, deep or rapid breathing empties the bag quickly, while slow or shallow breathing

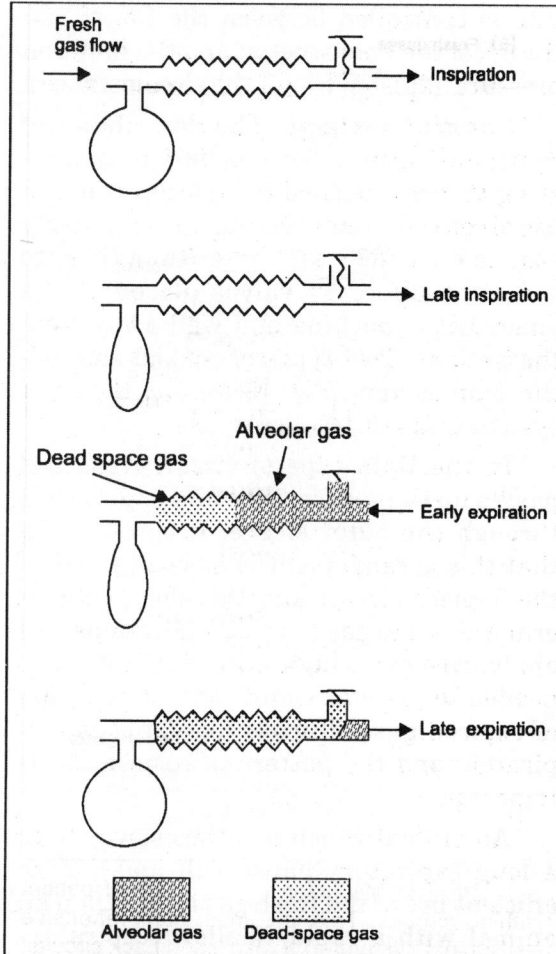

Fresh gas flow → Inspiration

Late inspiration

Dead space gas

Alveolar gas

← Early expiration

Late expiration

Alveolar gas   Dead-space gas

Fig. 15.11: The Magill circuit spontaneous breathing showing rebreathing of exhaled gas

allows the bag to become overdistended. These non-return valves can, therefore, be used to measure the minute volume of respiration, for if the gas flow rates are adjusted to maintain the bag at a constant average size at the end of expiration the total gas flow rate as read at the flowmeters will equal the respiratory minute volume. In practice, to avoid the necessity for repeated adjustments of the total gas flow rate, an excessive flow is employed and a spill valve is incorporated in the circuit between the reservoir bag and the non-return valve.

T-piece systems: The low resistance and small dead-space make the T-piece system, first described by Ayre suitable for use with cats and small dogs.

As shown in Fig. 15.12, an open tube acts as a reservoir and there are no valves. The exhaled gases are swept out of the open end of the reservoir tube by fresh gases flowing in from the anaesthetic apparatus during the expiratory phase. Unless the capacity of the reservoir tube is at least equal to the tidal volume of the animal the terminal part of the inspired gases will be air but if this will only enter the dead-space no dilution of the anaesthetic gases will take place.

The modifications of the T-piece system can be divided into three types. In the first there is no expiratory limb, in the second the capacity of the expiratory limb is greater than the tidal volume, the most convenient system is one in which the expiratory limb volume is greater than the tidal volume and which has an open-ended bag attached to the distal end of the expiratory limb (Jackson-Rees modification of the T-piece, see below). With such an arrangement fresh gas flows of up to 2.5–3 times the minute volume of respiration are required to eliminate rebreathing.

Using the basic T-piece system IPPV may be applied by intermittently blocking the open end of the reservoir tube thus directing the fresh gas into the animal's lungs. However, the inflation pressure, being that supplied by the anaesthetic machine, may be so high as to cause massive pulmonary damage if overinflation is allowed to occur. Ventilation may be controlled more safely by squeezing a bag attached to the end of the expiratory limb — the Jackson-Rees modification — because this bag has an open tail, the orifice of which

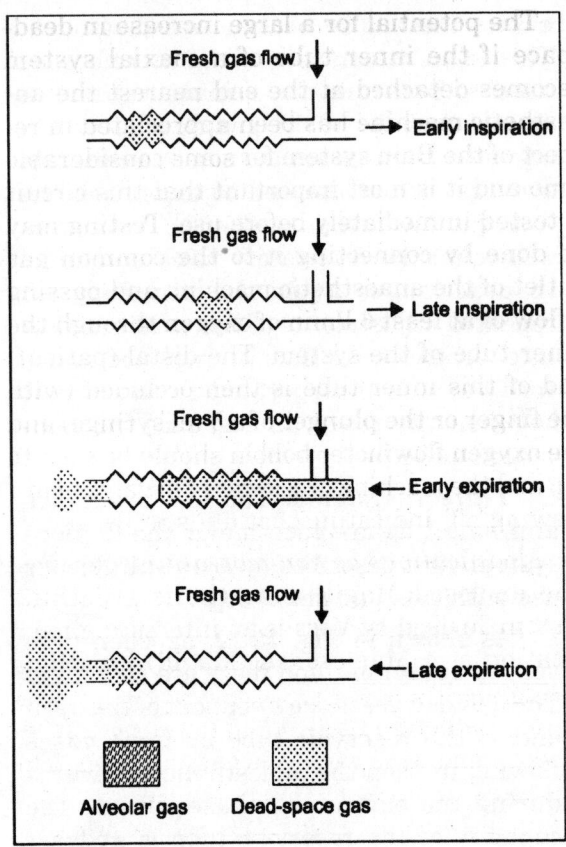

Fig. 15.12: T-piece circuit preventing rebreathing provided the fresh gas flow exceeds about twice the patient's minute volume

can be controlled between the finger and thumb of the anaesthetist and the inflation pressure adjusted to suit the circumstances.

Coaxial systems: The desirability of controlling atmospheric pollution in operating theatres has led to an interest in the use of coaxial circuits because it is relatively easy to duct the waste gases from them to the atmosphere by valves placed at the anaesthetic machine and well away from the patient. Two types of coaxial circuits, the Bain system (Fig. 15.13) and the Lack system (Fig. 15.14) are in use.

In the Bain type of circuit fresh gas passes up the central tube and expired gas through the outer sleeve. It can be seen that this arrangement is basically that of the T-piece circuit and therefore, in general, the same gas flow considerations will apply. However, higher gas flow rates are needed to prevent significant rebreathing of expired gases during spontaneous respiration and the pattern of respiration is important.

An animal which breathes slowly with a long expiratory pause will make more efficient use of the fresh gas inflow than an animal with a rapid, shallow respiratory pattern.

The Lack circuit uses the alternative arrangement in which the fresh gas flows up the outer sleeve and expiration takes place down the inner tube. This arrangement was designed to aid scavenging of expired gas and is more satisfactory than the conventional Mapleson A system in this respect. The Lack circuit cannot be used with controlled ventilation in the same way as the Bain circuit without excessive rebreathing so its use is restricted to spontaneously breathing animals.

The modified Bain circuit (Fig. 15.13) has proved reasonably satisfactory for use in dogs over 10 kg body weight and was the circuit used with very good results for IPPV in dogs over 20 kg body weight.

Use of these circuits in veterinary anaesthesia has revealed a number of problems. In some cases the internal or external tubing has been of too small a bore so that excessive demands were made on the animal's inspiratory or expiratory efforts. More serious, perhaps, the inner tube has become detached from the anaesthetic machine or patient, resulting in a very large dead-space.

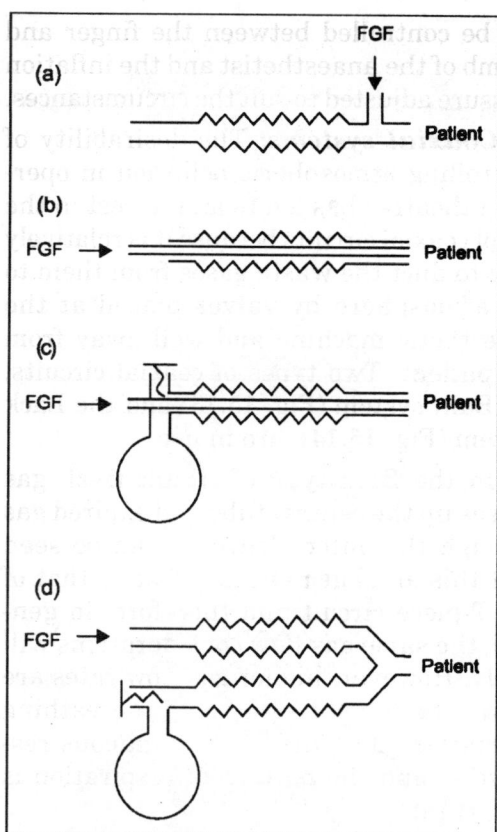

Fig. 15.13: The T-piece circuit, a. compared to the original Bain coaxial circuit, b. the modified Bain coaxial circuit, c. and the modified, parallel Bain circuit, d. In the modified circuits the bag is on the expiratory limb

The potential for a large increase in deadspace if the inner tube of a coaxial system becomes detached at the end nearest the anaesthetic machine has been appreciated in respect of the Bain system for some considerable time and it is most important that this circuit is tested immediately before use. Testing may be done by connecting it to the common gas outlet of the anaesthetic machine and passing a flow of at least 6 l/min of oxygen through the inner tube of the system. The distal (patient) end of this inner tube is then occluded (with the finger or the plunger of a 5 ml syringe) and the oxygen flowmeter bobbin should be seen to dip and the machine pressure relief valve heard blowing off, indicating that all is well.

Modifications of non-rebreathing systems: The enclosed Magill anaesthetic breathing system devised by Voss is an interesting modification of a Mapleson A (Magill) breathing system. In this configuration the fresh gas flow needed for normocapnia is similar in both spontaneous and controlled ventilation modes. The fresh gas flow passes into a bag, the enclosed reservoir, on the inspiratory limb of the system. This bag is enclosed in a rigid, transparent-walled bottle. The expiratory tube leads back to this bottle and there is a one-way valve proximal to its entrance into the bottle. The expiratory limb is thus continuous with the bottle and there is a Heidbrink valve and an open reservoir bag, situated distally.

Humphrey's ADE system is designed to facilitate changing from a Mapleson D or E configuration during controlled ventilation to a Mapleson A mode for spontaneous ventilation and is another, perhaps more commonly used, modification of an earlier system. It is not very efficient in conserving anaesthetic gases, the Bain system is 24% better.

Parallel circuits which operate in the same manner as the Bain and Lack circuits have two tubes running alongside one another rather than one inside the other (Figs 15.13 and 15.14).

Rebreathing Circuits

In anaesthesia, the carbon dioxide is usually removed by directing the exhaled mixture over the surface of soda lime. This is a mixture of 90% calcium hydroxide and 5% sodium hydroxide together with 5% of silicate and water to prevent powdering. It is used in a granular form, the granules being 4–8 mesh in size, and is packed into a canister so that, ideally, the space between the granules is at least equal to the tidal volume of the animal. Some brands of soda lime contain an indicator dye which changes colour when the carbon dioxide absorbing capacity is exhausted. Absence of visible cold change is no guarantee that the soda lime is capable of absorbing more carbon dioxide — a small quantity should be wrapped in gauze and a brisk flow of carbon dioxide directed through it. When this is done active soda lime becomes very hot but exhausted absorbent remains cool.

1. The 'to-and-fro' system
2. The 'circle system'

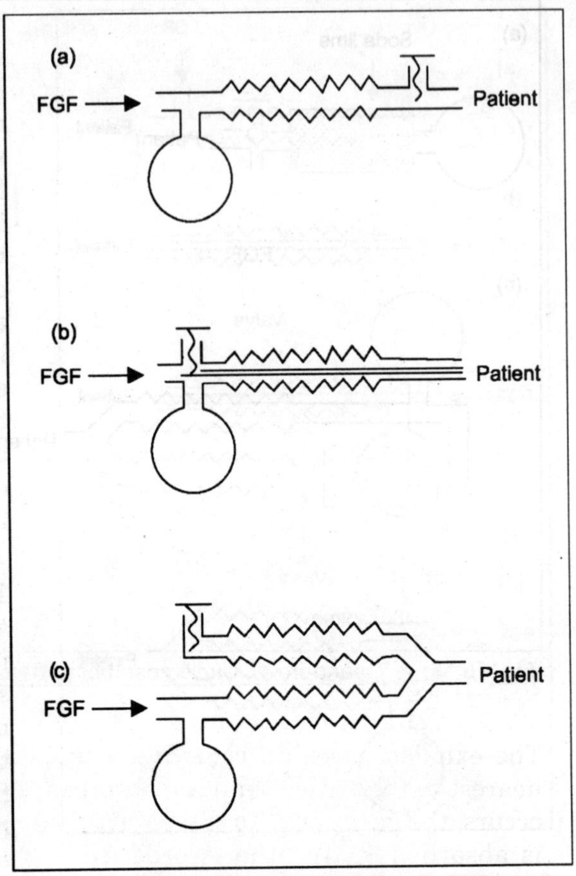

The 'to-and-fro' system: A canister full of soda lime is interposed between the animal and the rebreathing bag, fresh gases being fed into the system as close to the animal as possible to effect changes in the mixture rapidly (Fig.15.15). This system is simple and efficient but has several drawbacks. It is difficult to maintain the heavy, awkward apparatus in a gas-tight condition and the inspired gases become undesirably hot due to the chemical action between the soda lime and the carbon dioxide. Furthermore, irritating dust may

Fig. 15.14: The Lack coaxial circuit (b) compared to the standard Magill circuit (a) and the parallel Lack circuit (c) In all these circuits there is a reservoir bag on the inspiratory limb of the circuit

be inhaled from the soda lime and give rise to a bronchitis. Nevertheless the system is the one most commonly used in veterinary anaesthesia for the necessary apparatus is relatively inexpensive and may be improvised.

For small animal anaesthesia (dogs, sheep and goats, young calves, young foals and small pigs) the standard soda lime canisters used in man, which are known as Water's canisters after their designer, are quite satisfactory. They are available in various sizes and one canister to contain about 0.5 kg and a second one to contain about 0.3 kg of soda lime are adequate for most veterinary purposes. These canisters are used horizontally and unless the soda lime is tightly packed when the canister is filled it tends to settle, leaving a channel along the top through which gases pass without being subjected to the action of the soda lime.

Adult horses, cattle and large pigs need much larger soda lime canisters. They are designed on the principle that for efficient absorption of carbon dioxide the whole of the

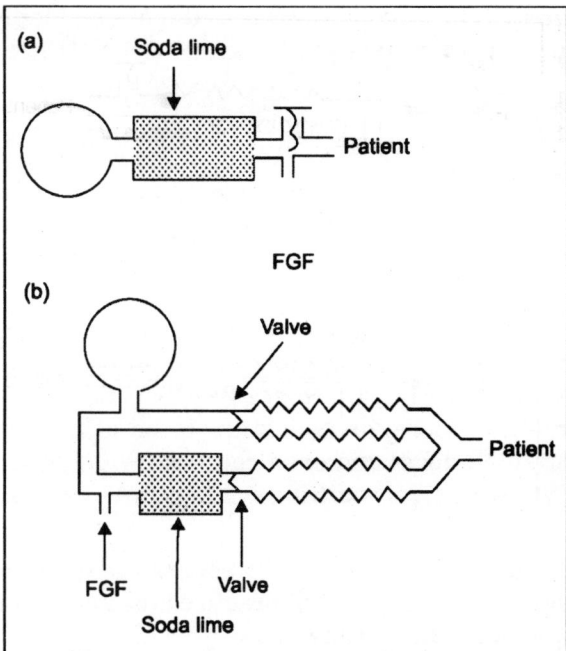

Fig. 15.15: a. To-and-fro, b. Circle absorber systems

animal's tidal volume should be accommodated in the spaces between the soda lime granules. It measures approximately 20 cm in length and 81 cm in diameter (internal measurements) and contains about 4.5 kg of soda lime. The connections to the rebreathing bag and to the expiratory mount are of 5 cm internal diameter. Because of the difficulty experienced in packing this canister sufficiently tightly with soda lime, special to-and-fro canisters have been designed and developed for large animals. The vertical position of these soda lime canisters means that tight packing is not necessary, and their cross-sectional area is large to ensure that the respired gases move through the absorbent slowly.

For adult horses and cattle a rebreathing bag having a capacity of about 15 litres is used.

The to-and-fro systems can never be really efficient absorbers of carbon dioxide. The exhaled gases all come into contact with the soda lime at the end of the canister nearest to the patient and the absorbent in this region is quickly exhausted. Thus, as this occurs, the gases have to travel further and further into the canister before carbon dioxide is absorbed or, in other words, the apparatus dead-space steadily increases during anaesthesia.

The 'circle' system: The circle system for carbon dioxide absorption incorporates an inspiratory and an expiratory tube with unidirectional valves to ensure a one-way flow of gases; the rebreathing bag and soda lime canister are placed between these tubes. The valves and tubing offer an appreciable resistance to breathing and unless the apparatus is carefully designed with regard to the diameter of airways in relation to flow rates, breathing through the apparatus can impose a considerable strain on the animal. Cycle-type absorber units are not, as a general rule, suitable for cats and small dogs of less than about 15 kg body weight because of the resistance offered by even the best-designed units and because of the inevitable degree of rebreathing which occurs at the T-piece connection to the patient. This rebreathing can be prevented by placing the unidirectional valves at the face-piece or connection to the endotracheal tube, but it is difficult to design robust, competent valves for use in this situation. In the majority of modern circle-type units the unidirectional valves are of the turret type; some, however, employ rubber flaps. The turret type is robust and competent but it has the disadvantage that it must be kept upright and of necessity, therefore, has to be mounted on the apparatus at some distance away from the animal. Circle absorber units are more efficient absorbers of carbon dioxide than arc to-and-fro units because their dead-space is constant since all the charge of soda lime is available to the respired gases. Exhaustion of soda lime is noticed more suddenly than in to-and-fro absorbers and once it occurs the inspired carbon dioxide concentration may soon become excessive.

To avoid this sudden exhaustion of the soda lime and for economy in its use, canisters are now often made with two compartments. The compartment of the canister which first receives the inspired gases and, therefore, whose soda lime is first used, can be refilled and the position of the canister reversed, so that the expired gases pass through the remaining partially used soda lime, using this to complete exhaustion before reaching the newly filled compartment.

Standard circle absorbers designed for man are satisfactory for young foals, young calves, sheep, goats, most pigs, and dogs over 15 kg body weight. Circle absorbers for large animal patients are now commercially available but there are few reports of their efficiency in terms of carbon dioxide absorbing capacity or resistance to breathing. In North America, circle absorbers designed for small dogs (and even cats) are widely used but they have never found favour in the UK where non-rebreathing systems are preferred for patients of this size.

All circle absorption systems for large animals are relatively cumbersome and expensive and are only likely to find favour for use in hospitals. For general practice a large animal to-and-fro system, in spite of its limitations, is much more convenient.

Practical Problems involved in the use of Closed Rebreathing Circuit

When anaesthesia is first induced with an inhalation anaesthetic the animal takes up the anaesthetic and the expired gases contain a lower concentration of the anaesthetic than the inspired gases. Thus, the concentration of anaesthetic in a completely closed circuit will become diluted. The speed of uptake of the anaesthetic depends on many factors but obviously the larger the animal, the greater the dilution, and the longer the time before equilibrium is attained. Also, during induction, nitrogen from the patient accumulates in the anaesthetic circuit and decreases the concentration of oxygen therein.

The problems of denitrogenation and of maintaining an adequate concentration of anaesthetic for the induction of anaesthesias are best overcome by increasing the fresh gas flow rate, opening overspill valves, frequently emptying the rebreathing bag ('dumping') and thus converting the system to a semi-closed circuit for the duration of the induction period.

The problems involved in rapidly decreasing the depth of anaesthesia are similar to those of induction but the gases exhaled by the patient will contain anaesthetic in higher concentrations than the inspired gas, so that the concentration of anaesthetic in the circuit will tend to increase, and the depth of anaesthesia will only lighten very slowly. Again, this can be overcome by increasing the gas inflow rates and emptying the rebreathing bag at frequent intervals.

Maintenance of a stable depth of anaesthesia also poses problems when a completely closed rebreathing circuit is employed.

A method of overcoming the problem of vaporization of the anaesthetic at low fresh gas flow rates is to place the vaporizer inside the breathing circuit. If the vaporizer is placed in the fresh gas supply line outside the breathing circuit the circuit receives a steady supply of anaesthetic. When the vaporizer is placed in the breathing circuit, however, the flow through it depends on the respiratory efforts of the patient so that vaporization of the anaesthetic depends on this rather than the fresh gas flow rate.

FACE-MASKS AND ENDOTRACHEAL TUBES

Anaesthetics given by the closed- and semi-closed-circuit methods must be delivered to the animal through a well-fitting face mask or endotracheal tube otherwise the anaesthetic agent will be diluted and inhaled with an unknown quantity of air.

Anaesthetic Face-masks

In domestic animals there are wide variations in the configuration and size of the face, so that it is difficult to obtain an accurate airtight fit between the face and the mask. However, this difficulty can be overcome by the use of malleable latex rubber masks (Fig. 15.16) which can be moulded around the face and held in position with a simple headstrap. The lower jaw must be pushed forward into the mask for if it is displaced backwards the airway may become obstructed by the base of the tongue coming into contact with the posterior wall of the pharynx.

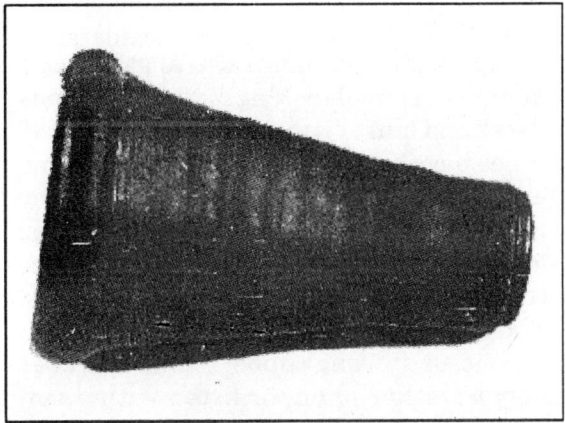

Fig. 15.16: Commercially available malleable face-mask

After use these masks should be thoroughly washed with soap and hot water and then disinfected.

Whenever a face mask is used care must be taken not to cause damage to the eyes and, in species of animal that breathe through the nose rather than the mouth, it is most important to ensure that the nostrils are not obstructed by coming into contact with the mask. Some patterns of face mask are made of transparent material to allow the anaesthetist to observe the position of the mouth and nostrils.

Endotracheal Intubation

There are two methods by which inhalation anaesthetics can be administered through an endotracheal tube, and the first to be used was that of 'insufflation' in which the anaesthetic agents are blown through a narrow-bore tube, the distal end which lies in the trachea near to the carina. Respiration and the return flow of gases and vapours takes place around the tube. The insufflation technique is said to render respiratory movements unnecessary but has the great disadvantage of causing a considerable loss of heat and water vapour from the body. It has fallen into disuse but has given rise to the technique of intermittent entrainment of air to produce ventilation of the lungs of small mammal patients during bronchoscopy under general anaesthesia with muscle relaxants. A line-bore tube (usually an 18 s.w.g. needle) mounted at the eyepiece end of a rigid bronchoscope has oxygen or a mixture of oxygen and nitrous oxide (Entonox) blown through it inter-mittently. The jet of gas entrains air and generates enough pressure to inflate the animal's lungs which deflate as soon as the gas flow through the fine-bore tube is stopped (Fig. 15.17). In the second endotracheal method to-and-fro respiration takes place through one large-bore tube.

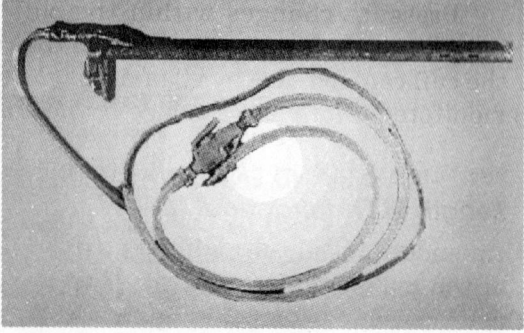

Fig. 15.17: Entrainer on rigid bronchoscope to allow ventilation of the lungs of the apnoeic patient during bronchoscopy

The standard endotracheal tubes used in man designed by Magill and two kinds ('oral' and 'nasal') are available. The 'oral' tubes have comparatively thick walls and are intended for intubation through the mouth, while the 'nasal' tubes, designed for passage through the nostril into the trachea, have comparatively thin walls. The tubes are obtainable in red rubber, plastic, or silicone rubber. The oral tubes may be either plain, or fitted with a cuff which can be inflated with air after the tube has been passed into the trachea. The inflated cuff provides an airtight seal between the wall of the trachea and the tube so that all the respired gases must pass through the lumen of the tube. A good seal between the trachea and cuffs reduces the danger of inhalation of for-eign material, but overinflation must be avoided as this may result either in pres-sure damage to the mucous membrane of the trachea or to respiratory obstruction by pressing the wall of the tube into its

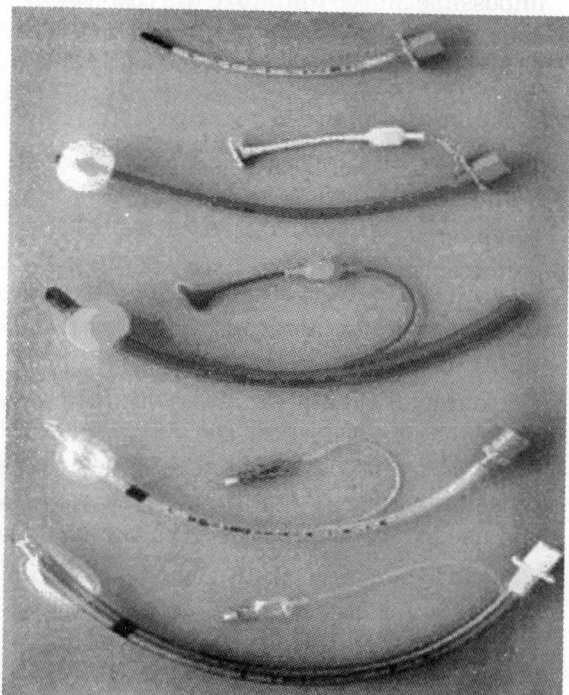

Fig. 15.18: Various types of endotracheal tubes

lumen. Some of these problems may be overcome by the use of tubes which have high-volume, low-pressure cuffs but, in general, production through the larynx may be dif-ficult. Cuffed tubes a pilot balloon connected to the cuff gives some guidance to the degree of inflation but does not show when an airtight seal has been obtained. The cuff should be inflated with air until compression of the reservoir bag of the anaesthetic circuit to which the patient is connected no longer causes an audible leak of gas around the tube, (Fig. 15.18).

Pressure changes within the cuff may be caused by diffusion of gases, the most important gas is oxygen and when the respired gases contain 30% oxygen the pressure in the cuff can increase by 90 mmHg (12 kPa).[1] Ideally, the pressure inside the cuff should be monitored to prevent damage to the tracheal mucosa.

Length of Endotracheal Tubes

An endotracheal tube which is too long may be inadvertently introduced into one or other of the main bronchi, and the lung on the non-intubated side will then act as a venous-arterial shunt. This may give rise to persistent cyanosis and endobronchial intubation should always be suspected if an animal shows cyanosis when breathing an oxygen-rich mixture through an endotracheal tube.

Magill tubes must be of correct length both to ensure that endobronchial intubation is impossible and to minimize the respiratory dead-space. Their bevelled tip lies in the trachea about midway-between the larynx and carina; their cut end is immediately below the nostrils. Also, the connecting piece between the tube and any closed or semi-closed anaesthetic apparatus should be as short as possible.

Reinforced Endotracheal Tubes

Frequent use, with the associated cleaning and sterilizing processes, makes red-rubber endotracheal tubes soft, and plastic tubes may soften when warmed to body temperature. Soft tubes flatten out when bent, and are easily compressed by pressure. Obliteration of the lumen from either of these causes may give rise to serious obstruction of the airway. Patency of the airway, when the animal has to be placed in any position which may cause flattening or kinking of the tube, can be assured by the use of an armoured, or reinforced, endotracheal tube. These special tubes are made of silicone rubber and incorporate a wire or nylon spiral in their walls. They are more expensive than the standard tubes. On the occasions when compression or kinking of the endotrapheal tube is likely to be encountered the use of a new red-rubber tube is usually satisfactory.[2]

Laryngoscopes

Although not strictly essential, a laryngoscope greatly facilitates the process of intubation in many animals and is a piece of equipment which is most desirable if endotracheal intubation is to bewidely practised. A suitable laryngoscope is one which holds a dry electric battery in the handle and has a detachable blade in order that blades of different sizes can be fitted to the instrument. The blades should be designed so as to enable the passage of a large-bore endotracheal tube to be made as easily as possible.[3] For veterinary purposes one standard human adult and one child-size 'Magill pattern' blades and one special blade are the minimum requirements. The special blade should be of the Macintosh pattern, 1.9 cm wide, and between 9 and 12 inches (23 and 30 cm) long. The blades should be separate from the lamp and its electrical connections so that they can be sterilized by boiling without risk of damage to the electrical system. Various types are available and one suitable instrument is shown in Fig. 15.19.

For small animal use, a modified penlight torch car provide an inexpensive light source which, although less satisfactory than a laryngoscope, may prove adequate in an emergency. For large animals, special laryngoscope blades are required and the Rowson blade has greatly simplified the intubation of cattle, sheep and large pigs. Wide-bore tubes may be introduced into the trachea in various ways and the method to be adopted in any particular case is decided by the skill and experience of the anaesthetist and the kind of animal in which the tube is to be passed. In the chapters on anaesthesia for the various species of animals, descriptions will be found on techniques which undergraduate students and anaesthetists in training have found relatively easy to master.

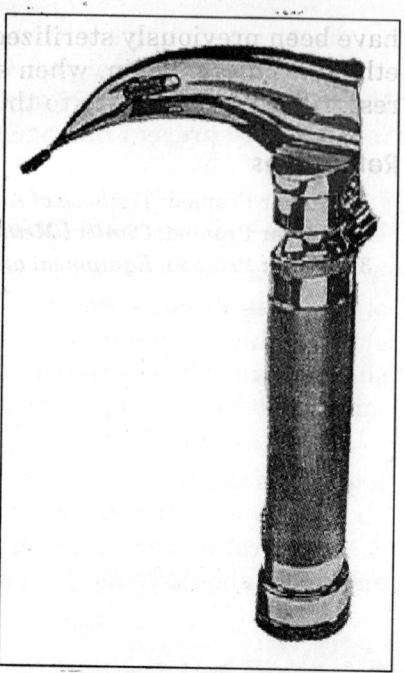

Fig. 15.19: Laryngoscope with Macintosh blade. Laryngoscopes such as the one illustrated have detachable blades and a wide variety of patterns of blade are available

CLEANING AND STERILIZATION OF ANAESTHETIC EQUIPMENT

Anaesthetic equipment is obviously a potential source of cross-infection from one patient to the next; ideally, all parts of the breathing circuits should be sterilized between each use. Unfortunately, this is not very practical as parts of the apparatus do not tolerate many of the possible methods of sterilization and, where they do, most of the methods shorten their life.
The nearer the part of the circuit to the patient, the greater the risk of cross infection from organisms associated with the previous patient. The compromise usually adopted with anaesthetic equipment is, therefore, to sterilize the components close to the patient such as endotracheal tubes or face-masks, whilst the rest of the equipment is only regularly cleaned. This equipment is sterilized periodically, or following its use on a patient thought or known to be suffering from an infectious disease.

Whatever method of sterilization is to be employed, the apparatus must first be thoroughly cleaned by washing in hot water with a detergent or soap. Many parts of the breathing circuit may be damaged if subjected to autoclaving. Heat sterilization by boiling may be used for endotracheal tubes although regular treatment of this nature does shorten their life. The various means of chemical sterilization rarely damage equipment but when they are used the apparatus must be thoroughly washed afterwards because traces of chemical, particularly if remaining on face-masks or endotracheal tubes, may prove very irritant indeed to the next patient. The use of ethylene oxide gas is now a practical method of sterilization in veterinary practice and although it causes no damage to anaesthetic equipment a sufficient time (up to 7 days) must be allowed to elapse before the equipment is used again in order to allow all traces of gas to disappear. Also, it must be remembered that some plastics which have been previously sterilized by γ irradiation produce an extremely toxic substance, ethylene chlorohydrin, when subjected to ethylene oxide gas so they should never be resterilized by exposure to this agent.

References

1. Kumar Pramod, *Textbook of Anaesthesiology,* 1st ed., Paras Med. Publishers, Hyderabad, 2008.
2. Kumar Pramod, *Clinical Methods of Anaesthesia,* 1st ed., Paras Med. Publishers, Mumbai, 2008.
3. Kumar Pramod, *Equipment and Drugs in Anaesthesia,* 1st ed., CBS Publishers, New Delhi, 2009.

16

Artificial Ventilation of Lungs

COMPLIANCE

Volume changes per unit pressure changes: Its measurements cannot be compared unless related to a lung volume such as the functional residual capacity (FRC). Unfortunately, measurement of FRC is not a simple procedure and such measurements as have been made in large animals have omitted this refinement. As normally measured, compliance has two components and compliance values can be found for both the lungs themselves and the thoracic cage but, of course, during thoracotomy the total compliance measured approaches that of the lungs alone. During anaesthesia the compliance may be altered by assistants resting their weight on the chest, by the use of retractors and by the degree of muscle relaxation. Airway resistance has to be overcome to deliver air to the alveoli at inspiration and to expel it during expiration. Unlike compliance, airway resistance must be measured during air flow. It becomes less as lung volume increases and is less during inspiration than expiration.

Airway resistance during anaesthesia is increased by the resistance of apparatus, such as endotracheal tubes, which may be used. Animals with pulmonary disease may also have increased resistance and, for example, 'broken-winded' horses have a rapid increase in airway resistance at the end of expiration. The effects of a sudden increase in airway resistance at the end of expiration must be clearly understood by the anaesthetist if trouble is to be avoided during IPPV. If the expiratory period of the IPPV is too short the lungs may not have time to empty completely because the increase in resistance will delay the expulsion of air from the lungs. This will mean that the lung volume will be greater at the start of the next inspiration. Thus, there will be a steady increase in FRC until the retroactive force of the lungs, which increases with increase in lung volume becomes sufficient to empty the lungs to a new FRC in the time available and the inspiratory and expiratory tidal volumes become equal. While conscious, the 'broken-winded' horse empties the lungs by active expiratory movements but when anaesthetized and under the influence of a muscle relaxant expiration may become passive and, consequently, longer in duration. The pattern of IPPV used must make allowance for this, and large tidal volumes should be delivered with long expiratory pauses between each inspiration.

Airway resistance is frictional in nature due to the movement of gas molecules through the air passages, but the tissues of the lungs and chest wall must also offer a resistance to movement due to their displacement during the breathing cycle. However, the magnitude of this resistance is seldom likely to interfere with pulmonary function.

To overcome pulmonary resistance a driving force has to be applied to the upper airway to produce an airflow through the respiratory passages. An analogy can be drawn with Ohm's Law, where, $R = E/I$, and the formula written: Resistance = Driving pressure/ Flow. During spontaneous breathing the driving pressure must be atmospheric less the alveolar pressure during inspiration and, during expiration, the alveolar pressure less atmospheric pressure. During IPPV the driving pressure or force during inspiration will be atmospheric pressure plus the pressure exerted on the reservoir bag less the alveolar pressure, but during expiration the driving pressure will be alveolar less atmospheric pressure unless a subatmospheric pressure is applied at the mouth.

Consideration of the 'flow formula' where Resistance = Driving pressure/Flow, shows that if the resistance is low and a small volume has to be delivered only a small driving pressure is required. If, however, the resistance is increased and/or a greater flow is required, the driving pressure must be greater. This is important, for registration of the pressure in the upper airway is often used to monitor the tidal volume delivered by a ventilator, increasing the pressure is assumed to increase the tidal volume delivered. While this may be so if the pulmonary resistance is low, considerable caution must be exercised in translating a pressure reading taken somewhere in the upper airway into a volume of gas actually reaching the alveoli high gas flow into the lungs, or a high airway resistance, can lead to the peak pressures recorded in the upper airways being much higher than the final peak alveolar pressure so that lung compliance cannot be easily calculated from upper airway pressures and consequently, related changes in lung volume cannot be assumed.

Airway resistance also depends on the nature of the airflow through the airway. With a clear airway and a low gas flow rate, flow is laminar (streamlined) and airway resistance is also low, but obstruction or a high flow velocity will give rise to turbulence and a greatly increased resistance. The many branches of the tracheobronchial tree tend to cause turbulent flow patterns, especially where there are irregularities in the bronchial tubes, i.e. blebs of mucus, foreign bodies, and the effect will be greater at high gas flow rates. Thus, during IPPV, attempts to produce large gas flows to minimize the duration of inspiration may necessitate the use of high driving pressures but, of course, the airway resistance will normally prevent the direct transmission of these pressures to the alveoli.

Mean intrathoracic pressure may be above or below atmospheric pressure as a result of apparatus resistance. For example, if the expiratory flow through a piece of apparatus with a high resistance is great enough to produce turbulence whilst the inspiratory rate is lower (as it often seems to be in horses) so that the flow is laminar, the mean intrathoracic pressure will be above atmospheric. Conversely, if the inspiratory flow rate is greater there may be a subatmospheric mean intrathoracic pressure. Mean intrathoracic pressures above atmospheric pressure may cause cardiovascular failure in hypovolaemic states. High subatmospheric mean pressures may be equally dangerous, perhaps by producing pulmonary oedema, but probably more importantly by reducing lung volume. Trapping of gas in the lungs occurs more readily at low lung volumes and in man, for example, an alveolar pressure of 5 cmH$_2$0 (0.5 kPa) below atmospheric produces widespread airway obstruction with quite serious impairment of respiratory function.[1]

Differences between IPPV and Spontaneous Respiration

In a spontaneously breathing animal active contraction of the inspiratory muscles lowers the normally subatmospheric intrapleural pressure still further by enlarging the thoracic cavity. The decrease in intrapleural pressure lowers the alveolar pressure so that a pressure gradient or driving force is set up between the exterior and the alveoli to overcome the airway resistance. Airflows into the alveoli until at the end of inspiration the alveolar pressure becomes equal to the atmospheric pressure. During expiration the pressure gradient is reversed and air flows out of the alveoli.

The pressure gradient between the pleural cavity and the exterior is largely open up in overcoming the retractive forces of the lungs and provided the airway is clear, the remaining small alveolar-exterior pressure gradient set up during inspiration is quite adequate to overcome the airway resistance and produce airflow into the lungs. The concept of intrapleural pressure is, however, difficult to explain. The pleural cavity is under the influence of gravity and if two bubbles of air are introduced into it, one some distance above the other, the pressure which can be measured in them will not be the same, the pressure in the lower bubble will be found to be greater. In man, the pressure of the pleural fluid facing the lowest part of the lungs is probably about 5 cm H$_2$O (–0.5 kPa), or just enough to keep the lung expanded and hence equal to the pleural surface pressure.

The pressure in the upper part of the pleural cavity should be much more below atmospheric, but it is not at all certain how uniform the pressure on the pleural surface of the lung really is; the hilar forces, the buoyancy of the lung in the pleural cavity and the different shapes of the lung and chest wall are all possible sources of local pressure differences. Because, therefore, there is no one intrapleural pressure it is now customary to measure the intra-oesophageal pressure instead. The changes in intrapleural (oesophageal) pressure in relation to changes in upper airway (mouth) pressure during spontaneous breathing and IPPV are compared and contrasted in Fig. 16.1

The most obvious effect of IPPV is on the circulatory system. During spontaneous breathing, inspiration, by lowering intrathoracic pressure, augments the venous return to the heart and in many animals, as can

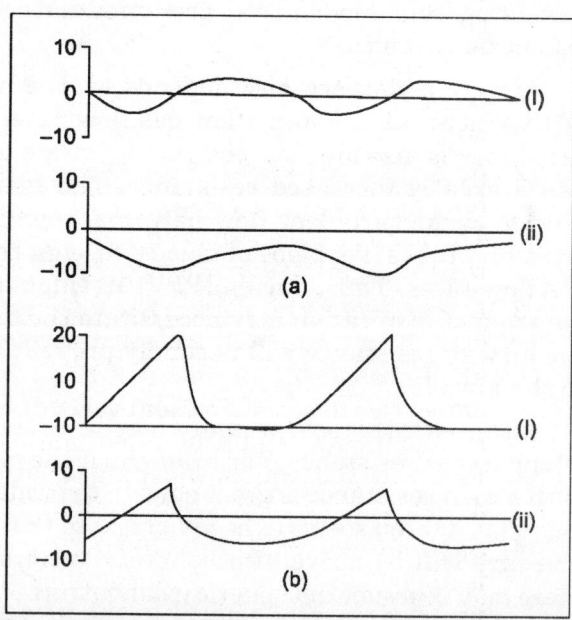

Fig. 16.1: Pressure changes (i) at the mouth end of endotracheal tube and (ii) in the thoracic oesophagus during (a) spontaneous breathing and (b) During IPPV

often be seen on a tracing of continuously recorded blood pressure, there are indications that an increase in stroke volume is produced. During controlled respiration, however, the intrathoracic pressure rises during inspiration, blood is dammed back from the thorax, venous return and stroke volume decrease; blood flows freely into the thoracic vessels during the expiratory period. Fortunately, this damming back of blood during inspiration by causing distension of veins produces a reflex increase in venous tone which in normal animals appears to compensate for the changed intrathoracic conditions during the inspiratory period and restores the venous return towards normality. Obviously, the extent to which an increase in venous tone can compensate will depend on the degree of venomotor integrity (which can probably be affected by drugs), on the blood volume, the magnitude of the intrathoracic pressure rise and its duration.[1]

The magnitude and duration of the increased pressure within the thorax during the inspiratory phase of IPPV are critical and are reflected in the 'mean intrathoracic pressure'. This mean pressure, like the mean arterial blood pressure, is not the simple arithmetical mean between the highest and lowest pressures reached in the system and its calculation is not always easy for the non-mathematician. It is clearly important to keep this mean pressure as low as possible during the respiratory cycle and this can be attempted in a variety of ways:

1. *Short application of positive pressure:* The shorter the inspiratory period during IPPV the lower the resulting mean intrathoracic pressure will be for any given applied pressure. Theoretically, it might seem that the peak pressure should never be maintained, expiration should commence as soon as the peak pressure is achieved, or the circulation will suffer. However, the short application of a positive pressure to the airway may not result in very good distribution of fresh gas within the lungs.

   A compromise seems to be necessary here, but exactly what it is likely to be for any one animal of any one species remains pure speculation.

2. *Rapid gas flow rate:* If the necessary tidal volume of gas is to be delivered to the lungs in a short inspiratory period it is clear that the flow rate will need to be high. The rate at which gas can flow into the lungs, however, is largely dictated by the resistance offered by the apparatus used and the airway resistance.

3. *Low expiratory resistance:* Because any resistance to the air flow created by the passive expiratory phase of IPPV will delay the fall in intrathoracic pressure it will result in an increase in the mean intrathoracic pressure and possibly in circulatory embarrassment. In patients with obstructive emphysema the use of expiratory resistance will result in a more orderly emptying of the alveoli and an increase in FRC with consequent widening of the airways. Thus, at least in some circumstances, a higher expiratory resistance may in fact be advantageous to an animal.

4. *Subatmospheric pressure during the expiratory phase:* If a subatmospheric pressure is applied to the airway during the expiratory part of the IPPV cycle the inspiratory pressure will be applied to the airway from a lower baseline. Hence the pressure gradient necessary to produce the required volume change in the lungs can be achieved with a lower peak pressure. A subatmospheric phase in the cycle may therefore help

to maintain cardiac output, but the changes in arterial pressure and cardiac output are proportional to the duration of the increased airway pressure and not necessarily simply to the peak pressures reached so that merely decreasing the peak pressure may have only little effect if the inspiratory phase is long.

5. *Cardiovascular effects: It* might be expected that most of the potentially harmful effects of IPPV on the circulatory system would be absent during thoracotomy. An opening in the chest wall should prevent compression of pulmonary capillaries when positive pressure is applied to the airway, leading to less interference with blood flow through the lungs. Nevertheless, it has been demonstrated in dogs that thoracotomy reduces the cardiac output to below levels which might be expected from the application of IPPV alone apparently by causing a further reduction in venous return to the heart.

6. *Ventilation perfusion:* Any uneven distribution of gas must have the effect of disturbing the normal ventilation/perfusion relationships within the lungs. It appears that these are often upset by anaesthesia itself and if IPPV producers more uneven gas distribution, it will probably fail to affect any improvement in the alveolar arterial oxygen tension gradient found during anaesthesia, in spite of any improvement in tidal exchange which it may produce. For example, in laterally recumbent horses it is possible that the gravitational force gradient from the top to the bottom of the lungs acting on the low-pressure pulmonary circulation may, by reducing the circulation to the upper lung, cause this lung to be overventilated in relation to its perfusion. Due to the weight of the horse's abdominal viscera acting on the lower cone of the diaphragm, IPPV is more successful in inflating the upper than the lower lung and hence the upper lung receives an even more disproportionately large part of the ventilation to the further detriment of its ventilation/perfusion relationships. Certainly, in the laterally recumbent horse controlled ventilation appears to produce very little improvement in the alveolar-arterial oxygen tension gradient found during general anaesthesia. Other situations in which the normal relationships between ventilation and perfusion may be upset occur in all animals where the expansion of one lung or part of a lung is limited by surgical procedures such as 'packing off' and retraction of lung lobes during intrathoracic surgery.

7. *Acid-Base:* IPPV should remove carbon dioxide from the animal's lungs and it is possible, over a period of time, to remove either too much or too little causing the animal to suffer from either respiratory alkalosis or acidosis. Respiratory acidosis (hypercapnia) is characterized by sympathetic over activity, cutaneous vasodilatation, a rise in arterial blood pressure and a bounding pulse. Respiratory alkalosis (hypocapnia) may, it has been claimed, lead to cerebral damage from cerebral vasoconstriction because the calibre of the cerebral blood vessels depends on the arterial carbon dioxide tension. However, convincing evidence of cerebral damage due to hypocapnia has yet to be produced. Moreover, although it has been demonstrated that hypocapnia has reduced cardiac output in man and in horses, at least in normovolaemic states no disaster appears to result and it seems to be generally agreed that hypocapnia is much less harmful than hypercapnia.

IPPV carried out with a face mask instead of an endotracheal tube can be harmful unless care is taken to avoid forcing gases down the oesophagus into the stomach. This entails careful limiting of the pressure applied at the mouth and nostrils and observations of the epigastric region to detect any inflation of the stomach. An inflated stomach not only hinders intra-abdominal surgery, if it becomes sufficiently distended with gas regurgitation of gastric fluid is a distinct possibility. Gas accidentally forced into the stomach should be removed as soon as possible by passing a stomach tube.

Positive End Expiratory Pressure (PEEP) and Continuous Positive Airway Pressure (CPAP)

In many conditions of advanced lung disease the imposition of an expiratory threshold resistance has been shown to have beneficial effects on the PaO_2 of an expiratory resistor during IPPV known as PEEP (positive end-expiratory pressure) and during spontaneous breathing as CPAP (continuous positive airway pressure). The respiratory benefits of an expiratory resistor include an overall reduction in airway resistance due to an increase in FRC, movement of the tidal volume to above the airway closing volume, a tendency towards reexpansion of any collapsed lung and, possibly, a reduction in total lung water. The net result is that ventilation/perfusion relationships are improved. However, these advantages are, in some circumstances, counterbalanced by circulatory disadvantages due to the inevitable rise in mean intrathoracic pressure which will impede venous return and decrease cardiac output. Although the venous return can be restored with an α-adrenergic stimulator such as metaraminol or by over-transfusion in clinical practice the situation is more complicated.

Both disease and drugs have profound effects on the circulatory response to a rise in mean intrathoracic pressure due to PEEP (or CPAP). Certain conditions may aggravate the reduction in cardiac output but others actually oppose it and it is in these latter conditions that PEEP or CPAP is likely to be of benefit. In animals with poor lung compliance much of the applied end-expiratory pressure will be opposed by the excessive pulmonary transmural pressure thus minimizing the increase in intrathoracic pressure. Thus, the stiffer the lungs, the safer is the application of PEEP (or CPAP) likely to be.

To PEEP (and CPAP) may corner respiratory advantages and circulatory disadvantages which interact in a complicated manner rendering it necessary to make direct measurements of the relevant physiological functions to ensure that overall benefit results. In veterinary practice, even in intensive care units, such measurements are seldom possible and the use of expiratory threshold resistors is, therefore, unlikely to gain wide acceptance in the treatment of sick animals. Moreover, the results of PEEP and CPAP during routine anaesthesia are disappointing.

MANAGEMENT OF CONTROLLED RESPIRATION

Before IPPV can be applied all spontaneous breathing movements have to be abolished if the animal is not to 'fight' the imposed ventilation. This is usually accomplished by:

1. Depressing the respiratory centres by relative overdoses of anaesthetics or agents such as morphine or fentanyl.
2. Paralysis of the respiratory muscles by neuromuscular block.

3. Lowering the carbon dioxide tension in the body by hyperventilation. This may be done by squeezing the reservoir bag at the end of each spontaneous inspiration to force a little more gas into the lungs, or by ventilating between spontaneous breaths.

4. Reflexly inhibiting the respiratory centres by regular rhythmical lung inflation. This inhibition does not depend on changes in blood pH and carbon dioxide tension. For example, in the cat subjected to IPPV it is known that respiratory neuronal activity usually synchronizes with the ventilator cycle within two to three respiratory cycles; this is too rapid for significant changes in the arterial blood gases to occur. It is believed that if the lungs are slightly overdistended at each inspiration, afferent impulses from pulmonary receptors inhibit the medullary centres.

When IPPV is carried out by manual squeezing of the reservoir bag this should be done gently and rhythmically. Once the desired degree of lung inflation has been produced the bag should be released and the lungs allowed to empty freely. The rate of lung ventilation should be faster than the normal respiratory rate of the animal and the chest wall movement produced should be more obvious than in normal breathing. During thoracotomy, expansion of the lung beyond the limits of the wound indicates that excessive inflation on the lungs is being produced. Simple observations such as these ensure that ventilation is being carried out in a manner which will result in no harm to the animal.

The end tidal concentration of carbon dioxide may be monitored continuously by a rapid infrared analyser and, once the endtidal to arterial tension difference has been derived from blood gas analysis, the ventilation may be adjusted to yield a normal $PaCO_2$, although it is important to note that the end-tidal to arterial carbon dioxide gradient may change during the course of anaesthesia. In practice, facilities for rapid gas and blood analysis are limited by financial and other constraints and it is usually necessary to perform IPPV without such assistance.

For small animal patients, where non-rebreathing systems can be employed, it is relatively easy to ensure the maintenance of satisfactory blood gas tension by hyperventilating with a gas mixture containing 4% carbon dioxide and at least 30% oxygen. Using such a gas mixture in this way it is only necessary to ensure that large tidal and minute volumes are being imposed and this can be done from observation of the frequency of lung inflation and the amplitude of the chest wall excursions. In large animals, where for reasons of economy in the use of gases it is essential to employ rebreathing systems, it is much less easy to ensure satisfactory blood gas levels and, in the absence of monitoring facilities, the anaesthetist has to rely on experience and aim to err, if at all, on the side of providing a degree of hyperventilation. In general, it is better to ventilate at slower rates with large tidal volumes than to achieve the same minute volumes by faster rates and smaller tidal volumes.

Return of Spontaneous Breathing

It is important to note that while in most animals apnoea may be established with the aid of relaxant drugs, in all cases at the end of operation, apnoea should be mainly due to reflex inhibition of respiration by the rhythmical slight overinflation of the lungs and, possibly, hypocapnia. Thus, prompt resumption of spontaneous breathing usually follows if:

1. The rhythm of lung inflation is broken.
2. Some accumulation of carbon dioxide is allowed by either removing the soda lime canister or, in non-rebreathing systems, adding more carbon dioxide to the inspired gases.

Residual neuromuscular block should be counteracted where appropriate by the intravenous administration of anticholinergic and anticholinesterase drugs. This should be done before any carbon dioxide accumulation is encouraged because anticholinesterases appear to be less likely to produce cardiac irregularities when the arterial carbon dioxide tension is low. When inhalation anaesthetics have been used the anaesthetic mixture should be diluted with oxygen. Provided only minimal central depression by anaesthetic agents is present animals will resume spontaneous breathing at very low arterial carbon dioxide tensions and dogs have been observed to start breathing with carbon dioxide tensions as low as 18–20 mmHg (about 2.2 kPa).

VENTILATORS

1. The inspiratory phase.
2. The changeover from the inspiratory to the expiratory phase.
3. The expiratory phase.
4. The changeover from the expiratory to the inspiratory phase.

Very briefly the inspiratory phase can be provided by either flow generators or pressure generators. With flow generators the tidal volume delivered is independent of factors outside the ventilator, if, for example, the patient's airway resistance rises then the inflation pressure increases. The flow is not necessarily constant and can be generated by a bellows compressed by a cam mechanism or by pneumatic compression of the anaesthetic reservoir bag situated in a bottle. Pressure generators maintain a constant pressure during the inspiratory phase of the respiratory cycle, often by a weight acting on a concertina bag[2] (as in the Manley ventilator). The volume delivered by a pressure ventilator will depend on such factors as the airway resistance (Fig. 16.2).

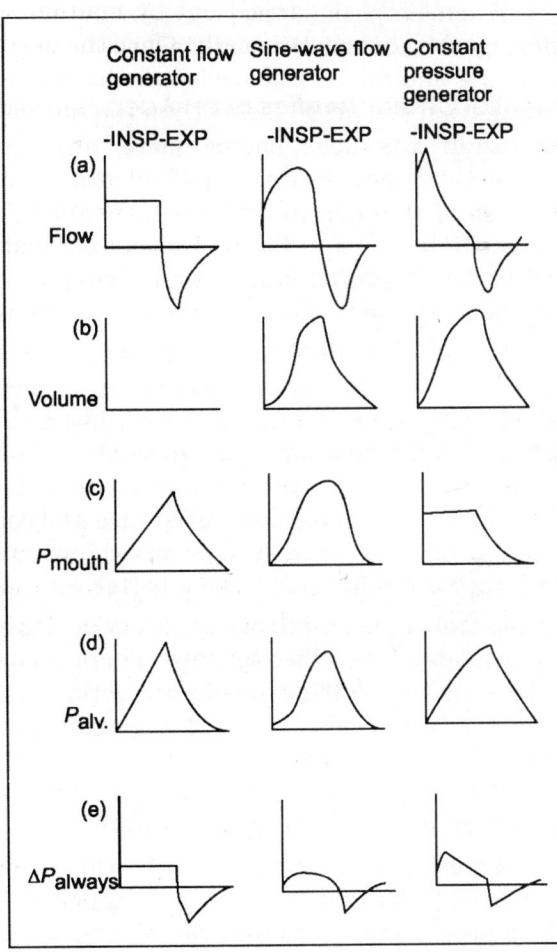

Fig. 16.2: Characteristics of three types of lung ventilator, a. Flow pattern, b. volume change in the lung, c. pressure change at the mouth, d. pressure changes in the alveoli, e. pressure gradient across the airway. Physiology of the Lungs by W. W. Mushin, el at., Blackwell Scientific, Oxford, 1976

Changeover from inspiration to expiration, i.e. the manner in which the ventilator cycles, may be:

1. Time cycled, in which inspiration is terminated after and preset time.
2. Volume cycled, where inspiration is terminated after a preset volume has been delivered.
3. Pressure cycled, in which case inspiration ceases once a preset pressure is reached.

In the expiratory phase a machine may act as a flow generator (e.g. an injector) or a pressure generator and the commonest arrangement is to expose the patient's airway to atmospheric pressure. The changeover from the expiatory to the inspiratory phase may be time cycled patient triggered. In the patient-triggered ventilator a slight inspiratory effort by the patient triggers the changeover to the inspiratory phase.

Essential Characteristics of an Adequate Ventilator

For use in cats, dogs, sheep, goats, small calves and small pigs, a ventilator needs to provide tidal volumes up to 1000 ml at a cycling rate of from 8 to about 40 cycles/min. The duration of the inspiratory phase should be variable, independent of the other settings and range from about 0.5 to 3 seconds' duration. Whenever possible the expired volume should be monitored since due to leaks the 'stroke volume' of the ventilator may not represent the tidal volume delivered to the animal.

Difficulty is experienced in using most commercially available ventilators in cats and small dogs. The problems seem to be similar to those encountered in infants and small babies, with high respiratory rates, low tidal volumes and, possibly (although in small animals no information appears to be available), high airway resistance. Adaptation of adult ventilators for infants and small babies has been accomplished by employing a controlled leak or a parallel resistance and compliance used in conjunction with an Ayre's T-piece. However, such systems are complicated and a ventilator designed specifically for the purpose would seem to be a better solution to the problem.

Control of the length of expiratory period should, like that of the inspiratory period, be independent of the other settings. There is no need to adjust all the controls of a ventilator when only one setting needs correction. It should be possible to obtain inspiratory: expiratory ratios of at least 1:3, the expiratory period beginning immediately the desired tidal volume has been delivered to the lungs. Resistance to expiration should be low although, as already mentioned, in certain circumstances it may be to an animal's advantage if the expiratory resistance can be increased.

A high peak gas flow rate during the inspiratory phase is always desirable if the lungs are to be inflated in a short inspiratory period. It is comparatively easy to adapt a ventilator which gives a high peak flow rate to give a lower flow, but it is impossible to obtain a high peak flow rate from a machine which is not designed to achieve this.

It is essential that provision is made for change to manual squeezing of a reservoir bag should any mechanical fault develop during the course of an operation. Secondly, if electrically driven, the machine must be electrically safe and explosion proof. Possibly less important, the machinery should not be noisy and if free standing it should occupy the minimum of floor space. In practice, the choice of ventilator is largely one of personal preference, convenience of operation for the particular circumstances in which it is to be used and the financial resources available.

Ventilators designed for use in man have given very satisfactory results when used on smaller animals and there is probably no need to develop special machines except, as already mentioned, for cats and very small dogs. Among the very many commercially available machines which have performed consistently are the Bird, the Manley and the Flowmaster. The three small, inexpensive ventilators (Minivent, Automatic Vent, and Microvent) are suitable for small animal practice whenever supplies of compressed air or oxygen are available. They are small, simple ventilators which fit onto any continuous flow apparatus and act as minute volume dividers. The distended reservoir bag provides the driving force of inspiration and the compliance of this bag must be low if they are to operate correctly; bags made of neoprene are much less satisfactory than those made from natural rubber.

The basic clinical criteria for ventilators for adult horses, cattle and large pigs are similar to those for the other animals described above. A useful ventilator has a tidal volume of between 2 and 20 litres with a cycling rate of between 4 and 15 cycles/min and an inspiratory phase of 2–3 seconds. It should be capable of sustaining pressures of up to 60 cm H_2O (6 kPa) in the upper airway during inspiration while the inspiratory: expiratory ratio should be at least 1:2.

Special machines have had to be developed for use with large animals and, until recently, most workers used machines constructed to their own specifications. Ventilators for adult horses and cattle have been available from commercial sources for only a very few years and proper data on their performance is scarce.

References

1. Kumar P., *Textbook of Anaesthesiology,* 1st ed., Paras Med. Publishers, Hyderabad, 2008.
2. Mashin W.W., *Physiology of the Lungs,* 1st ed., Blackwell Scientific, Oxford, 1976.
3. Kumar P., Equipment and Drugs in Anaesthesia, 1st ed., CBS Publishers, New Delhi, 2009.

17

Monitoring

CLINICAL ASSESSMENT

1. *The pulse volume* reflects cardiac output; urine output parallels visceral perfusion; skin temperature indicates peripheral resistance. If, in addition, central venous pressure is monitored, the adequacy of the circulatory volume' can be demonstrated. Pulse volume and skin temperature may be assessed by palpation; measurement of urinary output requires only the timed collection of urine voided or obtained by catheterization of the urinary bladder; measurement of the central venous pressure has been greatly simplified by the introduction of disposable, sterile packs prepared for transfusions.[1] All these procedures can be carried out on the conscious animal prior to anaesthesia; their value during operation and in the immediate postoperative period cannot be overestimated, and all are well within the capability of veterinarians working with the minimum of assistance outside of large hospitals.

2. The direct determination of arterial blood pressure cannot always be carried out on conscious animals but is reasonably easy when they are unconscious or anaesthetized. Indirect measurement, using a cuff and flow detector (Fig. 17.1), is nearly always possible in conscious animals.

3. The sound from the simple bell stethoscope placed over the region of the apex beat of the heart may be amplified by suitable electronic means to give a signal audible throughout a room, but most useful for monitoring during anaesthesia is the oesophageal stethoscope, where the sounds can be heard only by the anaesthetist. This instrument consists of a blinder led, plastic or rubber tube with side holes over an area 1–3 cm from the blind end (Fig. 17.2) covered by a thin rubber or plastic sleeve to prevent fluid from entering the tube. The instrument is passed into the oesophagus of the anaesthetized animal until the blind end lies over the heart and the open end is attached either to an ordinary stethoscope headpiece, or to a single earpiece which can be worn continuously by the

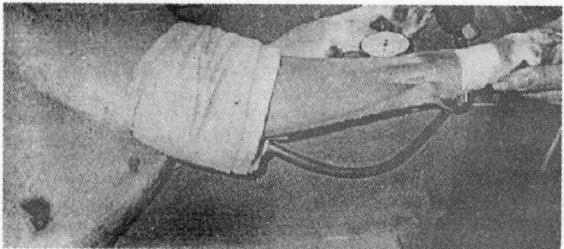

Fig. 17.1: Indirect measurement of the arterial blood pressure using an inflatable cuff and a flow detector

anaesthetist. Oesophageal stetho-
scopes suitable for dogs and cats are
commercially available and ones for
large animals can be constructed from
stomach tubes. It might well be
claimed that the instrument provides
one of the simplest, most inexpensive
yet effective monitors of the heart
beat and respiration. There are some
situations in which it is safer to use
an oesophageal stethoscope rather
than a vast array of more complicated devices but, unfortunately, the prolonged use of a binaural stethoscope
is uncomfortable and repeated use of
a monaural moulded earpiece may
lead to the anaesthetist developing
otitis external.

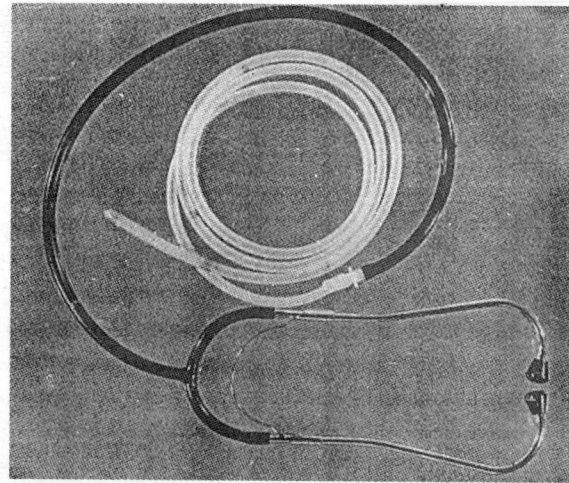

Fig. 17.2: The oesophageal stethoscope. It may be used with a single earpiece or with a conventional stethoscope headpiece

4. Determination of the central venous pressure can be made quite rapidly but the circumstances of anaesthesia can profoundly affect it. If it is allowed to rise unduly, the difficulty of certain operations can be greatly increased. It rises in the presence of respiratory obstruction or raised mean intrathoracic pressure, and a close correlation between the central venous pressure and the degree of bleeding at the site of operation is easily demonstrable.

While such observations are simple to make, their interpretation may not be so easy. Palpation of the pulse allows knowledge of its rate, rhythm and volume as well as giving an indication of cardiac output and of the adequacy of the circulation to the region of the body where the pulse is being monitored. Difficulty in feeling the pulse in a major artery suggests severe vasoconstriction and/or hypotension.

In normal subjects standing quietly the central venous pressure varies from animal to animal and, at the moment, the variations of normal resting central venous pressure seem to be as inexplicable as the normal variations of normal resting arterial pressure. In the dog and cat the value is relatively constant between 3 and 7.5 cmH$_2$O (0.3 and 0.75), no matter what the position of the animal's body; but in normal horses in lateral recumbency it is usually recorded as being between 25 and 35 cm H$_2$O (2.5 and 3.5 kPa), whilst in dorsal recumbency the reading may fall below the reference level. A single central venous pressure reading may indicate that all is not well but it is the change in pressure during the intravenous administration of fluid which is most informative. When the administration of fluid improves the animal's condition (improved pulse volume, increase in skin temperature and urine production), therapy should be continued until the central venous pressure remains steady in the normal range. Excessive administration of fluid with overloading of the heart is extremely unlikely to occur if the central venous pressure is not allowed to exceed the upper limit of normality. If the apparent beneficial effects of fluid administration are short lived and the central venous pressure falls quickly after an initial rise, it is likely that the blood is pooling in dilated peripheral vessels, i.e. the abnormality present is an increase in the vascular bed, and more fluids should be given. If an infusion or transfusion increases the central venous pressure without improving the animal's condition, then the cardiac pump mechanism is at fault.

5. The colour of the mucous membranes can be a very deceptive guide to the state of the patient, for while pink membranes suggest adequate oxygenation of the blood, a brighter pink or red colour may indicate hypercapnia. White coloration may be due to anaemia, peripheral vasoconstriction, or lack of circulating fluid. Cyanosis can only be seen where there is adequate blood flow to carry the deoxygenated haemoglobin to the mucous membranes and, in practice, except when α_2-adrenoceptor agonists are used, is it rarely observed during anaesthesia unless there is a marked oxygen lack due to severe lung disease or failure of the oxygen supply to the breathing circuit. The more usual causes of inadequate oxygenation such as respiratory obstruction, or respiratory depression induced by overdose of anaesthetic drugs, often result in concurrent circulatory failure so that the mucous membranes appear white. Abnormal coloration of the mucous membranes is also seen in dehydrated animals, in animals with a raised venous pressure and from the presence of fetal haemoglobin in young animals.

6. *Respiratory:* Efficiency is particularly difficult to judge from clinical observation. Chest movement indicates the rate of breathing but gives no indication of tidal volume and, in fact, where severe respiratory obstruction exists the patient may make violent respiratory efforts which result in no movement of air into and out of the lungs. With anaesthetic breathing circuits that include a reservoir bag the volume change in the bag produced by the respiratory efforts of the patient is a good guide to tidal volume but where a reservoir bag is not included it is almost impossible to be certain that tidal volume is adequate.

7. Colour of the mucous membranes may give a guide to the respiratory efficiency but, as already mentioned, the various factors influencing this colour often makes it difficult.

Assessment of the depth of unconsciousness is based mainly on reflex suppression, both somatic and autonomic, and the reflex suppression which occurs at different depths is discussed in another chapter, but this does not form more than a rough guide. Variations occur depending on the species of animal concerned and the drugs used, while it must also be remembered that the level of unconsciousness depends not only on the amount of drugs administered but also on the level of stimulation at the moment when the observation is made. Evoked reflex responses may be difficult to elicit because of lack of ready access to the patient, and may be modified by drugs (e.g. analgesics) which have been administered. Even the respiratory response to painful stimulation applied to the body may be difficult to assess and, while during general anaesthesia increasing depth of central nervous depression usually results in a decreased respiratory minute volume, this is often due to a decreased tidal volume and the rate may be increased or decreased. Hypercapnia, whether due to faulty equipment or respiratory depression from overdose of anaesthetic agent, causes increased muscle tone and may even result in muscular twitches which can lead to the erroneous assumption that the depth of anaesthesia is insufficient. When neuromuscular blocking agents are used, all reflexes involving somatic muscle are abolished and judgement of the depth of unconsciousness becomes more difficult still.

METHODS OF ELECTRONIC SURVEILLANCE

Heart Rate Monitors

It works by detection of the electrical signal of the electrocardiogram (ECG), the signal being processed in various ways, to give a digital readout of heart rate, an audible signal ('bleep') and/or a flash of light with each heart beat, or to sound a warning alarm when the heart rate ceases to lie within certain preset limits. At least one monitor allows the actual form of the ECG to be displayed, thus enabling abnormalities of rhythm as well as of rate to be observed. Although potentially useful, all such monitors suffer from various disadvantages in clinical use. The greatest problem encountered is that of electrical noise, for whilst this is easily identified when the signal is displayed on an oscilloscope or on a written trace, rate meters tend to incorporate it with the signal and give a false reading. In addition, unless the electrodes are correctly placed, some counters may be triggered by both the R and T waves of the electrocardiogram and display double the true heart rate. For their proper use there must be good contact between the leads and patient, and this is not always easy to maintain throughout surgery. Some instruments are incapable of handling the wide range of heart rates encountered in veterinary practice; instruments designed for use in man and small animals may 'double count' when receiving the greater amplitude signal from the hearts of large animals. All these problems are well recognized and newer instruments are often claimed to incorporate features to overcome them but in practice not all such claims are justified.

The most serious disadvantage associated with the use of heart rate monitors is that their use may engender a false sense of security in the surgical team. Derivation from the ECG means they only indicate a measure of electrical activity in the heart and the presence of such activity certainly does not guarantee that the heart is functioning adequately as a pump.

Electrocardiography

For monitoring purposes, display of the electrocardiograph signal, the ECG, on an oscilloscope screen is preferable to a pen write-out, for the pen may be damaged by interference from the high frequencies of surgical diathermy and the continuous consumption of recording paper is expensive.[2] Versatile machines are available in which an oscilloscope is provided for monitoring purposes, but a pen recorder is available if the record is needed for diagnostic inspection of any abnormality seen in the oscilloscope display (Fig. 17.3).

For monitoring during anaesthesia it is quite unnecessary to use the standard Eindhoven limb leads in which the right hind-leg lead is earthed. For safety when other electrical apparatus is connected to the patient, modern ECG machines do not require the patient to be earthed, so that all that is required is two leads spanning the heart and in positions where they do not interfere with the operation site. In the dog and cat the maximal signal is obtained if the 'right-arm' lead is placed on the brisket and the 'left-arm lead' between the xiphisternum and the umbilicus. In horses and ruminants leads placed as in dogs and cats give an inverted appearance to the ECG complex. Thus, to obtain a 'normal' ECG tracing it is necessary to reverse the lead positions. The difference between the lead positions needed in different species of animal is most significant if a heart rate monitor which counts deflections is included because if the deflection is in the reverse direction to 'normal' the machine may ignore it.

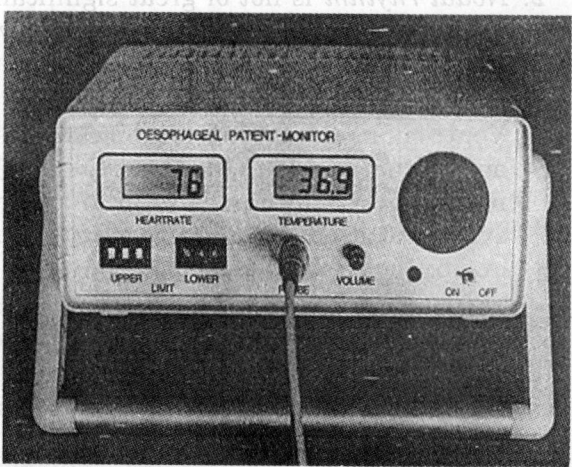

Fig. 17.3: The Aacomonitor monitors core body temperature, heart sound, respiratory sounds and cardiac frequency from one oesphageal probe. A standard ECG monitor can be connected to the rear panel

The majority of avoidable 50 Hz electrical interference results from poor electrode contact with the patient. For monitoring purposes, needle electrodes may be inserted sub-cutaneously or intramuscularly; equally satisfactory is the use of crocodile clips with electrode jelly to ensure good contact with the skin. This jelly may need to be renewed during the course of a long operation. Many substances, including surgical spirit, have been recommended as alternatives to electrode jelly, but most dry or evaporate too rapidly to be useful for long-term monitoring.

Ideally, electrodes should be silver plated to eliminate polarization and electrochemical currents, but stainless steel is an acceptable although imperfect alternative. Artifacts in the ECG occur through movement of the leads by the patient or by the surgeon and with heart movement due to respiration. Although many modern electrocardiographs are reputed not to be affected by diathermy, with most instruments the ECG is completely obliterated when this surgical apparatus is in use. Other electrical equipment or mains power lines in close proximity to the patient may also be sources of interference. The value of the information obtained from the ECG increases with the anaesthetist's ability to interpret the tracing obtained. Changes in rate and rhythm of the heart are most easily recognized.

1. *Sinus tachycardia* is frequently encountered during anaesthesia and is usually observed after the administration of atropine. An increase in heart rate may also result from surgical stimulation in an inadequately anaesthetized animal, or from sympathoadrenal stimulation due to carbon dioxide retention. Sinus bradycardia is a normal consequence of some types of anaesthesia, but extreme bradycardia which cannot be overcome by the administration of atropine is usually only seen just before death.

2. *Nodal rhythm* is not of great significance and atrioventricular block is uncommon during anaesthesia. Ventricular extrasystoles, on the other hand, are common. They may be isolated or occur alternately with sinus beats as in bigeminal rhythm; they may be unifocal or multifocal in origin.

3. Ventricular extrasystoles are seen most commonly in animals anaesthetized with agents that sensitize the heart to the effects of adrenaline, which may be exogenous in origin (e.g. injected with local analgesic solutions), or endogenous due to reflex sympathoadrenal activity. Sympathoadrenal stimulation occurs during hypercapnia and hypoxia and thus is usually due to respiratory inadequacy.

Frequently in dogs the pulse and heart rates may differ considerably. If an extrasystole occurs during a period when the heart is empty (ventricular bigeminy — ventricular premature depolarization coupled to the preceding sinus beat), no peripheral pulse will be produced. Thus, the heart rate is twice that of the pulse and this will not be diagnosed by palpation of the peripheral pulse. Single extrasystoles are of no significance, and bigeminy is only important in that it may precede more serious events. Ventricular tachycardia is usually considered to be the immediate precursor of ventricular fibrillation and its occurrence must be regarded as a serious portent. Because these changes frequently result from sympathetic activity on the sensitized myocardium, they often disappear if the depth of anaesthesia is reduced and adequate alveolar ventilation restored.

4. Changes in amplitude of the ECG are more difficult to interpret, as they may be significant or simply due to changing electrical conditions such as an alteration in the impedance of the skin-electrode contact. However, the anaesthetist should note that whilst S-T segment depression or elevation is considered by some to be normal in dogs, changes of more than a few millimetres are indicative of myocardial hypoxia and must not, therefore, be ignored. Changes in the amplitude in certain components of the ECG trace may be due to changes in blood electrolyte levels (especially of potassium) but considerable experience is required before interpretation of these changes can be made easily.

5. Asystole and ventricular fibrillation indicate extreme myocardial changes "rendering the heart incapable of acting as a pump. On occasion, QRS deflections, which may appear to be almost normal, are recorded from animals long after the onset of circulatory arrest. These terminal signs of electrical activity are not associated with mechanical activity (Fig. 17.4).

Pulse Monitors

An efficient monitor of a peripheral pulse would be invaluable to the anaesthetist as it would demonstrate the presence of a peripheral circulation and, if capable of measuring pulse volume, would also give some guide as to the cardiac output. Unfortunately, as yet, no such perfect monitor exists and there is no adequate substitute for the anaesthetist's finger on the pulse. It is, however, difficult to palpate the pulse continuously for long periods. Pulse monitors involving carbon microphone detectors were tested in dogs but artifacts, particularly those due to movement of the limbs, caused problems. Ultrasonic monitors based on detection of blood flow by the Doppler-shift principle are now being successfully used in animals. The flow detector consists of two crystals. One sends a beam of ultrasound energy into the skin through an aqueous gel applied to the skin. The other crystal receives the reflected waves from underlying tissue and the moving red blood cells (Fig.17.4). Since the underlying tissue is stationary, the frequency of the reflected waves is exactly the same as the frequency of the transmitted waves. However, the reflected waves from anything in motion, in this situation the red blood cells, are of a different frequency, due to the Doppler effect. The frequency difference is made audible by the monitor and the sound heard is the frequency difference between the transmitted and reflected sound waves. Because the red blood cells are moving at different (random) velocities, the sound is not a pure one but is best described as a hissing noise, the pitch being proportional to the velocity of the moving blood. The Doppler probe is fixed to the tail or to a limb (usually after clipping of the hair) over a palpable pulse, with an air-free coupling medium between it and the skin, and its position optimized to give the loudest blood flow signal, a pulsing, hissing noise. The transducer is taped in place, remembering that the sound beam is only about 1 cm wide and loose skin can shift it off the artery. These ultrasonic flow detectors do not suffer from problems due to movement of the extremity to which they are attached; they will detect blood flow when the arterial pressure is as low as 40 mm Hg (5.3 kPa) and the vessel constricted. All pulse monitors, including even the anaesthetist's finger, fail to detect the pulse when the arterial blood pressure falls below a certain level.

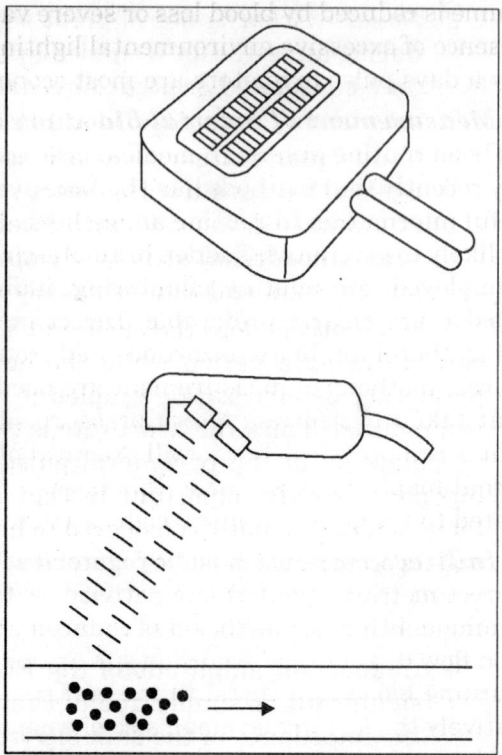

Fig. 17.4: Doppler-shift pulse detector. One piezoelectric crystal emits incident ultrasound signal whilst the other receives the reflected signal from the moving blood cells. The frequency shift between the incident and reflected sound is used to measure the velocity of the blood flow in the vessel. This is the best flow detector for the indirect measurement of arterial blood pressure (Parks Electronics, Oregon, USA)

Pulse Oximetry

The recent development of pulse oximeters, which both monitor the pulse rate and provide a continuous measurement of arterial oxygen saturation, represents a tremendous advance in monitoring. These devices may be placed on an animal's tongue or nasal septum and differ from all previous oximeters in that they are able to eliminate the background absorption attributable to tissue by measuring the light absorption at two different wavelengths at frequent intervals during each pulse. It is thus possible to derive an absolute measure of oxygen saturation of the arterial blood without precalibration. They are very sensitive to movement artifacts and may give inaccurate oxygen saturation readings when the pulse volume is reduced by blood loss or severe vasoconstriction. They may also be affected by the presence of excessive environmental lighting, bilirubinaemia or marked venous pulsations, now a days pulse oximeters are most economic monitors available.

Measurement of arterial blood pressure: Measurement of arterial blood pressure has been routine in human medical practice for many years but in veterinary practice it is only recently that methods have become available for its easy determination. It can provide useful information in routine anaesthesia and is mandatory in surgical procedures which are likely to precipitate sudden dramatic changes in pressure, or when induced hypotension is employed. For routine monitoring, indirect methods of measurement which are non-invasive are clearly preferable. Direct measurement requires cannulation of an artery and is, therefore, more hazardous and troublesome in clinical practice. Whether direct or indirect methods of measurement are used, the value obtained depends on the reference point taken to represent zero pressure. Probably the best reference point is the mean right atrial pressure, but for all practical purposes the most appropriate appears to be the sternal manubrium, because this is easily located and seems to be relatively constantly related to the position of the right atrium in most animals, irrespective of body position.

Indirect measurement of arterial blood pressure (sphygmomanometry): All indirect methods of measuring arterial blood pressure are modifications of the Riva-Rocci technique, involving occlusion of an artery by an inflatable cuff and detection of returning blood flow distal to the occlusion site as the pressure in the cuff is reduced. The detection of returning blood flow distal to the cuff presents especial difficulties in animals due to the relatively thick skin and small size of easily accessible arteries. The auscultatory technique of sphygmomanometry is the most widely used method of indirect measurement in man and determines both systolic and diastolic pressures. A stethoscope is placed over a limb artery distal to the occluding cuff which encircles the limb. The cuff is inflated to a pressure greater than the systolic pressure and then slowly deflated. When the first Korotkoff sound is heard through the stethoscope the cuff pressure is assumed to equal the systolic blood pressure and when the Korotkoff sounds either become muffled or disappear the cuff pressure is taken to be equal to the diastolic pressure. The detection of the Korotkoff sounds in animals is eased by the use of microphone detectors, but today in veterinary practice the ultrasonic Doppler technique for the demonstration of blood flow in the artery is usually employed, thus avoiding all difficulties in sound detection. The cuff pressure at which the first, tapping, audible sound is produced is taken as the systolic pressure and the pressure at which the sound first becomes a continuous hissing noise is related to the diastolic pressure. Determination of the systolic pressure is relatively easy and reproducible from one observer to another but the diastolic point is very observer subjective.

Both the length and width of the inflatable bladder in the occluding cuff are critical for accurate measurement of blood pressure. The optimum size of cuff for each species of animal remains controversial, although it has been suggested that a bladder which fully encircles the extremity compensates for any disproportion between bladder width and extremity circumference. The effect of varying the cuff width can be explained on the basis of efficiency of the transmission of the cuff pressure to the artery and the resistance which the cuff offers to the pulse travelling underneath it. Pressure is transmitted more efficiently as the cuff width is increased but after an optimum width is reached the frictional resistance offered to blood flow reduces the energy of the pulse and the occluding pressure has to be lowered excessively to allow blood flow through the compressed segment of artery and the pulse to become detectable in the distal region of the extremity. Combination of these two factors means that when the cuff width is below optimum for a given animal, readings will be erroneously high, and when the cuff width is too great the readings will be below the true value.

Horses: Auscultation of the Korotkoff sounds has been used in horses, the occluding cuff being placed above the hock of the anaesthetized animal or on the tail. For accuracy the cuff should be at the same level as the heart, which is not possible in conscious animals. The method may be made more sensitive if the Korotkoff sounds are amplified and displayed on a printer or oscilloscope from a microphone mounted inside the occluding *cuff.* This oscillation technique is combined with an instrument which automatically provides a digital readout of the pressure at the point of maximum pressure oscillation in the 'Dinamap Although continuous readings cannot be obtained, with practice the systolic pressure can easily be measured with accuracy every 30–60 seconds.

Cattle: Indirect blood pressure measurements are seldom made in cattle but they can be obtained from the coccygeal artery by very similar ways to those used in horses. In general, the tail circumference is less than in a horse of comparable weight so that a narrower occluding cuff is adequate and because the middle coccygeal artery is protected to some extent by the ventral spinous processes the cuff needs to be applied in an intervertebral region in order to ensure compression of the artery.

Sheep and goats: In sheep and goats the occluding cuff may be placed above the elbow and an ultrasonic Doppler-shift flow detector just below the carpus or, alternatively, the occluding cuff may be sited around the tibia just proximal to the hock joint and the flow detector over the perforating metarsal artery.

Pigs: For experimental purposes the occluding cuff may be wrapped around the limb above the elbow and the pulse detected on the medial aspect of the limb just above the first phalanx. If the head end of the animal is not accessible to the anaesthetist the cuff may be applied just above the hock and the sensor over the anterior metatarsal artery.

Dogs: The development of the ultrasonic Doppler-shift pulse detector has enabled systolic blood pressure readings, sufficiently accurate for all clinical purposes, to be readily made in all dogs by the use of an inflatable occluding cuff and associated pressure manometer. A 2.5 cm wide cuff is used for dogs up to about 15 kg bodyweight, and one 3.75 cm wide for those above this weight, but it is essential that the cuff is always long enough to completely encircle the limb and so they need to be 20–25 cm in length. For the best correlation with directly measured arterial pressures the cuff should be placed around the median artery above the elbow and it is usually convenient to site the detector over the subcarpal arch just below the stopper pad. It is most important to ensure an air-free contact between the detector and skin by clipping the hair and using adequate amounts of coupling gel while the detector is moved around to establish the clearest possible signal.

Direct measurement of arterial blood pressure: The mean arterial pressure can be measured with simple in-expensive apparatus but for accurate determination of the systolic and diastolic pressures more expensive pressure transducers and electronic amplifiers are necessary. Although direct measurement is invasive, it provides continuous monitoring for use in routine surgery, during the immediate postoperative period and for research purposes. It may be used in any animal where a suitable superficial artery is available for cannuation (Fig. 17.5).

Cannulation is most simply performed percutaneously and stringent aseptic precautions must be observed. After cleansing of the skin and, if the animal is conscious, following local infiltration analgesia of the site, a small nick with a pointed scalpel blade is made in the skin just over the proposed site of arterial puncture (Fig. 17.6). A plastic over-the-needle type of catheter is introduced through the nick in the skin into the lumen of the artery. As soon as the catheter enters the arterial lumen the needle is partially withdrawn and the catheter introduced fully into the vessel. Next, after complete withdrawal of the needle part, a sterile stopcock is attached to the hub of the catheter and the system flushed with previously prepared heparinsaline solution (2 units/ml). The catheter is fixed in position by suturing it to the skin. Loss of blood during the withdrawal of the needle part can usually be prevented by applying pressure over the artery proximal to the tip of the catheter until the stopcock is secured.

Haematoma formation following withdrawal of the catheter, but this can be minimized by applying firm digital pressure to the puncture site for 3 minutes (by the clock) after removal of the catheter.

The apparatus for measuring the mean arterial blood pressure is shown in Fig. 17.7. A number of variations are possible but the basic pattern is as shown. A standard type of anaeroid manometer has connected to it a 6 or 8 cm length of plastic drip tubing ending in a male Luer connection. This assembly

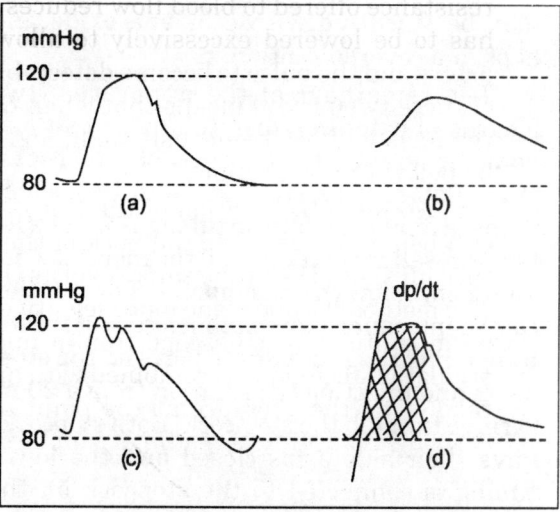

Fig. 17.5: Waveforms from direct measurement of the arterial pressure: (a), good trace; (b), recording of the same pressures but with excessive damping, systolic pressure low, diastolic pressure high, mean arterial pressure unchanged; (c), recording of same pressures but with resonance, systolic pressure apparently increased while diastolic pressure reduced, mean pressure unchanged; (d), illustration of how left ventricular contractility may be estimated from the rate of rise of pressure during early systole (dP/dt) while the shaded area gives an index of stroke volume

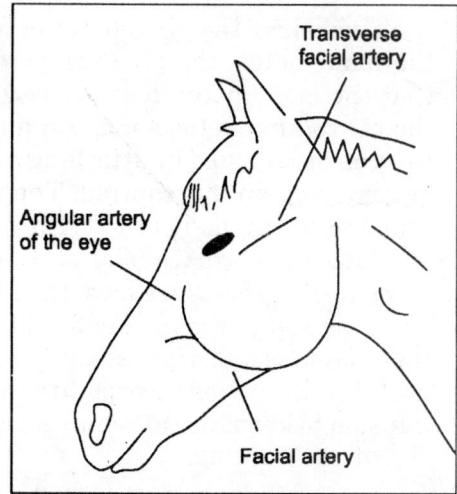

Fig. 17.6: Sites for arterial puncture or catheterization about the horse's head

may be sterilized with ethylene oxide and kept in a covered container.

The remainder of the apparatus (two lengths of extension drip tubing or two manometer lines and two disposable stopcocks) is available as presterilized and disposable items. After assembly the tubing is filled with heparin-saline solution until the meniscus lies 10–12 cm below the manometer. The solution can be introduced into both lengths of tubing by opening the appropriate ports on the stopcocks and injecting the solution from a 20 ml syringe through the stop-cock. Both stopcocks have their side arms closed and the lower tubing is connected to the stopcock on the arterial catheter. This stopcock is opened and pressure readings should be obtained. There is an initial flow of blood into the lower tube as the air in the upper tube and manometer is compressed. This blood is flushed back into the animal by injection of heparin-saline solution through the middle stopcock. After this, flushing is only needed at infrequent intervals. The stopcock on the arterial catheter can be used for obtaining arterial blood

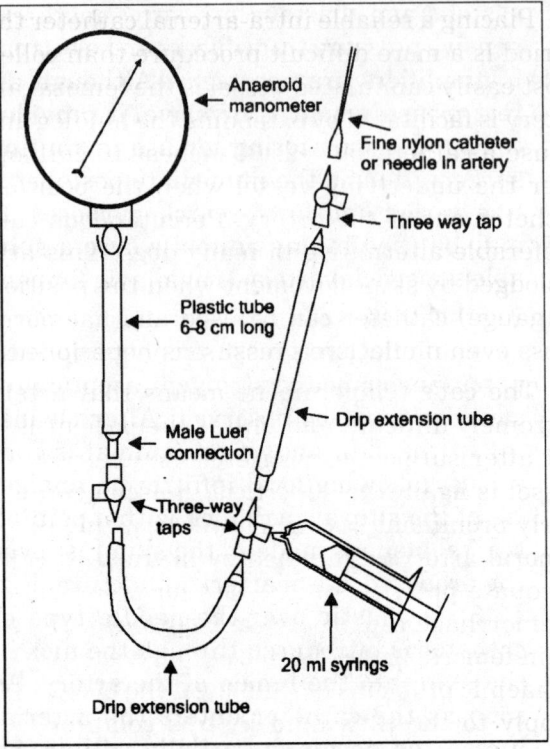

Fig. 17.7: Direct measurement of mean arterial blood pressure

samples and adds greatly to the convenience of setting up the apparatus and during transport of the animal from place to place.

The longer the air column between the meniscus of the heparin-saline solution and the manometer, the greater the damping, but care should always be taken to ensure that the manometer does not become contaminated by heparin-saline solution because the air column is too short. An air column of about 8 cm seems to be the optimum, and this can be adjusted by attaching a syringe full of air to the upper stopcock and introducing or removing air as required. The manometer must be attached to a suitable support so that the meniscus is at heart level. The air column can be replaced by a commercially available pressure transfer unit, in which a latex diaphragm inside a saline-filled barrel transmits the pressure from the saline column to the anaeroid manometer with minimal damping and prevents any fluid from entering the manometer. The reduced damping in the system is a distinct advantage when the pressures to be measured are low. Another useful modification incorporates a continuous infusion valve which regulates a pressure infusion to keep the catheter flushed continuously with heparin-saline solution to prevent clots from forming.

A pressure transducer may be used instead of the anaeroid manometer so that systolic and diastolic pressures may be determined. The pressure transducer is connected to a recorder and/or an oscilloscope to give a continuous display of the pressure waveform.

Placing a reliable intra-arterial catheter that is to remain in position for a considerable period is a more difficult procedure than collecting an arterial blood sample. In dogs, the most easily cannulated vessel is the femoral artery. Percutaneous puncture of the femoral artery is facilitated by extending the hindleg and rotating it slightly outwards. It is essential to use a catheter at least 4 inches (10 cm) long in dogs otherwise movement of the skin over the underlying vessel when the position of the hind limb is altered will pull the catheter out of the artery. Percutaneous catheterization of the metatarsal artery is a preferable alternative in many dogs. This artery is small but the catheter is less easily dislodged by skin movement when the position of the limb is altered. A small (21 or even 23 gauge) catheter can be used and haemorrhage after its removal does not tend to be gross even if effective pressure is not applied to the puncture site.

The cat's temperament means that arterial cannulation in the conscious animal is extremely difficult, and unless the patient is moribund, this procedure is usually carried out after surgical exposure of the artery under general anaesthesia. The most suitable vessel is again the superficial musculocutaneous branch of the femoral artery, which is fairly prominent in cats. However, owing to its small size it is often missed and the main femoral artery cannulated by mistake. If this happens, care must be taken to maintain adequate pressure on the site for a sufficient time after withdrawal of the catheter, as haemorrhage can otherwise be profuse. The catheter must not be too large nor must the main femoral artery be tied off, for serious ischaemic problems may follow if the blood supply to the cat's hind limb is compromised for any length of time.

In cattle, pressures may be recorded from the middle coccygeal or median auricular arteries. Cannulation of the middle coccygeal artery under caudal epidural block is not difficult in most conscious animals and complications arising after its use are most unlikely to have serious consequences. Cannulation of the median auricular artery with an 18 or 20 gauge indwelling catheter has been recorded in pigs.

Measurement of the Central Venous Pressure

Disposable venous manometer sets are available, but the complete apparatus for the measurement of central venous pressure can be made more cheaply from plastic three-way stopcocks, disposable giving sets and extension tubes (Fig. 17.8). A catheter of sufficient length is introduced

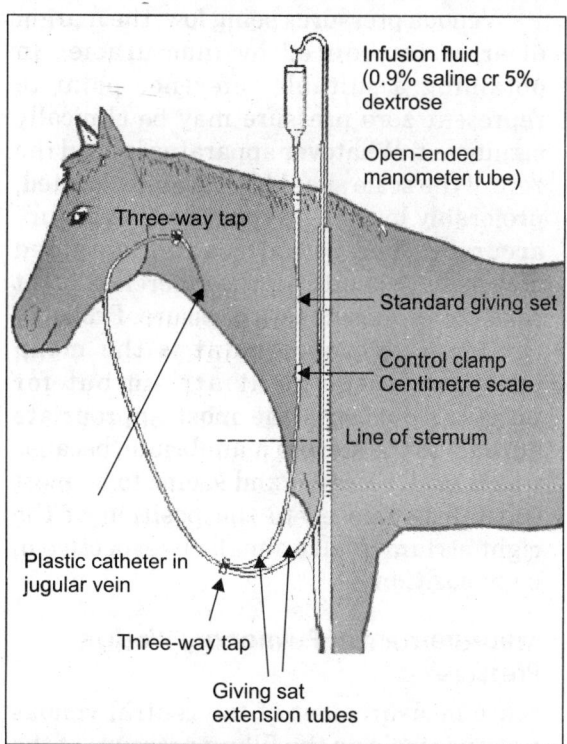

Fig. 17.8: Apparatus for the measurement of central venous pressure

Infusion fluid (0.9% saline cr 5% dextrose

Open-ended manometer tube)

Three-way tap

Standard giving set

Control clamp
Centimetre scale

Line of sternum

Plastic catheter in jugular vein

Three-way tap

Giving sat extension tubes

into the jugular vein and advanced until its tip lies in the anterior vena cava. The distance the catheter tip has to be introduced is, initially, estimated by measurement of length, but once the catheter is connected to the manometer its position may be adjusted until the level of fluid in the manometer tube moves in time with the animal's respiratory movements. In dogs and cats the introduction of a catheter into the jugular vein is often greatly facilitated by laying the animal on its side and extending its head and neck over a pillow or sandbag. If the catheter is to be left in position for a longtime it is kept patent with a drip infusion through a three-way stopcock or the catheter is kept filled with heparinsaline solution (10 units/ml) between measurements. Readings may be taken at any time. If an intravenous drip is used it is turned full on and the stopcock manipulated first to fill the manometer tube from the fluid reservoir and then to connect the manometer tube to the catheter. The fall of fluid in the manometer is observed and should be 'step-like' in response to respiratory pressure changes. The central venous pressure is read off when fluid fall ceases.

The central venous pressure may also be measured in the way previously described for arterial pressure if a suitably sensitive anaeroid manometer is used, but because low pressures are to be measured this system is only satisfactory when the damping is kept to a minimum by the use of commercially available pressure transfer units, e.g. 'Pressurveil'. (Fig. 17.9).

Venous pressures being low, the margin of error introduced by inaccuracies in obtaining a suitable reference point to represent zero pressure may be clinically significant. Whatever apparatus is used the zero of the scale should be carefully located, preferably by using a spirit level to ensure accuracy. The actual reading obtained obviously depends on the reference point taken to represent zero pressure. Probably the ideal reference point is the mean pressure in the right atrium but for practical purposes the most appropriate appears to the sternal manubrium, because this is easily located and seems to be most constantly related to the position of the right atrium in all animals, irrespective of body position.

Measurement of Pulmonary Wedge Pressure

Since measurement of the central venous pressure reflects the filling pressure of the right side of the heart, it is possible that left heart failure could precede that of the

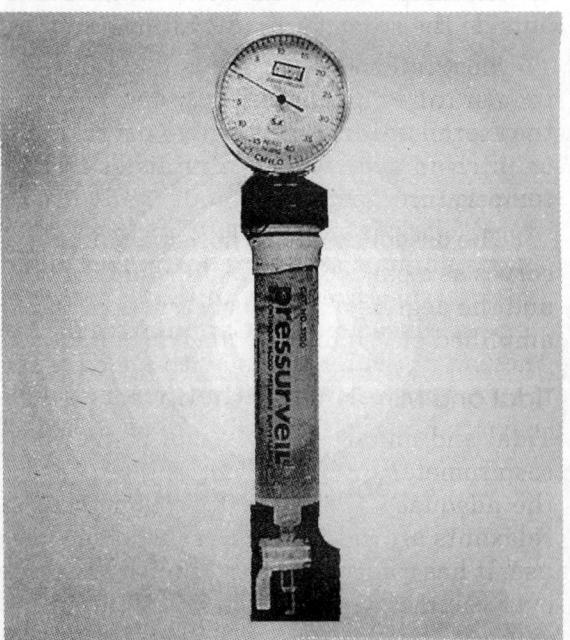

Fig. 17.9: Pressure transfer unit in which a latex diaphragm isolates the anaeroid manometer from the fluid-filled catheter line. These units are presterilized and disposable ('Pressurveil')

right side and precipitate pulmonary oedema without a rise in central venous pressure. For this reason the pulmonary wedge pressure is used as a measure of the left atrial filling pressure.

Soft catheters can easily be floated in the bloodstream from the jugular vein through the right side of the heart into the pulmonary artery and advanced until they wedge; balloon catheters and/or radiological control are not essential. The measurement is made using the same apparatus as is used for the measurement of central venous pressure but care must be taken to ensure that vessel occlusion is not maintained between measurements or pulmonary infarction may occur.

Measurement of Cardiac Output

Dye or thermal dilution are used for accurate measurement of cardiac output but both these methods are invasive. Another method which may be regarded as almost non-invasive and has been used during anaesthesia is aortic velography using an oesophageal ultrasound probe. A probe on which piezoelectric crystals are mounted is introduced into the thoracic oesophagus and rotated until the maximum signal strength is obtained. Its use during clinical canine anaesthesia has also been used in horses. Aortic velography is not claimed to give an accurate measurement of cardiac output but the technique yields a quantitative measurement of blood velocity in the aorta and, with certain assumptions, changes in both cardiac output and the inotropic state of the myocardium can be assessed."

All three methods of measuring cardiac output requires expensive equipment and are outside the scope of routine monitoring during veterinary anaesthesia.

Most rate monitors and apnoea alarms use a thermistor placed in the airway to detect temperature differences between the inspired and exhaled gases. The signal derived from the thermistor is used to drive a digital rate meter, to make a noise which varies in intensity or pitch in time with the animal's breathing, or to sound an alarm if a constant gas temperature is detected.

The oesophageal stethoscope not only enables cardiac action to be monitored but also serves as a particularly useful simple monitor for the presence of respiration, its character and the degree, if any, of obstruction. Its main disadvantage is that unless the sounds are amplified electronically, the freedom of movement of the anaesthetist is restricted.

Tidal and Minute Volume Monitor

Tidal and minute volumes can be measured in small animals by introducing a Wright's respirometer into the breathing circuit. This instrument gives useful information as to the adequacy of tidal volume and readings taken before the administration of muscle relaxants are valuable guides when spontaneous respiration is being restored after their use. It has a dead-space of 25 ml, a low resistance to breathing, and is reasonably accurate over volumes ranging from 4 to 15 l/min. It underreads below 4 l/min and is said to be fail-safe.

For horses and cattle the dry gas meter maybe used to measure tidal and minute volumes but this instrument is unlikely to be available for routine clinical monitoring unless it is built into a circle absorber circuit.

Arterial Blood Gas Tension

The most effective way of monitoring respiratory efficiency is to measure the levels of oxygen and carbon dioxide in the arterial blood and these blood gas measurements also give the anaesthetist valuable information as to the acid-base status of the animal. This information is essential if a veterinary surgeon wishes to perform complicated cardiac surgery, or to operate on very sick patients (e.g. equine 'colic' cases). Unfortunately, the equipment needed for these measurements is expensive.

The blood should be collected in glass syringes, as although disposable plastic syringes may be adequate if analysis is to be carried out immediately, the gas tensions may change if analysis is delayed. The dead-space of the hub of the syringe (and needle, if used) should be filled with heparin solution before collection of the sample and any gas bubbles in the syringe afterwards should be expelled before sealing the hub with a cap.

Capnography

In animals with healthy lungs, the level of carbon dioxide contained in the air which is last expired (endtidal air) approximates to that of the arterial blood. Infrared carbon dioxide analysers can be used to sample gas in the endotracheal tube and give a continuous record of carbon dioxide levels at this site throughout the respiratory cycle. Infrared analysers suffer from having a relatively slow response time so they are not satisfactory when respiratory rates are high. Collision broadening is produced by nitrous oxide but, provided the nitrous oxide concentration remains stable and the instrument is calibrated with mixtures of gases containing nitrous oxide in appropriate concentrations, the carbon dioxide measurement can be relied upon. The loss of the sample volume (which may, with some instruments, be up to 500 ml/min) may seriously affect the dynamics of low-flow circle systems.

Continuous measurement of carbon dioxide concentrations is a useful monitor for pulmonary embolism and may warn of changes in cardiac output. An acute reduction in the end-tidal carbon dioxide concentration occurs when there is a sudden decrease in cardiac output or a large pulmonary embolus of air or blood clot.

Temperature

The standard mercury-in-glass thermometer may be used to obtain a reading of rectal temperature but under anaesthesia the reading obtained from this site is often artificially low because of the presence of faeces and/or ballooning of the rectum precludes good contact with the thermometer. Simple electronic thermometers with thermistor probes are now available for application at various sites in the body. Body core temperature is best measured in the lower oesophagus at heart level because upper oesophageal temperature may be influenced by the temperature of the respired gases. Peripheral body temperature correlated sell with blood lactated levels and cardiac output and may be influenced by the temperature of the respired gases. Peripheral body temperature correlates well with blood lactate levels and cardiac output and may be measured from the skin. The peripheral to core temperature gradient may be a good index of cardiac output and is often claimed to be an invaluable simple measurement of the adequacy of tissue perfusion.

Monitoring Urinary Output

The urinary output depends on the renal blood flow which, in turn, depends on cardiac output and circulating blood volume, and thus it is a relatively sensitive indicator of the circulatory state during anaesthesia and at other times. Catheterization of the urinary bladder is a simple operation in most domestic animals and the urine may be drained into a plastic bag for collection and subsequent measurement. Either self-retaining catheters should be used or, once inserted, the catheter should be fixed in place with a suture or adhesive plaster. In restless animals where continuous draining is difficult, the open end of the indwelling catheter may be clamped, the clamp being released every hour to drain the accumulated urine.

Monitoring Metabolic Changes

Estimation of the acid-base status of the animal provides a useful guide on which further treatment can be based in a rational manner. Venous blood samples suffice for other measurements such as those of serum sodium and potassium concentrations.

In the diabetic patient, blood glucose estimations may be necessary before, during and, perhaps most important, after surgery. Major changes in the level of certain blood electrolytes, in particular sodium, potassium and chloride, may occur in gastrointestinal disturbances, and accurate measurements of these ionic concentrations may be essential if therapy is to be appropriate. Blood urea measurement and liver function tests may be useful prior to anaesthesia in order to enable the fitness of the patient to be assessed.

Monitoring of Neuromuscular Blockade

The mechanical response to nerve stimulation (i.e. muscular contraction) may be observed following the application of supramaximal single, tetanic or 'train-of-four' electrical stimuli to a suitable peripheral motor nerve. During general anaesthesia the response obtained may be influenced by the anaesthetic agents and any neuromuscular blocking drugs which have been used. Observation of the muscle contraction to a tetanic stimulus will give a crude indication of the state of any neuromuscular blockade. The long-lasting block due to a non-depolarizing muscle relaxant is characterized by a non-sustained response (fade) and post-tetanic facilitation. A pure depolarizing block shows no fade or post-tetanic facilitation. The train-of-four technique is useful both experimentally and clinically. Four single 'twitch' stimuli are applied to the nerve at 0.5 second intervals. This rate of stimulation produces a depletion of acetylcholine at the nerve endings during stimulation but, at the same time, the 'tetanus' does not cause post-tetanic facilitation. Comparison between the first and fourth twitch response gives an index of the extent of the neuromuscular blockade. Following non-depolarizing block satisfactory relaxation for abdominal surgery is achieved at 95% suppression, i.e. when the fourth twitch is 25% of the first of the train-of-four.

Expired concentrations of all the halogenated volatile anaesthetics can also be monitored by infrared analysers (e.g. Normac, Datex). One halothane analyser (Narkotest, Drager) which works on the principle of relaxation of silicone rubber bands in the presence of halothane vapour can be used with other volatile agents after appropriate calibration. All the halogenated hydrocarbon anaesthetic vapours can be measured by the Engstrom

Multigas Monitor for Anaesthesia (EMMA) which utilizes a quartz crystal detector. The detector comprises a quartz crystal coated with a layer of silicone oil, whose frequency of oscillation alters as a result of increases in mass of the organic layer in the presence of anaesthetic vapours. The change in oscillation frequency is proportional to the vapour concentration and an electrical signal is generated in such a way that its magnitude is linearly related to the vapour concentration. The instrument is said to have minimal zero drift, sufficient sensitivity and a response which is rapid and accurate enough to permit continuous monitoring.

References

1. Kumar P., *Clincal Methods in Anaesthesia,* 1st ed., National, Mumbai, 2008
2. Kuram P., *Textbook of Anaesthesia,* 1st ed., Paras Med. Publishers, Hyderabad, 2008.

18

Regional Anaesthesia Practice

DIFFERENT METHODS OF PRODUCING LOCAL ANALGESIA

Various methods producing local anaesthesia are as under:

Surface Analgesia

Agents which cause freezing of the superficial layers of the skin are sometimes used for analgesia. Ice is the simplest but, generally, volatile substances which cause freezing by the rapid volatilization from the surface of the skin are used. Ethyl chloride spray, ether spray and carbonic acid snow are examples. Their action is very superficial and transient, and their use is limited to the simplest forms of surgical interference, such as the incision of small superficial abscesses. Used too freely, they may cause considerable necrosis. In man, the thawing out after their use is known to be painful. Decicaine and lignocaine are sometimes incorporated in ointments and applied with friction to the skin. Some slight absorption occurs producing a local numbing which is useful for the relief of pruritis. Aqueous solutions of 2% lignocaine or 4% procaine may be applied topically for the relief of pain from superficial abraded or eczematous areas. The application is made by soaking a piece of absorbent wool or gauze in the solution and placing it on the affected area for about 5 minutes. For analgesia of the mucous membrane of the glans penis and the vulva, solutions of lignocaine may be applied in a similar manner. However, perhaps the most satisfactory agent to use on the glans penis and vulva is the preparation of lignocaine made for use in the urethra — a sterile carboxymethylcellulose gel containing 2% of the analgesic agent. This gel possesses very good lubricating properties and is an excellent lubricant for urethral catheters.

For procedures in the nasal chambers of the horse, or the transnasal passage of a stomach tube in dogs, spraying with 4% lignocaine provides satisfactory analgesia. In ophthalmic surgery 4% lignocaine is quite safe in the eye but perhaps the agent of choice for topical analgesia of the cornea is proxymetacaine hydrochloride 2-diethylaminoethyl-3-amino-4-propoxybenzoate hydrochloride), known by the trade name 'Ophthaine'. The commercial preparation is a 0.5% solution which contains 2.45% glycerin as a stabilizer, and 0.2% chlorobutanol together with 1:10 000 benzalkonium chloride as preservatives. Using a single drop, the onset of corneal analgesia occurs in about 15 seconds and persists for about 15 minutes. This compound does not produce pupillary dilatation and is non-irritant, but its solution is rather unstable, having a shelf-life of only 12 months.

Intrasynovial Analgesia

Surface analgesia is also employed for the relief of pain arising from pathological processes involving joints and tendon sheaths. A solution of local analgesic is injected into the synovial cavity and then dispersed throughout the cavity by manipulation of the limb. If the synovial cavity is distended with fluid, it is first drained to ensure that the injected solution is not excessively diluted. Analgesia develops within 5–10 minutes after injection and persists for about 1 hour. The injection renders the synovial membrane insensitive but it is not known whether the nerve endings in the underlying structures are affected.

A needle can be introduced into synovial sheath™ quite easily when they are distended with synovia™ fluid, but entry into a normal sheath is not easy. When searching for a synovial sheath the exploring needle should be connected to a syringe containing local analgesic solution and a slight pressure maintained on the syringe plunger. As soon as the needle enters the sheath the resistance to injection disappears and some of the solution enters the synovial cavity, lifting its wall away from the underlying tendon.

Infiltration Analgesia

By this method the nerve endings are affected at the actual site of operation. Most minor surgical procedures not involving the digits or teats can be performed under infiltration analgesia and the technique is also useful, in conjunction with light basal narcosis, for major operations in animals which are bad operative risks. Infiltration should, however, never be carried out through, or into, infected or inflamed tissues.

Suitable concentrations of lignocaine are 0.2–0.5% and stronger solutions than 0.5% should never be necessary. It is usual to add adrenaline 1:400 000–1:200 0000 to the solution, but this vasoconstrictor should be omitted when there are circumstances present which may interfere with healing, e.g. damaged tissue, possible contamination. A hypodermic syringe and needle is all the apparatus necessary for the administration of local infiltration analgesia.

1. The limits of the area to be infiltrated are conveniently defined and marked for subsequent recognition by the use of intradermal weal. To produce an intradermal weal a short needle is held almost parallel the skin surface with the bevel of its point innermost away from the skin. The needle is thrust into the skin until the bevel is no longer visible and by exerting considerable pressure on the plunger of the syringe 0.5–1 ml of local analgesic solution is injected. The resulting weal is insensitive as soon as it is formed and if punctures are repeatedly made at the periphery of such weals, a continuous weal can be produced along the proposed line of incision without an animal feeling more than the initial needle prick. Such intradermal infiltration is only easily performed in thick-skinned animals; in horses and cattle it is usual to simply mark the proposed line of infiltration by raising a weal at either end of the line.

2. Subcutaneous tissues are infiltrated by introducing needle through the skin at the site of an intradermal weal. For infiltration of a straight-line incision a needle about 10 cm long is introduced almost parallel to the skin surface and pushed through the subcutaneous tissue along the proposed line. Before injecting any local analgesic

solution, aspiration is attempted to ascertain that the needle point has not entered a blood vessel. If blood is aspirated back into the syringe, the needle is partially withdrawn and reinserted in a slightly different direction. If no blood is aspirated, injection of the local analgesic is carried out as the needle is slowly drawn out of the tissues so that a stream of solution is deposited subcutaneously. About 1 ml of solution is required for every centimetre of incision.

3. To infiltrate several layers of tissue, the procedure is to inject, from one puncture site, first the subcutaneous tissue and then, in succession by further advancing the needle, the deeper tissues. Field block consists of making walls of analgesia enclosing the operation field. It is accomplished by making fanwise injections in certain planes of the body so as to soak all the nerves which cross these planes on their way to the operation field, but no attempt is made to pick out the nerves individually. Usually the entire thickness of the soft tissue in which the nerves run is involved. Generally, walls of analgesia are created obliquely to the skin surface, involving only part of the tissues around the region, but meeting below so that the operation area is held in a sort of cup of infiltrated tissue (Fig. 18.1).

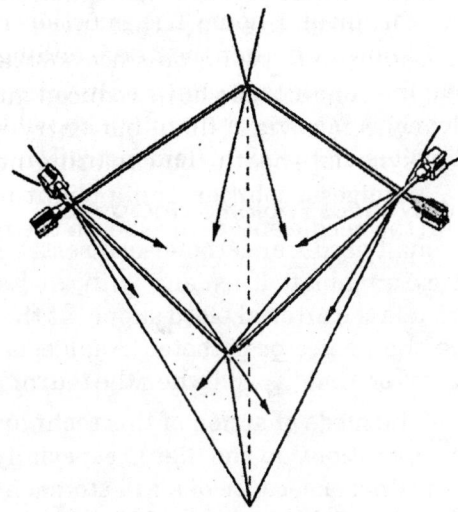

Fig. 18.1: Technique of infiltrating a 'cup' of tissue to include the operation site

Vasoconstrictor is incorporated in the solution of local analgesia the principal advantages of field block are:

1. Absence of distortion of the anatomical features in the line of incision.
2. Ischaemia of the tissues within the blocked area.
3. Muscular relaxation.
4. Absence of interference with the healing of the wound which is often claimed to be the chief objection to direct local infiltration analgesia.

The field block most commonly used in veterinary practice is probably that for rumenotomy and this block differs from the type of field block described above. Because of the course and distribution of the nerves supplying the operation site it can be accomplished by two linear infiltrations of the whole thickness of the body wall, one anterior to, and one above, the line of incision. Up to 200 ml of local analgesic solution may be required for this block.

Ring block of an extremity is another special type of field block in which a transverse plane through the whole extremity is infiltrated with local analgesic solution and particular attention is given to the sites of large nerve trunks. The technique is more effective when the injection is made distal to a tourniquet. It is a type of block which is particularly useful for amputation of digits in cattle and may also be used for operations on lows' teats. Vasoconstrictors should not be added to solutions used to produce ring block in teats, for prolonged vasoconstriction may result in ischaemic necrosis of the end of the teat.

Regional Analgesia

Regional analgesia is brought about by blocking conduction in the sensory nerve or nerves innervating the region where an operation is to be performed. The operative field itself is not touched while its sensitivity is being abolished and good analgesia results from the use of small quantities of local analgesic solution. The solution must, however, be brought into the closest possible contact with the nerve which is to be blocked, and special care must be taken to ensure that there is no sheet of fascia between the nerve and the site of deposition of the solution since solutions do not diffuse through fascial sheets. Success in regional analgesia comes only from practice, as does success in other techniques, but clearly it requires a thorough knowledge of the topographical anatomy of the nerves and the sites of injection, demonstration and tuition by an experienced practitioner.

Intravenous Regional Analgesia

A small needle or catheter is inserted into a vein at the distal extremity of a limb. The limb is exsanguinated, usually with an Esmarch bandage, a tourniquet is inflated or tied to occlude the arterial blood supply at the top of the limb and local analgesic solution is injected via the needle or catheter. Analgesia of the limb up to the lower limit of the tourniquet comes on rapidly, and when the tourniquet is released it wears off with almost equal rapidity.

The mode of action of this technique is unclear but it seems to be both safe and simple for operations on the digits, especially in ruminant animals and in dogs unfit for general anaesthesia because of a full stomach or intercurrent disease. The good analgesia and the bloodless field are appreciated by the surgeon.

Local Analgesia for Fractures

The injection is made directly into the haematoma at the site of the fracture and deposition of the solution in the correct place is essential for success. The needle should be inserted as far into the haematoma and as near the bone ends as possible. The position of the needle should be verified by aspiration, when blood or blood clot should be drawn into the syringe. Lignocaine hydrochloride (1% solution without adrenaline) is the best agent to use. In small animal patients, 2–5 ml, and in large animals, 10–15 ml of solution are required. Analgesia follows 5–10 minutes after injection. Scrupulous asepsis must be observed when injecting into a fracture site as the consequences of infection are serious.

This technique is particularly suitable as a first-aid measure and in the relief of pain arising from fractured ribs.

1. Subarachnoid injection, in which the needle penetrates the dura mater and the arachnoid mater and the analgesic solution is introduced into the cerebrospinal fluid.
2. Epi-(extra) dural injection, in which the needle enters the spinal canal but does not penetrate the meninges, and the injected solution penetrates along the canal outside the dura mater.

Bibliography

1. Kumar P. *Textbook of Anaesthesiology,* 1st edn., Paras Med. Publishers, Hyderabad, 2008.
2. Kumar P. *Clinical Methods in Anaesthesia,* 1st edn., Mumbai, National, 2008.
3. Mc Donell W., Modern Veterinary Anaesthesia, Practice, 1972.

Section 3

Anaesthesia for Individual Species

19

Anaesthesia for Horse

SEDATION

In the search for a completely reliable, safe method of producing sedation in standing horses a number of mixtures of drugs have been used. Appropriate doses of many of these have proved to have a more certain and profound effect than can be regularly obtained from the use of any single drug. However, the possibility of untoward reactions and the appearance of as yet unrecognized drug interactions must always be considered when these mixtures are employed. The most popular drug combinations in use at the present time include those shown in Table 19.1.

Table 19.1: Drug combinations used by intravenous injection to sedate horses

Drug mixture	Dose of components (mg/kg)
Xylazine	0.6
Methadone	0.1
Xylazine	1.0
Morphine	0.1–0.2
Buprenorphine	0.004
Acepromazine	0.04
Xylazine	0.2
Buprenorphine	0.006
Detomidine	0.01–0.02
Butorphanol	0.03–0.05

Acepromazine/α_2-adrenoceptor Agonist Combinations

Acepromazine (0.02 mg/kg) and xylazine (0.5 mg/ kg) have often been used together for sedating horses. Originally the combination was used in an attempt to reduce the dose of the costly xylazine but it was soon realized that the prolonged calming action of acepromazine could be exploited in a variety of circumstances where the α_2-adrenoceptor agonists were used, particularly for premedication and in combination with opioids. However, many North American sources now state that acepromazine and the α_2-adrenoceptor agonists should not be used. If high doses of both agents are given to a horse it may collapse, but considers that carefully administered low doses may be safe. The pharmacological reasoning behind the suggestion that the two drugs should not be given together rests on the fact that acepromazine causes hypotension through a-blocking action and xylazine causes bradycardia. However, it must be noted that maximal bradycardia occurs 1–2 minutes after the intravenous injection of xylazine and at this time is accompanied by hypertension. If detomidine is given to horses already sedated with acepromazine, there is still a hypertensive response, albeit starting from a lower base.

The authors have administered xylazine or detomidine to over 2000 horses already sedated with acepromazine with no ill effects and agree with Short that providing both drugs are given at suitable doses there is no reason why the combination cannot be used.

Sedative/Opioid Combinations

The addition of the opioid, even at subanalgesic doses, appears to enhance sedation dramatically and, in particular, diminishes the response to touch, thus reducing the likelihood of provoking well-directed kicks from the sedated horse. The disadvantage is that ataxia is also increased (particularly with combinations involving methadone or butorphanol). Also, opioid excitement reactions such as aimless walking may occur when sedation becomes inadequate and it is irrational to combine a short-acting sedative such as xylazine with opioids with long actions such as buprenorphine or high doses of morphine. Acepromazine has a very long action so problems are less when this is part of the combination. The chance of the opioid-induced excitement occurring early on can be reduced by administering the sedatives first followed by the opioid once sedation is apparent, although if the opioid concerned is one which has a delayed onset of action (e.g. buprenorphine) this is neither necessary nor desirable.

Table 19.1 lists some of the sedative/opioid combinations that have been satisfactorily used. Morphine has been given in much higher doses than recommended here but although generally satisfactory a few animals show marked bradycardia and respiratory depression and the doses given in Table 19.1 are safer and generally adequate. The advantage of drug mixtures using butorphanol or buprenorphine is that they are not subject to such strict control regulations as the pure agonists and in the combination of intravenous detomidine (15 µg/kg) and butorphanol (0.03 mg/kg) has proved very successful, particularly for clipping fractious horses.

LOCAL ANALGESIA

Infraorbital Nerve Block

The infraorbital nerve is the continuation of the maxillary division of the fifth cranial nerve after it crosses the pterygopalatine fossa and enters the infraorbital canal. The nerve emerges on the face as a flat band about 1 cm broad, through the infraorbital foramen, where it is partly covered by the levator nasolabialis muscle. It is entirely sensory. During its course along the infraorbital canal it supplies branches to the upper molar, canine and incisor teeth on that side, and their alveoli and contiguous gum. The nerves supplying the first and second molars (PM1 and 2), the canine and incisors, arise within the canal about 2.5 cm from the infraorbital foramen and pass forwards in the maxilla and premaxilla to the teeth. The nerves to cheek teeth three to six (PM3, M1, 2) and 3) pass directly from the parent nerve trunk in the upper parts of the canal. After emerging from the foramen the nerve supplies sensory fibres to the upper lip and cheek, the nostrils and lower parts of the face.

It may be approached at two sites (Fig. 19.1):

1. At its point of emergence from the infraorbital foramen, the area desensitized will comprise the skin of the lip, nostril and face on that side up to the level of the foramen.

2. Within the canal, via the infraorbital foramen, when in addition the first and second premolars, the canine and incisor teeth with their alveoli and gum, and the skin as high as the level of the inner canthus of the eye, will be influenced.

The lip of the infraorbital foramen can be detected readily as a bony ridge lying beneath the edge of the flat levator nasolabialis muscle. When it is desired to block the nerve within the canal it is necessary to pass the needle up the canal about 2.5 cm. To do this the needle must be inserted through the skin about 2 cm in front of the foramen after reflecting the edge of the muscle upwards. An insensitive skin weal is an advantage. For the perineural injection a needle 19 gauge (1.1 mm), 5 cm long, is suitable. The quantity of local analgesic solution required will vary from 4 to 5 ml. For blocking the nerve at its point of emergence from the canal, the needle is introduced until its point can be felt beneath the bony lip of the foramen (Fig. 19.2).

A point is selected on the caudal border of the mandible about 3 cm below the temporomandibular articulation. After penetrating the skin the needle is allowed to lie in the depression between the wing of the atlas and the base of the ear. The needle is advanced as its point is depressed until it passes deep to the medial border of the ramus. It is then advanced further in the direction of the point of intersection of the previously mentioned lines, keeping as close as possible to the medial surface of the mandible but as the nerve lies medial

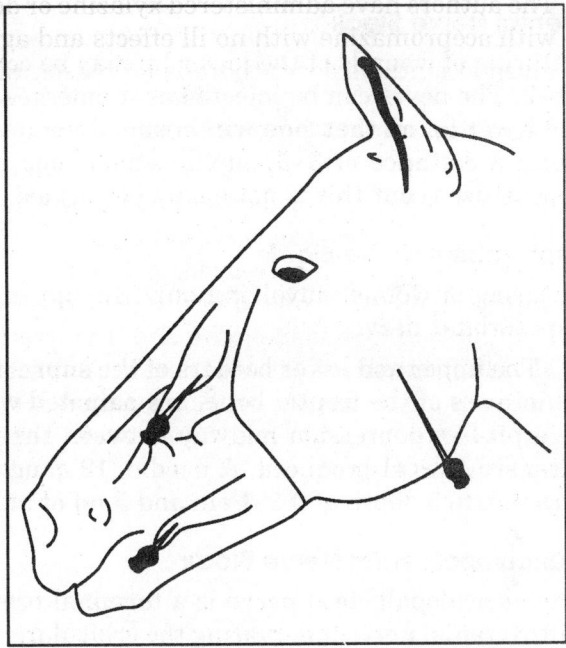

Fig. 19.1: Sites for insertion of the needle to block the supraorbital, infraorbital, mental and mandibular nerves

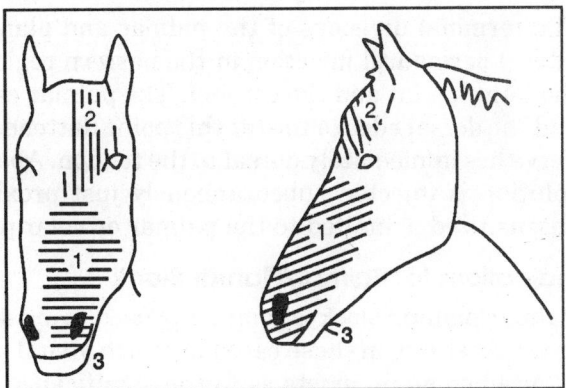

Fig. 19.2: Area of skin desensitization after blocking: the infraorbital nerve within the canal (1); the supraorbital nerve (2); the mental nerve (3)

to the accompanying artery and vein, the needle does not need to follow the bone closely. Following this method the needle should lie parallel with the nerve for a distance of 3–4 cm. About 5 ml of analgesic solution is injected along this length.

The chief indications are molar dental interferences in the lower jaw, but most surgeons today prefer to carry out all dental surgery under general anaesthesia and this nerve block will only be used when, for some reason, general anaesthesia is impracticable.

Mental Nerve Block

Suturing of wounds of the lower lip may be conveniently carried out under mental nerve block. The nerve can be injected as it emerges from the mental foramen and analgesia of the lower lip on that side will ensue. Attempts may be made to pass the needle along a canal a distance of 3–5 cm (in which case the canine and incisor teeth will also be desensitized) but this is not easily performed.

Supraorbital Nerve Block

Suturing of wounds involving only the upper eyelid is easily possible after block of the supraorbital nerve.

The upper and lower borders of the supraorbital process, close to its junction with the main mass of the frontal bone, are palpated with the fingers. The foramen is recognized as a pit-like depression midway between the two borders. The skin is prepared and an insensitive weal produced. A needle, 19 gauge (1.1 mm), 2.2 cm long, is passed into the foramen to a depth of 0.5–1 cm and 5 ml of analgesic solution injected.

Auriculopalpebral Nerve Block

The auriculopalpebral nerve is a terminal branch of the facial division of the trigeminal (fifth) cranial nerve innervating the orbicularis oculi muscles. Blocking this nerve prevents voluntary closure of the eyelids but does not in any way desensitize them. It is blocked by injecting 6 ml of 2% lignocaine at most dorsal point of zygomatic arch.

Technique of Blocking Palmar Terminal Digital Nerves

The terminal divisions of the palmar and plantar nerves may be subjected to medial and lateral perineural injection in the pastern region. The site for injection is midway between the fetlock joint and the coronet. The palmar or volar border of the first phalanx is located, and the dorsal edge of the (at this point flattened) deep digital flexor tendon is palpated. The nerve lies immediately dorsal to the tendon. About 2 ml 1% mepivacaine or 0.5% bupivacaine solution is injected subcutaneously just proximal to the collateral cartilages. The area desensitized is limited to the palmar or volar part of the foot and heel on that side.

Indications for Palmar/Plantar Block

Palmar/plantar block is commonly used to aid diagnosis of the site of lameness, particularly of the forelimb, in those cases in which visual and manipulative examination fail to reveal it, or when doubt exists as to the significance of some obvious lesion.

Apart from their use in the location of the site of lameness, these nerve blocks may be used to relieve pain and allow rest.

The nerve blocks may also allow the painless performance of palmar and plantar neurectomy and of operations about the foot, coronet and heel, such as exposure of a corn or gathered nail track, partial operations for quittor and sandcrack.

The Complete Desensitization of the Forelimb Below the Carpus

Simultaneous block of the median, ulnar and musculocutaneous (cutaneous branch) nerves desensitize the entire manus.

Median Nerve

With the animal standing squarely, the administrator stoops adjacent to and slightly behind the opposite forelimb. The caudal border of the radius where it meets the distal edge of the caudal superficial pectoral muscle is located with a finger. The point of insertion of the needle is immediately proximal to the finger. A needle, 19 gauge (1.1 mm), 2.5–3 cm long, is suitable. It is directed proximally and axially at an angle of 20° to the vertical, to ensure penetration of the pectoral muscle and the deep fascia; 7.5–10 ml of local analgesic solution are injected. To facilitate insertion of the needle to the proper depth it is best first to induce an insensitive skin weal.

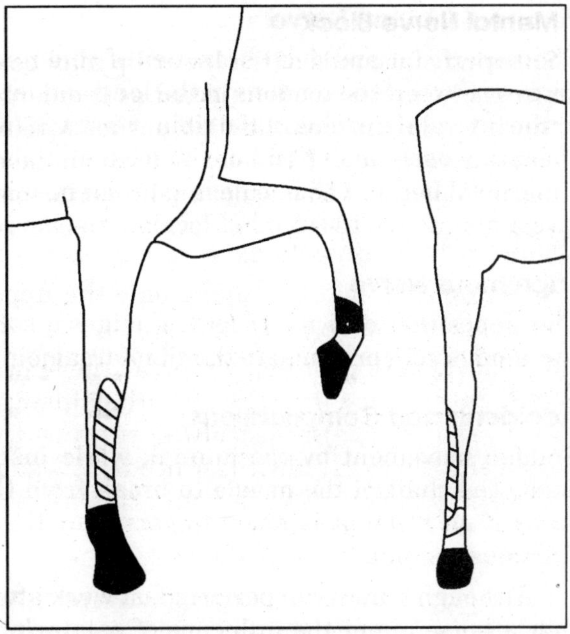

Fig 19.3: Area of skin desensitization after block of the ulnar (shaded) and medial nerves (spotted). Palma block (blue lines)

Ulnar Nerve

This nerve may be blocked (Fig. 19.3) by the injection of 10 ml of local analgesic solution in the centre of the caudal aspect of the limb about 10 cm proximal to the accessory carpal bone, in the groove between the tendons of the ulnaris lateralis and flexor carpi ulnaris, and beneath the deep fascia.

Musculocutaneous Nerve

This nerve is blocked on the medial aspect of the limb where it lies on the surface of the radius halfway between the elbow and carpus, immediately adjacent to the cephalic vein. At this site, it can easily be palpated just cranial to the cephalic vein and blocked by the injection of 10 ml of local analgesic solution.

The Complete Desensitization of the Distal Hind limb

The technique of nerve block of the hind limb sometimes works extremely well but is unreliable, especially for removal of cutaneous sensation.

Tibial Nerve

Injection is made about 10–15 cm above the point of the tarsus, in the groove between the gastrocnemius tendon and the deep digital flexor tendon. Palpation of the nerve at this site is facilitated by holding up the foot and slightly flexing the leg although the injection is best made with the limb bearing weight. Care must be taken to inject deep to the subcutaneous fascia or only the superficial branch of the nerve will be affected. Some 20 ml of local analgesic solution should be injected at this site through a 2.5 cm, 20 gauge (0.9 mm) needle that has been placed beneath the fascia.

Peroneal (fibular) Nerve

The superficial and deep branches of this nerve are best blocked simultaneously in the groove between the tendons of the long and lateral digital extensors about 10 cm proximal to the lateral malleolus of the tibia. First a 3.75 cm, 22 gauge (0.7 mm) needle is introduced subcutaneously and 10 ml of the local analgesic solution injected through it to block the superficial nerve. The needle must then be inserted another 2–3 cm to penetrate the deep fascia and about 10–15 ml of local analgesic solution injected around the deep branch.

Saphenous Nerve

The deposition of 5 ml of local analgesic solution on the dorsal aspect of the median saphenous vein proximal to the tibiotarsal joint will effectively block the saphenous nerve.

Accidents and Complications

Sudden movement by the animal, while inserting the needle or during injection, may cause the shaft of the needle to break from the hub. The accident is especially liable to occur if an attempt is made to carry out the operation without twitching a nervous or fractious animal.

Although horses can perform fast work after surgical neurectomy care should be taken that a horse under the influence of palmar/plantar block is not exercised vigorously, for incoordinate movement after the acute loss of sensation may result in bone fracture.

Local Analgesia for Castration

There are three methods in common use for desensitizing the scrotum, testicle and spermatic cord by injection of local analgesics but for all of them it is essential that the animal is properly restrained or sedated if the operator is not to be injured when carrying them out on the standing animal. The animal is placed with its right side against a wall or partition and if not sedated a twitch is applied to its upper lip. After preparation of the skin of the scrotum, prepuce and medial aspect of the thighs, the operator stands with his left shoulder pressed lightly against the caudal part of the animal's left chest wall. The neck of the scrotum on the right side is gripped with the left hand and the testicle drawn well down until the skin of the scrotum is tense.

Method 1

A 19 gauge (1.1 mm) needle is quickly thrust into the substance of the testicle to a depth of 3–4 cm and 30–35 ml of 2% lignocaine injected. When an adequate amount of lignocaine has been injected the testicle feels firm. The procedure is repeated for the left testicle, and local analgesic solution is injected along the median raphe of the scrotum. Castration can then be carried out painlessly after about 10 minutes has elapsed.

Method 2

The spermatic cord is grasped with the fingers just above the testicle and a 5 cm 19 gauge (1.1 mm) needle thrust into the subcutaneous tissues of that region. The needle is kept stationary to avoid penetration of blood vessels and about 20 ml of 2% lignocaine injected around each spermatic cord. The scrotal skin is injected along the line of the proposed incisions. This method does not seem as effective as the one described above.

Method 3

A long (12–15 cm) 19 gauge (1.1 mm) needle is thrust through the testicle and directed into the spermatic cord while 20–25 ml 2% lignocaine are being injected! After treatment of both spermatic cords the scrotal skin is infiltrated.

To infiltrate the scrotal skin it is important that the direction of the needle shall be almost parallel to the skin to ensure that its point lies in the subcutaneous connective tissue, for if it enters the dartos or the substance of the testicle itself, difficulty, may be experienced in injecting the solution and, what is more important, the skin does not become analgesic. The animal usually moves as the needle is inserted and the operator must be prepared for this recognized acupuncture point.

CAUDAL EPIDURAL ANALGESIA

In horses the caudal block is performed by entering between the first and second coc-cygeal vertebrae (Fig. 19.4) the spinal cord and its meninges ending in the midsacral region. The depression between the first and second coccygeal dorsal spinous pro-cesses can usually be felt with the finger when the tail is raised, even in the heavy breeds, about 2.5 cm cranial to the com-mencement of the tail hairs although in fat animals it may be impossible to detect any of the sacral or coccygeal dorsal spinous processes. Upward flexion at the sacrococ-cygeal articulation is seldom discernible; in fact, in many animals this joint is fused. A line drawn over the back joining the two coxofemoral joints crosses the midline at the level of the sacrococcygeal joint. Im-mediately behind this may be palpated the dorsal spinous process of the first coccygeal bone, and the site for insertion of the needle is the space immediately caudal to this. The interarcual space is smaller than in the ox and may be more difficult to locate with the needle, particularly in well-developed or fat animals in which the root of the tail is well covered by muscle or fat. Sometimes it is possible to detect a 'popping' sensation as the interarcual ligament is penetrated. The surest evidence, however, that the canal has been entered is the almost complete absence of resistance to injection of the local analgesic solution into the skin with a 25 gauge (0.5 mm) needle will prevent any painful reaction to the epidural (3–5 cm, 19 gauge or 1.1 mm) needle.

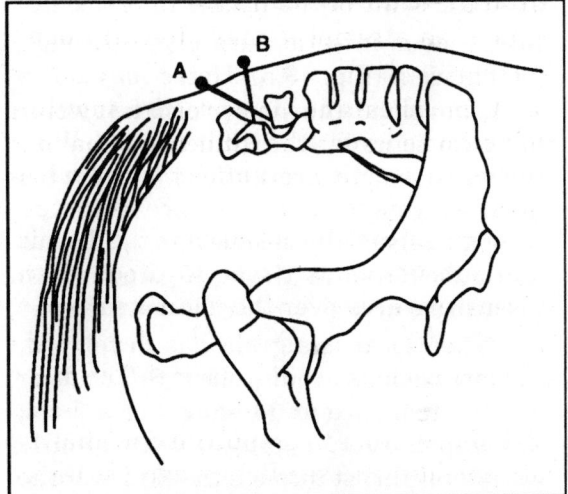

Fig. 19.4: Caudal block in the horse. The needle may be inserted at right angles to the skin surface between the first and second caudal vertebrae or it may be introduced further caudally over the cranial border of the second coccygeal vertebra and inclined at an angle of about 30° to the horizontal to run up the neural canal

Ten millilitres of 2% lignocaine or 0.5 % bupivacaine, with or without a vasoconstrictor, is usually sufficient to produce caudal block in the largest of horses. For extending the block cranially upto 100–150 mg 00.2% lignocaine is used. It does cause hypotension, needing fluids and vasopressors.

Indications

General

For amputation of the tail and for operations about the anus, perineum and vulva: suture of wounds, operation for prolapsed rectum, Caslick's operation for vaginal wind sucking.

Obstetrical

To overcome straining during manipulative correction of the simpler forms of malpresentation of the fetus, and for partial embryotomy.

INTRAVENOUS ANAESTHESIA

Intravenous infection are made through jugular vein (Fig. 19.5). Horse may tense neck muscles and obscure the jugular furrow whenever a twitch is applied. With the usual aseptic precautions 1 or 2 ml of local analgesic solution are injected through a short, fine needle into the dermis and subcutaneous tissue to produce an insensitive area over the jugular furrow.

When local analgesia has developed, the intravenous needle (about 6–7 cm long and 2.1 mm bore or 14 gauge) or a 5 cm, 2.4 mm bore (13 gauge) over-needle catheter is thrust through the skin over the vein with its point directed towards the head.

Catheters need to be introduced through a small skin incision made in the weal of local analgesic solution. The vein is distended by the application of pressure which is best applied by pressing the thumb into the jugular furrow just below the site of venepuncture. This tenses the skin and the distended vein is easily palpable. The point of the needle or catheter is directed towards the vein and thrust into it. It is important that a good length of needle or catheter shall be introduced into the vein otherwise

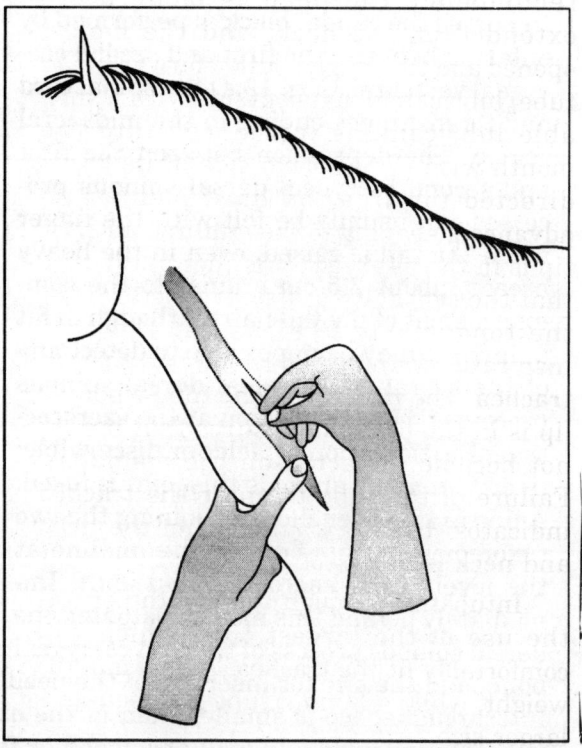

Fig. 19.5: Injection into the jugular vein of the horse. The vein is easily raised with simple digital pressure and 'neck ropes' should never be employed for this purpose because they invariably displace the skin, resulting in withdrawal of the needle or catheter when their compression is released

there is a risk that as the vein subsides, on the release of pressure, it will retract away from the needle or catheter whose position is fixed by the skin. Moreover, unless about 2–3 cm of the needle or catheter is in the lumen of the vein, the slightest movement is likely to cause it to leave the vessel. A free flow of blood indicates that it is well placed in the lumen of the vein. If only a few drops of blood fall it may be concluded that either (1) the needle or catheter is in a perivascular haematoma or (2) the needle or catheter is in the vein but its lumen is partially blocked. Once it is certain that a catheter is in the vein to its maximum length it should be secured in position with a partial skin thickness stitch of nylon or linen thread, and a stopcock attached. The catheter may be kept patent for many hours if its lumen is periodically flushed with heparin saline solution (10 units/ml). The skin suture should be laid before venepuncture is attempted so that it may be tied securely around the catheter without risk of displacing this from the vein.

Endotracheal Intubation

In horses the passage of a Magill-type endotracheal tube presents no great problem. With the anaesthetized horse in lateral recumbency the head is moderately extended on the neck, and the mouth opened and the tongue pulled forward. The tube, lubricated on its outside with a suitable lubricant, is introduced into the mouth with the concave side of its curve directed towards the hard palate and advanced, keeping to the midline, until its tip is in the pharynx. It is then rotated so that the concavity of its curve is towards the tongue (Fig.19.6) and at the next inspiration it is pushed rapidly on into the trachea. The rotation of the tube when its lip is in the pharynx ensures that it does not become impacted on the epiglottis. Failure of the tube to enter the trachea indicates that the alignment of the head and neck is incorrect.

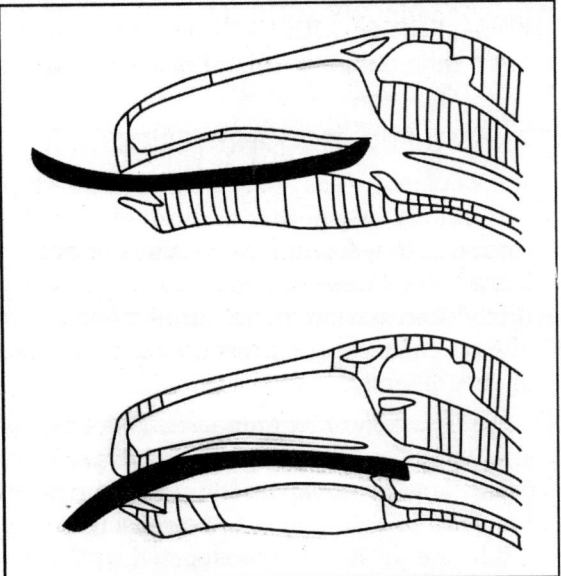

Fig. 19.6: Passage of an oral endotracheal tube in a horse

Intubation through the mouth permits the use of the largest tube which will comfortably fit the trachea. A 16.0 mm tube is suitable for ponies up to about 150 kg body weight, while a 30 mm tube is adequate for most thoroughbred. Heavy horses often take larger size.

The cuffs of endotracheal tubes are often damaged by contact with the horse's teeth even when a reliable mouth-gag is used to keep the mouth open during intubation and extubation. Cuffed tubes made of red rubber for use in horses are expensive and because of the relatively short life attempts have been made to produce them in much less expensive plastics.

PREMEDICATION

Premedication with acepromazine has been used in horses for many years to lessen, or to prevent, excitement during recovery from barbiturate anaesthesia, and to reduce the quantity of anaesthetic needed for maintenance (but not for induction) of anaesthesia. It may be given by intramuscular injection in doses of 0.03–0.05 mg/kg about 1 hour before anaesthesia is to be induced, or it may be given intravenously at half this dose rate. After intravenous injection it is necessary to allow 5–20 minutes to elapse to ensure it is producing its full effects.

α_2-Adrenoceptor agonists (xylazine and detomidine) are much more versatile agents for premedication. They contribute markedly to the anaesthetic and reduce the dose of both intravenous and inhalation anaesthetic agents. Xylazine may be given in a 10% solution by intramuscular injection in doses of 2 mg/kg about 15–20 minutes before induction of anaesthesia. Alternatively, it may be given by intravenous injection in doses of 1 mg/kg about 2–4 minutes beforehand. Detomidine may be used in a similar manner, the appropriate doses being 20–40 µg/kg and 10–20 µg/kg, respectively. After, premedication with these agents horses are reluctant' to walk, so whenever possible the drug should be administered in the place where anaesthesia is to be induced.

ANAESTHETIC RECOVERY PERIOD

It is not always easy to decide whether a horse is likely to recover from anaesthesia smoothly and quietly or whether additional drugs will be required to ensure this. Probably the best course is to wait and see; if signs of excitement do appear it is a simple matter to give an intravenous dose of about 0.1 mg/kg of xylazine, particularly if an intravenous cannula introduced earlier in the anaesthetic is still in place. This dose of xylazine will nearly always ensure a quiet recovery without causing circulatory problems or undue prolongation of recumbency.

As surgery or examination under anaesthesia nears completion the level of anaesthesia should be lightened as much as possible, even to the point where spontaneous movements occur. Horses do not suddenly get up and walk away at the end of anaesthesia and in the majority of cases there is no reason why anaesthesia should be maintained at deep levels while the animal is transported to the recovery area. An animal which has been supine should be placed on its left side in the recovery area, but animals which have been lying on their sides probably should not be turned over to lie on the side which was uppermost during anaesthesia.

Endotracheal tubes which have been passed through the mouth should be removed as soon as the anaesthetic is terminated because the recovering animal may occlude the tube by biting on it. Respiratory obstruction caused in this way can be difficult to relieve and expensive tubes may be ruined. In addition, stimulation of the trachea by the tube has been associated with cardiac arrest, presumably through a vagal mechanism, as anaesthesia lightens. Following prolonged anaesthesia, respiratory obstruction is frequently observed after removal of the endotracheal tube. It is probably due to hypostatic congestion of the nasal and pharynneal mucous membranes during anaesthesia and the horse makes a characteristic snoring noise. It may be relieved by passing a smallbore endotracheal tube through one nostril and this tube should be secured in place by a transfixing suture tied to the head collar or halter. Unless it is properly secured such a tube may be aspirated into the tracheobronchial tree.

It is probably advisable to administer oxygen to all horses recovering from general anaesthesia, but it is obligatory in critically ill animals. The oxygen should be given through a nasal endotracheal tube or a narrow-bore stomach tube passed into the trachea via the nostril. The endotracheal or stomach tube should be connected to a source of oxygen in such a manner that it will become disconnected if the horse moves or rolls during recovery. To produce any significant improvement of P_aO_2, oxygen must be administered into the trachea at a flow rate of at least 15 l/min.

In general, analgesics should not be given until the horse is standing because if given before this they may prolong recovery. However, doses of intramuscular pethidine of up to 0.5 g or intravenous flunixin (1 mg/ kg), do not seem to add to recovery time and may be given at the end of anaesthesia to control pain during the recovery period. Moreover, local nerve blocks given at the end of surgery on the digits for postoperative analgesia do not seem to cause problems for the horse attempting to stand up. Unless catheterized, the bladder of male animals given fluid intravenously during operation may become distended and cause considerable abdominal pain. Catheterization of the bladder produces immediate relief of this pain. This problem does not occur in female animals because urine will seep from the bladder during anaesthesia.

ANAESTHESIA IN THE FIELD

Although horses are most safely anaesthetized under controlled hospital conditions, there are times when it is necessary to perform short operations, such as castration, in the field. As anaesthetic apparatus is unlikely to be available, although some practitioners still use chloroform, anaesthesia is usually both induced and maintained with intravenous agents. Every effort should be made to ensure that a supply of oxygen under pressure is at hand, however, should respiratory arrest occur IPPV of the lungs can only be satisfactorily provided by the use of a stream of oxygen directed into the trachea for the Venturi effect.

The aims of anaesthesia in the field are much the same as in a hospital — to provide a quiet induction, adequate anaesthetic conditions for surgery (including analgesia and relaxation), an adequate time for the procedure, followed by a quick, calm recovery with minimal ataxia when the animal regains the standing position. In the field it is particularly important that the drugs used do not cause respiratory depression, for under the circumstances prevailing it will be found that this is difficult to manage. Almost any drug or combination of intravenous agents already discussed may be used but as yet there is no perfect combination — hence the multiplicity of methods employed, the number of clinical trials found in the literature and the many literature reviews relating to the subject (Table 19.2).

The anaesthetist must aim at maintaining an even plane of anaesthesia and this is best performed by giving chloroform anaesthesia. On completion of the operation the mask is removed and the nostrils wiped clean. Anaesthesia is followed by hypnosis, the horse lying quietly in a state of sleep which lasts for about 20–30 minutes, and no attempt should be made to induce it to rise during this period. As soon as the horse feels able to do so it will get to its feet — usually in a sluggish manner. There may be considerable incoordination, particularly of the hind limbs, but provided that the animal has not been made to get up before it was ready to do so, it will be able to maintain the standing position. Very occasionally anaesthesia is followed by a state of vigorous narcotic excitement and if all restraint has been removed the animal may sustain injury. Because of this occasional excitement it is probably wise to maintain control of the head and to continue restraint for 10 minutes after completion of the operation in every case. If no struggling occurs during this period, it may be taken as certain that recovery will be quiet.

Table 19.2: Drug combinations useful for colt

Premedication	Induction	Maintenance (increments)
Acepromazine i.v. (0.02 mg/kg)	Thiopentone (11 mg/kg)	Thiopentone (1 mg/kg)
Xylazine i.v. (1 mg/kg)	Thiopentone (5.5 mg/kg)	Thiopentone (1 mg/kg)
Xylazine i.v. (1 mg/kg)	Methohexitone (2.5 mg/kg)	Methohexitone (0.5 mg/kg)
Detomidine i.v. (20 µg/kg)	Thiopentone (5.5 mg/kg)	Thiopentone (1 mg/kg)
Acepromazine i.v. (0.03 mg/kg)	Chloral hydrate 10% i.v. until ataxic then thiopentone (5.5 mg/kg)	Thiopentone (1 mg/kg)
Acepromazine i.v. (0.03 mg/kg)	Guaiphenesin until ataxic (about 50 mg/kg) then thiopentone (5 mg/kg)	Thiopentone (1 mg/kg) ± further guaiphenesin
Xylazine i.v. (1 mg/kg)	Ketamine i.v. (2 mg/kg) (0.5 mg/kg) + ketamine (1 mg/kg)	Thiopentone (1 mg/kg) or xylazine
Detomidine (20 ug/kg)	Ketamine (2 mg/kg)	Thiopentone (1 mg/kg) or ketamine i.v. (1 mg/kg)
Acepromazine i.v.	Chloroform by	Chloroform by mask (0.03–0.05 mg/kg) mask

INDUCTION OF ANAESTHESIA

In the theatre the wheeled trolley may become the top of the operating table or the horse may have to be transferred from it to the table. An electrically operated overhead hoist is most helpful both for this and for maintaining the position of the animal on the table during surgery. This system can be operated with minimal, even relatively untrained assistants and mechanical failures are unlikely to be disastrous.

Induction Agents

General anaesthesia may be induced with either inhalation anaesthetics or intravenous agents but in most cases the intravenous route is used. The ease of induction with inhalation anaesthetics and the dose of intravenous agents needed are dependent on the sedation produced by premedication. Toxaemia and hypoproteinaemia also reduce the quantity of anaesthetic agent required.

Thiopentone

Thiopentone, at a dose of 10 mg/kg given as a bolus by intravenous injection into the jugular vein, has been found to be very satisfactory for the induction of anaesthesia in horses premedicated with 0.03–0.04 mg/kg of acepromazine 30–40 minutes previously. Unconsciousness is produced and the horse becomes recumbent 25–30 seconds after the thiopentone injection. For many years it has been the practice of some anaesthetists to inject a bolus dose of suxamethonium (0.12 mg/kg) immediately after the thiopentone to smooth the transition to an inhalation agent when anaesthesia is to be maintained for long periods. The use of intravenous xylaxine (1 mg/kg) or detomidine (15–20 µg/kg) premedication 4–5 minutes prior to induction reduces the dose of thiopentone to about 5.5 mg/kg and the use of suxamethonium to ease the induction of continuation inhalation anaesthesia is unnecessary.

Ketamine

A combination of an α_2-adrenoceptor agonist pre medication and injection of a ketamine bolus 2 mg will produce an excellent induction of anaesthesia followed by a spectacularly rapid, but usually very quiet, recovery. It appears to be safe, and possesses certain advantages over α_2-adrenoceptor agonists/thiopentone or methohexitone combinations. However, if consistently good results are to be obtained a very strict adherence to a set procedure is essential. This procedure has evolved by trial and error and almost all the possible variations of it which have been tried have been found to be less consistently successful. In detail the method is as follows.

Xylazine (1 mg/kg) over a 2 minute period or detomidine (20 µg/kg) as a bolus is given by intravenous route before ketamine dose.

MAINTENANCE OF ANAESTHESIA

During general anaesthesia the weight of the horse compresses blood vessels so that tissues become ischaemic. In the lateral position the brachial nerves and vessels may be trapped between the humerus and the rib cage, while venous congestion of the upper hind limb can result from its weight causing adduction to obstruct veins in the groin. It is not entirely certain that postanaesthetic lameness can be prevented by careful positioning of the horse during anaesthesia. The same horse may be anaesthetized under apparently similar conditions for the same length of time and develop lameness on one occasion and not on another. However, raising the limbs by a B hoist so that the shoulder region is clear of the table or ground surface and the upper hind limb does not adduct appears to reduce its incidence after periods of lateral recumbency. Similarly, partial suspension by the legs in conjunction with the use of a V-shaped back support seems to diminish the risk of serious damage to the back muscles (Fig. 19.7). Under field conditions, where these facilities are not available by a horse lying on its side may have adduction of the upper limbs prevailed by supporting them on straw bales, and the

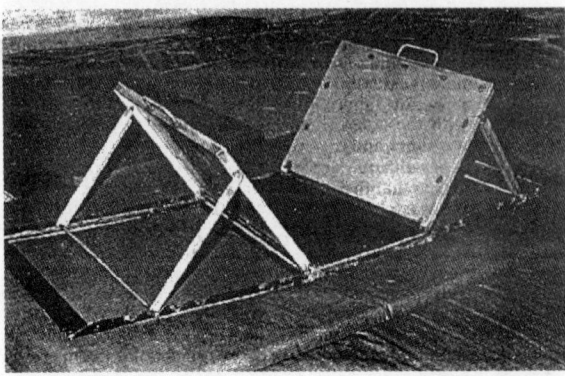

Fig. 19.7: Back support for supine horse. In use the support is covered with foam padding 3 inches (7.5 cm) thick. The weight of the horse is taken by the dorsal spines and the spines of the scapulae, thus avoiding pressure on the hack muscles

undermost foreleg may be drawn as far forward as possible to minimize pressure on the brachial vessels and nerves. A proper padding of the body by mattresses prevent vascular congestion and nerve damage.

Intravenous Agents

The advantages associated with the use of intravenous agents for the maintenance of anaesthesia are obvious. They are easy to administer using only the simplest of apparatus, there is no difficulty in instructing nursing staff or others to give controlled doses as needed during anaesthesia, and they do not pollute the atmosphere. The inhalation agents like halothane can be used safely for maintenance.

Ventilation (TPPV)

In hypovolaemic horses (e.g. many colic cases), and where the inhalation anaesthetic agents block the effect of sympathetic discharge, the peripheral venoconstriction may be inadequate to counter the rise in mean intrathoracic pressure due to IPPV so that venous return falls and the cardiac output declines. Diagnosis of hypovolaemia in horses is not always easy and even when correctly diagnosed there may be insufficient time for full replenishment of the blood volume by transfusion before anaesthesia has to be induced. For these reasons many anaesthetists claim that equine colic cases which may be hypovolaemic fare better if allowed to breathe spontaneously during anaesthesia even if their $PaCO_2$ rises to around 60 mmHg.

Experience is often the only reliable guide to proper pulmonary ventilation in any individual horse. Whenever possible, the arterial blood pressure should be monitored so that any embarrassment of the circulation can be recognized before too much harm results from an unsuitable pattern of lung inflation. Assisted ventilation, in which the horse triggers the ventilator which then delivers a prescribed tidal volume, cannot be recommended in equine anaesthesia. The horse determines the frequency and hence the minute volume of respiration, so under general anaesthesia alveolar hypoventilation and hypercapnia are to be expected.

Bibliography

1. Moller AW, In RW Kirk Ed., *Current Veterinary Therapy,* Vol. 3, Small Practice, p. 400–427, 1968.
2. Muir WW, Scarda, RT and Sheehan T, *Equine Pharmacology,* P. 18–173, 1987.
3. Soma LR, *Textbook of Veterinary Anaesthesia,* p. 121–621, 1978.

20

Anaesthesia for Cattle

LOCAL ANALGESIA

Any technique of local infiltration may be used in cattle. Although nerve blocks are simple to perform, many flank laparotomies are still carried out using clumsy, time-consuming and often inefficient T-block infiltration of the abdominal wall.

Cornual Nerve Block

The site for injection is the upper third of the temporal ridge, about 2.5 cm below the base of the horn (Fig. 20.1). The needle (19 gauge, 2.5 cm long) is inserted so that its point lies 0.7–1 cm deep, immediately behind the ridge, and 5 ml of local analgesic solution injected. The needle must not be inserted too deeply, otherwise injection will be made beneath the aponeurosis of the temporal muscle and the method will fail. In large animals with well-developed horns a second injec-

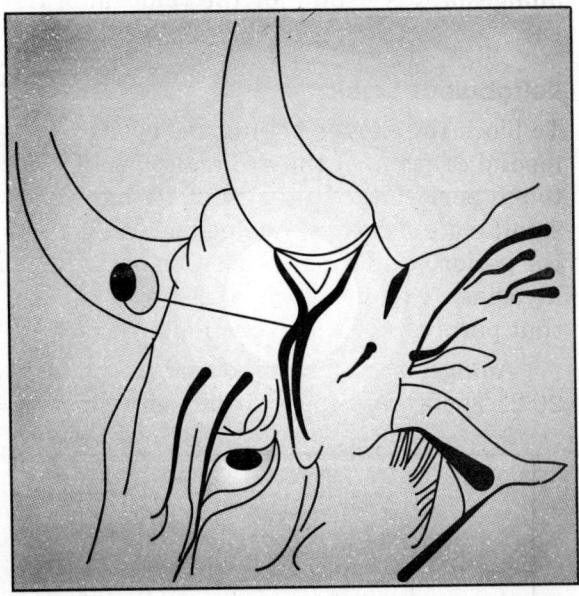

Fig. 20.1: Injection of the nerve to the horn core. In some animals the branch to the caudal part leaves the parent trunk cranial to the normal site for injection

tion should be made about 1 cm behind the first block in the posterior division of the nerve. Loss of sensation develops in 10–15 minutes and lasts about 1 hour. This form of nerve block has been widely used for the dishorning of adult cattle but under conditions of practice, it is not invariably successful. Variability in the curvature of the lateral ridge of the frontal bone makes exact determination of the site of the nerve difficult, while in a struggling' animal it may be difficult to ensure that the point of the needle is at the correct depth. A third injection may be required in adult cattle with well-developed horns; it is made posterior to the horn base to block cutaneous branches of the second cervical nerve.

Lignocaine hydrochloride, on account of its great power of diffusion in the tissues has come to be widely used for dishorning, generally as a 2% solution. Bupivacaine 0.5% has a longer duration of local anaesthetic action.

Auriculopalpebral Nerve Block

The nerve supplies motor fibres to the orbicularis oculi muscle. It runs from the base of the ear along the facial crest, past and ventral to the eye, giving off its branches on the way.

The needle is inserted in front of the base of the ear at the end of the zygomatic arch and is introduced until its point lies at the dorsal border of the arch.

About 10–15 ml of analgesic solution is injected beneath the fascia at this point.

This block is used to prevent eyelid closure during examination of, or interferences on, the eyeball. It does not produce analgesia of the eye or the lids. In conjunction with topical analgesia it is useful for the removal of foreign bodies from the cornea and conjunctival sac.

Retrobulbar Block

To block the nerves behind the eyeball a needle is introduced about 2.5 cm lateral to the medial canthus of the eye and pushed along the floor of the orbit until it penetrates the tough periorbita, 20–30 ml of 2% lignocaine solution (or its equivalent) being injected in small increments as the needle is advanced and the bulk of the injection is made beneath the periorbita. Proper deposition of the local analgesic solution produces corneal analgesia, mydriasis and proptosis of the eyeball. The nerves to the ocular muscles are blocked so that paralysis of the eyeball follows.

Analgesia may be produced in the forelimb by injection at the sites indicated in Fig. 20.2. The dorsal metacarpal nerve is located by palpation at about the middle of the

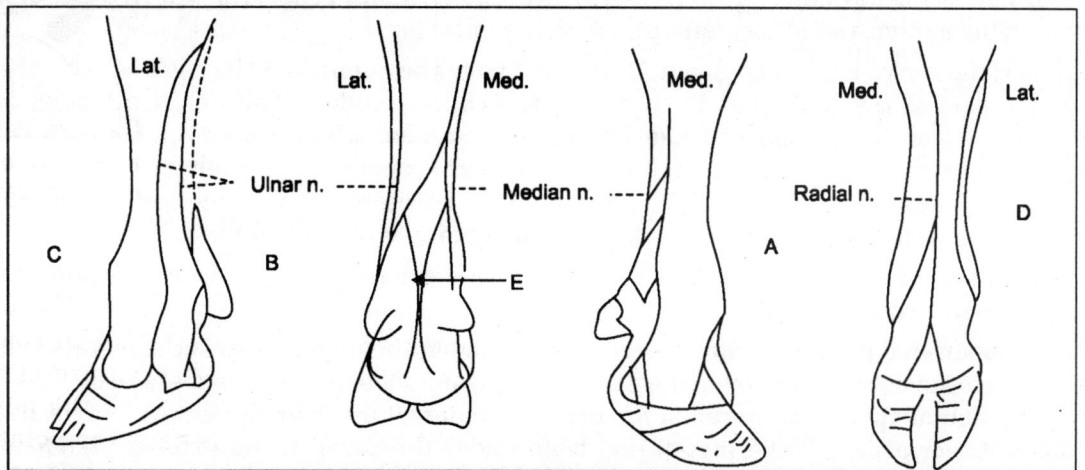

Fig. 20.2: Nerve block of the forlimb to block the whole of the digit, injections must be made at A, B, C, D and E. To block the medial digit, inject at A, D. and E. To block the lateral digit, inject at points B, C, D and E

metacarpus, medial to the extensor tendon. The dorsal branch of the ulnar is blocked about 5 cm above the fetlock on the lateral aspect of the limb, in the groove between the suspensory ligament and the metacarpal bone. At this point the volar branch of the ulnar nerve may also be blocked, the two nerves being respectively situated in front of, and behind, the suspensory ligament. The axial palmar aspect of the digits may be rendered analgesic by a single injection in the midline just above the fetlock. The injection will reach the lateral branch of the median nerve before it divides, or if it has already divided its two branches will still be close to each other. The two branches may also be simultaneously blocked on the midline just below the level of the dew-claws, i.e. after they have passed from below the fibrous plate of the dew-claws. The medial branch of the median nerve is blocked on the medial side of the limb in the groove between the suspensory ligament and the flexor tendons about 5 cm above the fetlock. As practically the whole of the palmar aspect, and a large part of the lateral aspect of the digits is supplied by the median nerve, the obvious point to make the injection is higher up the limb before the nerve divides. Unfortunately, at this point the nerve lies beneath the artery and vein and is not conveniently situated for injection.

The fibular (peroneal) nerve is blocked immediately behind the caudal edge of the lateral condyle of the tibia, over the fibula and before it dips down between the extensor pedis and flexor metatarsi muscles to divide into the deep and superficial fibular nerves. The bony prominence can easily be palpated in most animals, and in some the nerve itself can be rolled against the bone as it passes superficially, obliquely downwards and cranially, at this point. A narrow gauge needle about 2.5 cm long is inserted through the skin, the subcutaneous tissue and the aponeurotic sheet of the biceps femoris until its point just touches the bony landmark and 20 ml of lignocaine hydrochloride solution (or 0.5% bupivacain) are injected through it. Analgesia develops after 5–20 minutes. Paralysis of the nerve is shown by a loss of sensation in the exteroceptive area and a paralysis of the extensor muscles of the digit. The signs associated with this motor paralysis are that the animal can walk normally on a level surface but is inclined to stub the toe against obstructions so that the fetlock and phalangeal joints flex.

The tibial nerve is blocked about 10–12 cm above the summit of the calcaneus on the medial aspect of the limb, just in front of the Achilles tendon. The Achilles tendon is grasped between the thumb and index finger of one hand while a needle, about 2.5 cm long, is inserted immediately below the thumb until its point can be felt just under the skin by the index finger. About 15–20 ml of local analgesia solution is injected at this site and the block takes 5–15 minutes to develop, depending on the drug used.

When both nerves are blocked, (Fig. 20.3) there is complete loss of sensation from the fetlock downwards.

The superficial fibular (peroneal) nerve is blocked in the upper third of the metatarsus where it lies subcutaneously over the midline of the dorsal aspect of the metatarsal bone. The deep fibular (peroneal) nerve accompanies the dorsal metatarsal vessels in a groove on the anterior aspect of the metatarsal bone under the cover of the extensor tendons. Injection is made about half-way down the metatarsus beneath the extensor tendons. To facilitate this the needle is inserted from the lateral aspect of the bone and its point directed beneath the edge of the tendon. The plantar metatarsal nerves are blocked at the sites so familiar in the horse, i.e. in the depression on the medial and lateral sides of the limb between the suspensory ligament and the flexor tendons some 5 cm proximal to the fetlock joint and deep to the superficial fascia. About 5 ml of local analgesic solution is injected over each nerve.

Intravenous Regional Analgesia of the Digit

Lumbar segmental epidural injection results in a broad belt of analgesia encircling the abdomen and involving the whole depth of the wall including the parietal peritoneum. Analgesia develops some 10 minutes after injection and persists for about 3 hours.

GENERAL ANAESTHESIA

Because it is only safe when the trachea is intubated with a cuffed tube and the inspired gases are enriched with oxygen, general anaesthesia is seldom used when surgery has to be carried out on the farm. However, under hospital conditions where expert anaesthetists are available, general anaesthesia is often more convenient, more certain and less time consuming than methods of local analgesia.

Endotracheal Intubation

In adult cattle the larynx cannot be seen without the use of the Rowson laryngoscope and 'blind' intubation through the mouth is successful only on rare occasions unless manipulation of the tube is very gentle indeed. However, when the Rowson laryngoscope is not available, a tube may be introduced into the trachea with certainty if the procedure known as 'intubation by palpation' is adopted (Fig. 20.4).

For this, a wedge-shaped gag is insinuated between the molar teeth of the

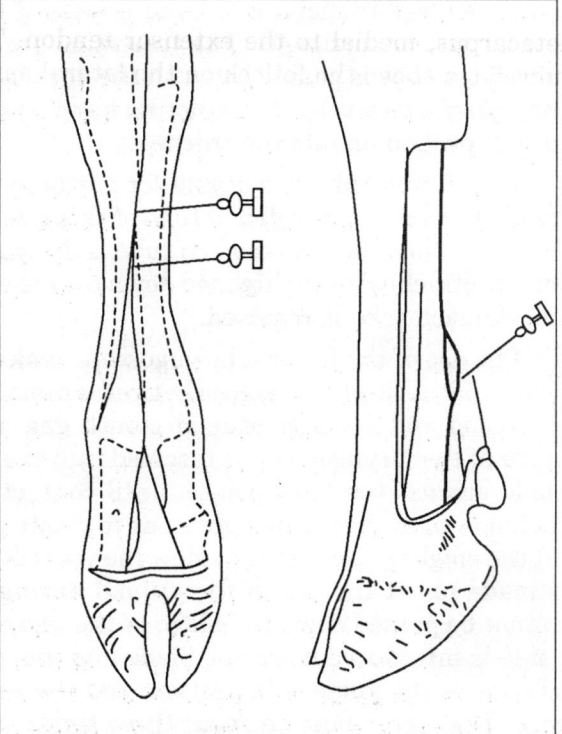

Fig. 20.3: Nerve block of the distal part of the hind-limb using Raker's technique: A. injection of the superficial peroneal nerve, B. Injection of the deep peroneal nerve, C. injection of the plantar metarsal nerves

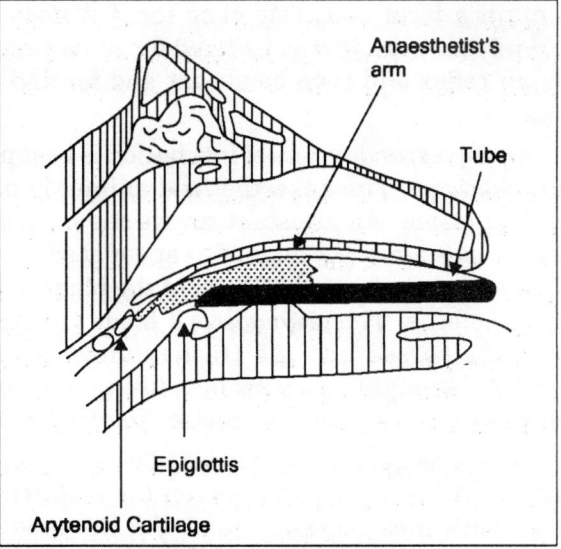

Fig. 20.4: Intubation by palpation

anaesthetized animal and a hand is passed through the mouth to identify the epiglottis and arytenoid cartilages. The fingertips are placed on the arytenoid cartilages and the lubricated tube is passed between the dorsum of the tongue and arm. The tube is directed through the glottis by the exploring hand which is then withdrawn from the mouth as the tube is pushed on into the trachea.

A 25.0 mm tube is suitable for cattle of about 450 kg body weight. It is sometimes impossible to accommodate a tube of this size and the forearm in the mouth cavity. Under these circumstances a stomach tube is directed into the trachea, the arm withdrawn and the endotracheal tube threaded down over the stomach tube and when it is correctly placed the stomach tube is removed.

The use of the Rowson laryngoscope makes intubation a relatively simple matter. The head and neck of the anaesthetized animal are positioned so that the head is in full extension and a wedge-shaped mouth gag is introduced between the molar teeth. The blade of the laryngoscope is inserted into the pharynx with the open side of the C-section blade against the hard palate, until contact is made with the epiglottis. The handle is then moved to the left or right so as to rotate the blade, when one of the two distal tips will lift the epiglottis, exposing to view the vocal cords and the interior of the larynx. No attempt is made to lift the jaw of the animal during this procedure. A large endotracheal tube cannot be passed down the blade of the instrument so a rubber-covered, fairly stout wire guide is introduced down the blade and into the trachea. The laryngoscope is withdrawn as soon as the guide is in position and the endotracheal tube is passed around the guide wire. The guide must be about three times as long as the endotracheal tube to avoid the possibility of its being lost into the trachea during this manoeuvre, and it is, of course, withdrawn from the lumen of the tube once this has been introduced. One problem is that the tube may catch on the epiglottis unless it is rotated at the appropriate moment.

The lubricant applied to any endotracheal tube used in ruminant animals should never contain a local analgesic drug for if it does the mucous membrane of the trachea and larynx may remain desensitized for some time after the tube is withdrawn. The protective cough reflex will then be absent and foreign material may be inhaled into the bronchial tree.

In calves, endotracheal intubation is best performed with the aid of a more conventional laryngoscope. The anaesthetized animal is placed on its back with its head and neck in full extension. An assistant draws the tongue well out of the mouth and fixes the upper jaw by pulling on the ends of a tape placed just behind the dental pad. The laryngoscope is then introduced so that the tip of the blade is behind the base of the tongue and in front of the epiglottis. The laryngoscope blade is lifted to expose the larynx and vocal cords and the tube passed into the trachea under direct vision. It is important to note that the larynx is brought into view by a lifting movement and not by employing the laryngoscope blade as a lever using the incisor teeth as a fulcrum.

Endotracheal tubes may also be passed through the mouth and 'threaded' through the larynx which is gripped between the anaesthetist's finger and thumb. Using this method it is sometimes necessary to stiffen the tube by passing down it a piece of straight brass rod of suitable length which is withdrawn as soon as the tube is in the trachea. It is difficult to pass tubes by this method unless the calf is quite deeply anaesthetized, but the method is useful if a laryngoscope is not available. Most newborn calves will accommodate tubes of 12 mm internal bore, and 16 mm tubes are adequate for animals of 3–4 months of age.

Intravenous Agents

Pentobarbitone Sodium

Satisfactory anaesthesia can be induced in small bovine animals by the slow intravenous injection of pentobarbitone sodium. The injection should occupy at least 4 minutes. Induction is quiet and the dose taken to induce light anaesthesia varies from 1–1.45 g/50 kg body weight. Surgical anaesthesia persists for about 30 minutes and is followed by a lightening narcosis. The animal will not be able to regain its feet in less than 3 hours. For the very young calf, animals up to 1 month old, pentobarbitone is unsuitable. Narcosis is prolonged for 2 days or even longer, and there is a grave danger that during this period the animal will succumb from oedema of the lungs, or that it may subsequently develop pneumonia.

Thiopentone Sodium

Thiopentone sodium has come to be used in adult cattle either alone to provide full anaesthesia for operations of short duration or to induce anaesthesia which is then maintained by inhalation agents. It enables anaesthesia to be induced in the standing animal so that casting tackle is unnecessary and only one assistant is required to hold the animal while the injection is being made.

Premedication is seldom indicated but if essential it must be remembered that its use may delay recovery from anaesthesia. Thiopentone sodium is injected rapidly into the jugular vein in a dose of 11 mg/kg estimated body weight; if xylazine premedication has been used a dose of 5–6 mg/kg is usually adequate. (The 5 g pack of the drug is particularly convenient. The dose should be dissolved in a maximum of 50 ml of water for larger volumes cannot be injected rapidly enough to produce unconsciousness when this minimal dose is employed. The animal sinks quietly to the ground within 20–30 seconds of injection and there is a brief period of apnoea. Apnoea seldom lasts for more than 15–20 seconds and artificial respiration is not required. Surgical anaesthesia of about 3–4 minutes' duration is followed by recovery which is usually complete within 45 minutes. Recovery is invariably quiet and free from excitement. The animal can be propped up, and will maintain a position of sternal recumbency, about 12–15 minutes after the injection of the drug. The period of surgical anaesthesia, although brief, is adequate for minor operations.

Bibliography

1. Moller A.W. In Kirk R.W., ed., Current veterinary Therapy, Vol. 3, Small Practice, P. 300, 1968.
2. Occupational Safety and Health Administration. New Publication of National Institute of Occupational Safety and Health (NIOSH). US Govt. Printing Office, Washington DC, 1992.
3. Soma L.R., *Textbook of Veterinary Anaesthesia,* P. 420, 1971.

21

Anaesthesia for Sheep and Goat

SEDATION OF THE SHEEP AND GOAT

α₂-Adrenoceptor Agonists and Antagonists

Most sheep can be sedated by the intramuscular injection of xylazine (0.2 mg/kg); some goats appear much more sensitive to this drug and doses of 0.05 mg/kg may result in profound sedation for 12 or more hours. Because results following intramuscular injection are unpredictable, in both sheep and goats it is probably best to administer the drug by very slow intravenous injection, assessing the degree of sedation as injection is made over some minutes. When given in this way doses of 0.1–0.15 mg/kg are usually required to sedate sheep, while 0.01 mg/kg are sufficient for most goats. In sheep, xylazine administration has occasionally been associated with the development of pulmonary oedema.

The intrathecal spinal injection of xylazine has been shown to result in analgesia and doses of 50 µg appear equivalent to an intravenous dose of 50 µg/kg but the duration of action is much shorter when the drug is given intravenously (45 minutes versus 120 minutes after intrathecal injection).

Medetomidine, in intravenous doses of 10–20 µg/kg, produces very deep sedation in sheep similar to that seen after the use of 0.2 mg/kg of xylazine.

Although little information is available, there is no reason why the α₂-adrenoceptor antagonists should not be used to counteract the effects of the α₂-adrenoceptor agonists in sheep and goats. In sheep, atipamezole given intravenously in doses of 25 or 50 µg/kg awakens animals sedated with 0.3 mg/kg of xylazine, but some animals given the lower dose relapse into a sedated state.

Benzodiazepines

Diazepam can be given by mouth in doses of about 15 mg/kg and wild sheep or aggressive male goats may be sedated by mixing this in a small meal of oats and bran, or a small quantity of concentrates. For procedures such as radiography or foot-trimmings, large rams or male goats may be given 2 mg/kg of diazepam by intramuscular injection, but these intramuscular injections appear to cause pain.

Midazolam may be given intravenously and a dose of 4 mg/kg produces, after about 3–5 minutes, very satisfactory sedation for most non-painful procedures.

Further increments of 1–2 mg/kg may be given intravenously to produce recumbency which lasts about 30 minutes, but it is difficult to produce full anaesthesia with this agent. A total dose of 1 mg of the antagonist, flumazenil, produces very rapid awakening when given by intravenous injection but relapse to deep sedation may follow.

Phenothiazine Derivatives

Only phenothiazine tranquillizer is likely to be used today for sedating sheep or goats. Acepromazine is usually used in sheep by intramuscular injection in doses of 0.05 mg/kg but the smaller breeds such as the soay may need up to 0.1 mg/kg for effective sedation. Most goats can be satisfactorily sedated by the intramuscular injection of 0.1 mg/kg. As in all ruminants, the phenothiazines relax the gastro-oesophageal junction and increase the risk of regurgitation of ruminal contents.

LOCAL ANALGESIA OF THE SHEEP AND GOAT

Nerve Blocking for Dishorning

Technique

The site for producing block of the cornual branch of the lacrimal nerve is caudal to the root of the supraorbital process (Fig. 21.1). The needle should be inserted as close as possible to the caudal ridge of the root of the supraorbital process to a depth of 1.0–1.5 cm.

The site for blocking the cornual branch of the infratrochlear nerve is at the dorsomedial margin of the orbit (Fig. 21.1). In some animals the nerve is palpable by applying slight pressure and moving the skin over this area. The needle should be inserted as close as possible to the margin of the orbit to a depth of about 0.5 cm. In adult animals, about 2–3 ml of local analgesic solution should be injected at each site.

These nerves may be blocked for the disbudding of kids, but kids are very small animals and it is all too easy to administer a toxic dose of local analgesic. A light general anaesthesia with halothane/oxygen is much safer for disbudding of these very young animals provided the oxygen mixture is switched off before any cautery is used.

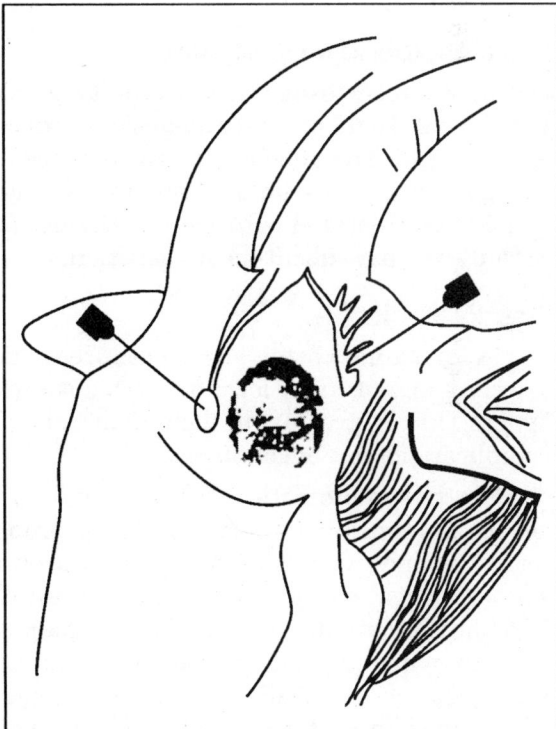

Fig. 21.1: Nerve blocks for dishorning of goats. The cornial branches of both the lacrimal and infratrochlear nerves must be blocked. Care must be taken in young kids to ensure that attempts to block both these nerves do not lead to the injection of toxic quantities of local analgesic solution

Paravertebral Block

For operations carried out through the flank the thirteenth thoracic and the first three lumbar nerves are blocked. For each of these nerves 5 ml of 1% lignocaine hydrochloride with 1:100, 000 adrenaline is injected ventral to the intertransverse ligament and a further 2 ml is injected dorsal to the ligament. An increase in the skin temperature due to hyperaemia can be detected very soon after injection and full analgesia is present about 5 minutes later. Analgesia persists for about 60 minutes.

Pudendal Block

After clipping and skin disinfection a finger is introduced into the rectum and the slit-like lesser ischiatic notch is located on one side (usually about finger depth from the anus). The needle is inserted at the corresponding site and 7 ml of local analgesic solution (e.g. 2% lignocaine hydrochloride with 1:100, 000 adrenaline) is injected at the notch. After massage through the rectal wall to distribute the solution, the other side is injected keeping the same finger in the rectum. Complete analgesia and in the ram, exposure of the penis follow within about 5 minutes of injection of the second side.

Local Analgesia for Castration

Dosage for intratesticular injection depends on the size and age of the animal concerned and from 2–10 ml of local analgesic solution (1% lignocaine hydrochloride) is injected into each testicle. The needle is plunged perpendicularly through the tensed scrotal skin into the testicle and the bulk of the dose is injected into its substance. The line of the skin incision is infiltrated with the remainder of the dose after the point of the needle has been withdrawn to a subcutaneous position.

Caudal Block

For intravaginal obstetrical procedures caudal epidural analgesia may be induced by the injection of 3–4 ml of local analgesic solution into the canal through the sacrococcygeal space. This is a valuable technique and if careful aseptic precautions are observed no complications are encountered.

For the symptomatic relief of painful conditions of the vagina and rectum which provoke severe and continuous straining the technique of continuous caudal block can be extremely useful. A fine nylon catheter is introduced into the canal through a Tuohy needle at the sacrococcygeal space and advanced cranially for 6–8 cm. The needle is then withdrawn leaving the catheter *in situ*. Local analgesic solution (3–4 ml) is injected through the catheter whenever the animal shows signs of sensation returning to the pelvic organs. If all injections are made with aseptic precautions and the free end of the catheter is maintained in a sterile condition — capped and bound up in a sterile gauze swab, for example — between injections, analgesia can be safely maintained for many hours by this technique

The injection of 0.75–1 ml of 1% lignocaine hydrochloride, or its equivalent, at the sacrococcygeal space provides excellent analgesia for the docking of lambs' tails but it must be remembered that analgesia takes about 5 minutes to develop after the injection is made.

Epidural and Subarachnoid Block

With full aseptic precautions, the site of the introduction of the epidural needle is infiltrated with 2 or 3 ml of local analgesic solution using a very fine needle. A large-bore needle is introduced through the insensitive zone made by this injection and then withdrawn to leave a clearly defined skin puncture. The epidural needle (6 cm long, 16 gauge with a fitted stilette) is inserted through the skin puncture and directed towards the lumbosacral space (Fig. 21.2). When the needle point is judged to have entered the tough ligamentum flavum the stilette is removed and a 20 ml syringe containing about 5 ml of air is attached to the needle. The needle is advanced cautiously with one hand while the thumb of the other hand maintains a continuous pressure on the plunger of the syringe. The sudden loss of resistance to injection of the air when the needle emerges from the ligamentum flavum is immediately apparent by

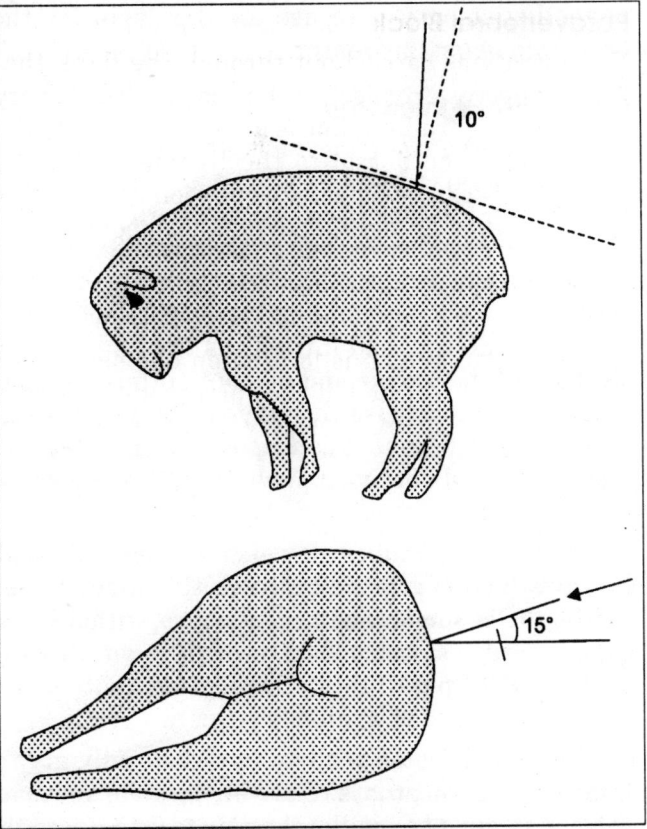

Fig. 21.2: Direction of insertion of needle for lumbar epidural injection in sheep in lateral recumbency

movement of the syringe piston. The loss of resistance indicates that the epidural space has been entered and the injection of air tends to force the dura away from the advancing needle point. Next, an attempt is made to aspirate cerebrospinal fluid into the syringe. If fluid is drawn into the syringe or drips from the needle when the syringe is detached it must be assumed that the dura has been punctured and in these circumstances either a subarachnoid injection is made or the whole procedure should be abandoned, for experience has shown that it is not safe merely to withdraw the needle slightly and proceed with the epidural injection. If all is well and the dura has not been punctured a syringe containing the local analgesic solution is attached to the needle and the injection made. If predominantly unilateral analgesia is required the sheep is maintained in lateral recumbency (the side to be desensitized being undermost) but if bilateral analgesia is desired the animal is turned on to its back as soon as the needle is removed. In either case it is an advantage to apply a 10° head-down tilt to the animal's body by raising the end of the table till LA is fixed with 1.5% of lignocaine 8–15 ml.

The ear veins, cephalic vein and jugular veins are used in sheep for infusion or for taking the sample, but the accurate intravenous injection of agents is not so easy. Most anaesthetists prefer to use another vein for the injection of tissue irritants such as thiopentone for this reason.

Endotracheal Intubation

In sheep and goats endotracheal intubation is best performed under direct vision with the aid of a laryngoscope. The anaesthetized animal is placed on its back with its head and neck in full extension. An assistant draws the tongue well out of the mouth, holding it in a gauze sponge for better grip, and fixes the upper jaw by pulling gently downwards on the ends of a tape placed just behind the dental pad. The anaesthetist uses a gauze sponge on a sponge-holding forceps to clear the mouth of saliva and any regurgitated ruminal contents, and introduces the laryngoscope so that the tip of its blade is behind the base of the tongue and in front of the epiglottis. The laryngoscope blade is then lifted horizontally to expose the larynx and vocal cords and the tube passed into the trachea under direct vision. It is important that the larynx is brought into view by a lifting movement and not by employing the laryngoscope blade as a lever using the dental pad as a fulcrum.

Endotracheal tubes may also be passed through the mouth and 'threaded' through the larynx which is gripped between the anaesthetist's finger and thumb. When using this method it is sometimes necessary to stiffen the tube by passing down a piece of thick copper wire of suitable length which is withdrawn as soon as the tube is in the trachea. It is difficult to pass tubes of really adequate size by this technique but it is useful if a laryngoscope is not available.

Tubes lubricated with an analgesic jelly may also be passed through the nostril. The inferior nasal meatus is relatively large in sheep and goats and although tubes passed via the nostril must be smaller than those introduced through the mouth reasonably adequately sized ones can be used. If the tube passed up the nostril cannot be introduced blindly through the larynx a laryngoscope is used to expose the tip of the tube in the pharynx and the vocal cords. The tip of the tube is grasped with Magill's intubation forceps and assisted into the laryngeal opening as it is advanced through the nostril.

For large sheep a 16 mm tube can be passed through the mouth and a 12 mm tube through the nostril. For intubation of adult goats by the oral route 11 and 12 mm tubes are usually adequate.

PREPARATION FOR ANAESTHESIA OF THE SHEEP AND GOAT

Most clinical surgery performed on sheep is carried out at short notice — e.g. caesarean section for dystocia — and there is no time to prepare the animal for anaesthesia. Experience of such situations suggests that there may be little need to withhold food and water before anaesthesia for non-emergency surgery since sheep do not regurgitate copiously at the time of induction of general anaesthesia and any ruminal tympany may be dealt with by passing a stomach tube or by needle paracentesis of the rumen. In goats, planned surgery (e.g. for the repair of fractures) is more common and for this preanaesthetic preparation is possible but, again, experience has shown there is no good reason for denying access to food and water right up to the time of operation. It is doubtful if atropine has any value in sheep and goats. The doses necessary to prevent salivation completely (0.2–0.8 mg/kg) produce undesirable tachycardia and ocular effects, while smaller doses merely make the saliva more viscid and hence more difficult to drain from the oropharynx. On the rare occasion when bradycardia develops during general anaesthesia an anticholinergic (e.g. atropine, 0.6–1.2 mg) may be given intravenously.

Sedative premedication is seldom necessary before general anaesthesia and, if given, can delay recovery. It may, however, be useful in counteracting some of the undesirable side-effects of the anaesthetic agents. Probably the best sedative premedication is diazepam given intravenously in doses of 1 mg/kg, or 2 mg/kg intramuscularly; it is particularly effective in both sheep and goats in countering the unwanted actions of ketamine.

GENERAL ANAESTHESIA OF THE SHEEP AND GOAT

Sheep and goats should not be maintained for any longer than is essential in the supine position during general anaesthesia. In this position the weight of the ruminal and intestinal contents compresses the aorta and posterior vena cava, leading to circulatory embarrassment (supine hypotensive syndrome) and restricts the free movement of the diaphragm, giving rise to respiratory acidosis with decreased tidal volume and alveolar collapse. Whenever possible-surgery should be carried out with the animal in lateral decubitus, or in the prone position with the pelvis supported in such a way as to allow free movement of the abdominal wall during breathing. A jointed operating table which is tilted so that the hind-quarters of the laterally recumbent or prone animal are about 15 cm below the level of the withers, to allow the abdominal viscera to fall away from the diaphragm, and the head is inclined downwards to allow saliva and any regurgitated ruminal contents to drain from the mouth, is highly desirable if much surgery is to be performed on sheep and goats.

A cuffed endotracheal tube should always be passed as soon as possible after the induction of anaesthesia to prevent the inhalation of saliva and regurgitated ruminal contents, and for all but the shortest anaesthetics a stomach tube should be introduced into the rumen to prevent the development of ruminal tympany. If the rumen still becomes distended with gas in spite of the presence of the stomach tube no time should be lost in performing paracentesis through the left flank with a 14 gauge needle.

Unconscious sheep and goats will continue to produce saliva and because this will not be swallowed and reabsorbed, progressive acidosis develops. These animals may lose up to 500 ml of saliva per hour and during long operations this loss should be replaced by the injection of sodium bicarbonate solution at a rate of 1 mmol/(kg/h).

Intravenous Anaesthesia of the Sheep and Goat

What little clinical surgery has to be performed on sheep and goats is probably best carried out under inhalation anaesthesia and the role of the intravenous drugs should only be that of inducing anaesthesia in particularly vigorous animals. Nevertheless, in certain situations, especially when only relatively minor surgery is contemplated, intravenous anaesthesia can be useful.

Pentobarbitone Sodium

In lambs up to 2 months old a dose of 29 mg/kg by slow intravenous pentobarbitone injection gave anesthesia of sufficient depth and duration for abdominal surgery. With adult sheep there was found great variation in response to the drug. In all cases the duration of anaesthesia was shorter than in lambs, about 15 minutes only. In adult sheep the dose for induction varied from 28 to 33 mg/kg.

Pentobarbitone sodium appears to be a satisfactory anaesthetic for minor operations of short duration in sheep but, in contrast to its effects in other species of animal, detoxication is rapid; the duration of anaesthesia from a single injection is short and thus it is not satisfactory for prolonged intra-abdominal surgery. Today, most workers prefer to use pentobarbitone simply as an induction agent and to maintain anaesthesia with an inhalation anaesthetic administered through the endotracheal tube.

Thiopentone Sodium

An initial dose of about 10 mg/kg of thiopentone in a 2.5% solution given by intravenous injection produces induction of anaesthesia and, often, 30–50 seconds of apnoea. During the period of apnoea, muscle relaxation is profound enough for the jaw to be opened widely and endotracheal intubation to be performed. Recovery from thiopentone is considerably quicker than from pentobarbitone and is usually quiet and uneventful. Defecation always occurs during anaesthesia and regurgitation of ruminal contents is not uncommon. Today, thiopentone sodium is extensively used to induce anaesthesia which is to be maintained by endotracheal inhalation methods.

Methohexitone Sodium

In both sheep and goats the intravenous injection of 4 mg/kg of a 2.5% solution of methohexitone sodium produces anaesthesia of 5–7 minutes' duration. Recovery to the standing position is complete within 10–14 minutes of the injection but the recovery is usually associated with violent jerking or convulsive movements and excitement if the animal is disturbed by noise during this period. Anaesthesia may be prolonged by the injection of 50–75 mg/min of the drug. It is used less frequently now-a-days.

INHALATIONAL AGENTS

Fluorinated Agents

Halothane is most commonly used. Enflurane, isoflurane and sevoflurane have apparently not been used to anaesthetize sheep or goats for clinical surgery. They are more expensive and are unlikely to offer any major advantages over halothane in these animals.

The Recovery Period

After general anaesthesia the endotracheal tube should be left in place until the animal has regained the swallowing and cough reflexes. As in all ruminants, sheep and goats should be propped up in the prone position, supported on either side by bales, so that eructation can take place during the recovery period. They should be kept under observation to ensure that company does not develop due to them slipping into lateral recumbency. Hypothermia is unlikely to occur unless the environment is exceptionally cold.

The relief of postoperative pain demands the same care in sheep and goats as in all other animals. Because they do not become violent when in pain it is often assumed that they are comfortable when in fact pain may be acute. The different, much more normal behaviour seen after the administration of a suitable analgesic is often remarkable. Up to 10 mg of morphine or 250 mg of pethidine by intramuscular injection is usually adequate for up to 4 hours in spite of experimental evidence of a much shorter period of effectiveness.

Camels (Camelus dromedarius)
Local and Regional Analgesia

Nerve blocks of the hindlimb in camels were reported by various workers. These workers described the topographical anatomy and technique of nerve blocks of the peroneal, tibial and plantar nerves with 2% lignocaine. However, it is probable that intravenous regional analgesia for foot operations, being easier to perform, will always be preferred for desensitization of the digit. Intravenous regional analgesia may be produced by the injection of 60 ml of 2% lignocaine (without adrenaline) distal to a tourniquet applied halfway down the limb without prior exsanguination.

Epidural block may be produced by the injection of 2% lignocaine or its equivalent at the sacrococcygeal or first intercoccygeal space. A 5 cm long, 19 gauge needle is inserted at an angle of about 45° with the horizontal in an animal restrained in the sitting position. For caudal block 12–15 ml of solution is adequate; 50 ml will produce sensory block caudally from the umbilicus.

Chloral Hydrate
Guaiphenesin and Thiopentone

Guaiphenesin (100–110 mg/kg) intravenously produces ataxia and intravenous thiopentone (4.5 mg/kg) may then be used to produce anaesthesia which can be maintained with halothane/oxygen administered by mask or through an endotracheal tube using a low-flow absorption method.

α_2-adrenoceptor Agonists

Xylazine given intramuscularly at a dosage rate of 0.4 mg/kg produces obvious sedation after about 9 minutes, followed quite quickly by recumbency. Recovery to the standing position occurs some 3 hours after injection. Arterial hypotension is not associated with elevated central venous pressure or bradycardia, but marked hyperglycaemia occurs. The vagal stimulation is responsible for first-degree atrioventricular block, sinoatrial block, sinus arrhythmia and wandering pacemaker in the sinoatrial node. This dose of xylazine is claimed to provide adequate/sedation and analgesia with sufficient muscle relaxation for minor surgery of short duration.

Intravenous xylazine 0.5 mg/kg produces a state bordering on full anaesthesia which lasts for approximately 30 minutes; the animals usually sit up after about 45 minutes and stand about 15 minutes later. The xylazine antagonist, tolazoline, given intravenously in doses of 0.4 mg/kg 15 minutes after the administration of the xylazine, enables the animals to stand 15 minutes later.

Detomidine in doses of 50 µg/kg by intramuscular injection usually produces recumbency within 10 minutes. As sedation develops the neck muscles relax and the head droops. Ataxia is followed by voluntary sternal recumbency. Preliminary studies indicate that analgesia can be expected to be present for the next hours. The heart rate, respiratory rate and rectal temperature show little change from preinjection levels during the period of sedation. Recovery is quiet and the animals stand about 3 hours from the time of injection. Although there are no reports of their use it is likely that the α_2-adrenoceptor antagonists can be given to hasten recovery from detomidine sedation.

Ketamine

Ketamine (1–2 mg/kg intravenously) may be used after xylazine (0.4–0.5 mg/kg intramuscularly) to produce anaesthesia of approximately 30 minutes' duration with good muscle relaxation. Full recovery takes about 3 hours from the time of the ketamine injection. Because intravenous ketamine injection may be followed by a rather long period of apnoea many workers prefer to give this drug intramuscularly. The doses of both xylazine and ketamine may be reduced in tame, working camels and in the very young.

Inhalation Anaesthesia

Inhalation anaesthesia is best administered through an endotracheal tube but intubation in male animals can be difficult due to the 'goola' pouches. Interference from the pouches can be minimized by ensuring free respiration through the nostrils during the intubation process; the tube is not likely to enter the pouch opening for this faces caudally and not cranially. It is advisable to induce complete relaxation of the jaw muscles with an intravenous or intramuscular agent so that the mouth can be opened widely. In the adult the technique of intubation is similar to that used in cattle but the male animal has prominent canine teeth and in both sexes the cheek teeth are usually very sharp. The use of a good mouth gag to protect the anaesthetist's arm is almost essential. Small, young animals are best intubated using a laryngoscope and difficulties arise when the animal has grown too large for this and the mouth cavity is too small to admit a palpating hand. Blind intubation is possible if the head and neck are extended and the tube is stiffened with a maleable stilette but can be more difficult than in cattle.

Halothane is the least expensive of the inhalation agents used today and is usually given after induction of unconsciousness with an intravenous or intramuscular agent. Respiratory depression is marked and it is a common practice to fast camels for 48 hours prior to general anaesthesia to minimize the weight of the forestomach and prevent tympany from developing. Respiratory function is best maintained when the animal is in sternal recumbency and this position should always be adopted for the recovery period.

It is generally agreed that regurgitation of stomach contents occurs more readily in camels than in cattle. In camels the oesophagus enters directly into the forestomach unlike in cattle where the oesophageal opening is at the junction of the rumen and the reticulum.

It is not known whether this difference accounts for the higher incidence of regurgitation in anaesthetized camels.

Buffaloes (Bubalus bubalis)

Most anaesthetic techniques for the buffalo have been adapted from those used in cattle but there are marked differences in the way in which they respond to some agents.

α_2-adrenoceptor Agonists

The effects of xylazine on buffalo calves have been reported. Intravenous doses of 0.22–0.44 mg/kg produce dose-related duration of sedation from to–130 minutes. Intramuscular doses of 0.44 mg/kg produce inability to stand for some 150 minutes while intramuscular administration of 0.22 mg/kg of xylazine produces excellent sedation, analgesia and moderate muscle relaxation with an onset time of 10–15 minutes and a duration of approximately 45–60 minutes.

Preliminary trials of detomidine indicate that 20 μg/kg by intramuscular injection produces deep sedation of about 30 minutes' duration. This dose may be associated with recumbency, but there is no evidence of cutaneous analgesia and the swallowing reflex is not abolished in the sedated animal. Intramuscular doses of 40 μg/kg cause the animal to lie down and saliva runs from the mouth but it is not clear whether this indicates increased production of saliva or inability to swallow the normal quantities; recovery is usually complete in 50–70 minutes. Micturition is usual as sedation develops and vocalization is not uncommon. Under deep detomidine sedation the P_aCO_2 is usually about 43 mmHg (5.7 kPa) and the P_aCb about 75 mmHg (10 kPa).

There appear to be no reports of α_2-adrenoceptor antagonists being used to hasten the awakening of buffaloes given xylazine or detomidine, but there is no obvious reason why they should not be given for this purpose.

Chloral Hydrate

Administered intravenously at doses of between 0.13 and 0.18 g/kg, chloral hydrate was found to be superior to the barbiturates. The drug has also been administered mixed with magnesium sulphate and a barbiturate in the proportions of 30 g chloral hydrate, 15 g magnesium sulphate and 2.5 g thiopentone per litre. Some 2 ml/kg of this mixture produce anaesthesia of 15–25 minutes' duration.

Guaiphenesin

The intravenous infusion of 165 mg/kg of guaiphenesin to buffalo calves has been found to produce unacceptable levels of arterial hypotension and respiratory depression. Smaller doses may be free from these disadvantages.

Ketamine

The ketamine has been used on its own and with chlorpromazine hydrochloride in buffalo calves on blood glucose, serum glutamic pyruvic transaminase, serum glutamic oxaloacetic transaminase and lactic dehydrogenase.

In buffalo calves up to 1.5 years old, 2 mg/kg of ketamine by intravenous injection produces an anaesthetic effect of 3–5 minutes' duration. This is characterized by rigidity of the limb muscles but analgesia seems profound. Intramuscular injection of 2 mg/kg of chlorpromazine 15 minutes prior to the intravenous injection of this dose of ketamine is given.

Elephant

Only the Indian or Asiatic elephant can be regarded as a domestic animal. Trained elephants are usually relatively quiet and intravenous injection into an ear vein presents no great difficulty but animals that are not so tame may need to be dosed by dartgun.

Xylazine (0.08–0.15 mg/kg) given by intravenous or intramuscular injection may be used to sedate elephants. They become somnolent but usually remain standing and recovery from a single dose takes about 3 hours.

Etorphine at a dose of 2 µg/kg will yield satisfactory sedation for the performance of venepuncture and the administration of drugs such as thiopentone to produce the desired depth of anaesthesia. Endotracheal intubation presents no difficulty for the mouth can usually be opened widely. Maintenance of anaesthesia is usually with halothane/oxygen and, at the end, the administration of diprenorphine at twice the etorphine dose hastens recovery. Some anaesthetists prefer the use of immobilon (2.45 mg etorphine plus 10 mg/ ml acepromazine per ml) to plain etorphine, claiming the mixture to be more effective than etorphine on its own.

At the University of Florida School, were sedated juvenile elephants (between 3 and 5 years old) weighing between 300 and 650 kg for transport with a xylazin/ketamine cocktail (0.1 and 0.6 mg/kg respectively by intramuscular injection), then induced anaesthesia with intramuscular etorphine 2 µg/kg which took about 20 minutes to produce recumbency and unconsciousness. Oral intubation with a cuffed endotracheal tube was performed by manual palpation, checking to exclude the presence of food residues in the mouth. Bivona, thick-walled, endotracheal tubes of 18 mm internal diameter i.d. were used for elephants up to 250 kg body weight, 22 mm i.d. for those up to 300 kg, 26 mm (i.d.) for up to 450 kg, and 30 mm i.d. tubes were used for any larger animals. Anaesthesia was maintained with halothane in oxygen, the initial vaporizer setting with a fresh gas flow rate of 3–5 l/min (i.e. a 'low-flow' setting) to a large animal circle absorber system being less than 1%, rising to 1–2% after the first 40–60 minutes. With spontaneous breathing blood gas values were in the region of 80–150 mmHg (10.7–20 kPa) for the P_aO_2 and 50–60 mmHg (6.7–8 kPa) for the P_aCO_2 with typical respiratory rates of 6–12 breaths/min. If the $PaCO_2$ climbed to around 60 mmHg (8 kPa) IPPV was performed using an equine ventilator set to deliver between 5 and 10 ml/kg. Heart rates were between 40–60 beats/min and the systolic blood pressure was well maintained at over 100 mmHg. Of 20 elephants, two developed episodes of ventricular arrhythmias and one showed second-degree heart block. Monitoring was via an ECG (lead 2 with the electrodes set for a base-apex system) and arterial blood pressure by intra-arterial pressure recording from an auricular artery or by using a Doppler-shift flow detector distal to a pressure cuff on the tail. At the end of anaesthesia the halothane was turned off and when good jaw muscle tone was present diprenorphine was given at twice the dose of etorphine used for the induction of anaesthesia. Extubation was carried out as soon as the animals rose to sternal recumbency. Because of hot weather conditions all the animals were given balanced electrolyte solutions at the rate of 10–20 ml/kg/h from the time of induction of anaesthesia until just before extubation. One animal collapsed when given the diprenorphine and ventilatory support was needed.

Bibliography

1. Grahm Jones *Small Animal Anaesthesia,* p. 151, 1964.
2. Kirk R. W. *Current Veterinary Therapy,* Vol. 3, Small Practice, 1968.
3. Soma L. R., *Textbook of Veterinary Aneasthesia,* p. 99, 1971.

22

Anaesthesia for Pig

SEDATION OF THE PIG

A rise in temperature is observed by anaesthetist alongwith spreading apart of the digits. Next, the body temperature starts to rise and the skin often shows blotchy reddening. If no attempt is made to treat the condition, the body temperature continues to rise (rectal temperatures of over 42°C have been recorded); eventually respiration ceases and death ensues. Presumably death is due to cellular hypoxia, for at temperatures over 42°C oxygen utilization exceeds oxygen supply.

Although various treatments have been described, there is no specific therapy for malignant hyperthermia and, at present, immediate cooling coupled with the administration of sodium bicarbonate provide the best chance of success. Dantrolene sodium, skeletal muscle relaxant, given orally before the induction of anaesthesia, may prevent the onset of the syndrome in susceptible pigs and in doses of between 2 and 10 mg/kg it has proved of some use in the treatment of the established condition. Induction of anaesthesia with saffan also affords a measure of protection against the development of the syndrome in some strains of susceptible animals.

The pig's reaction to restraint (struggling accompanied by ear-splitting squeals) is unpleasant for all concerned and, therefore, sedation is widely used to facilitate all handling and minor procedures, as well as for restraint prior to local or general anaesthesia. In the pig, α_2-adrenoceptor agonists may help in smoothing reactions to ketamine but, for reasons as yet unknown, they are generally ineffective as sedatives.

Azaperone

This butyrophenone drug is inexpensive and extremely safe and effective in pigs so that other sedatives are now seldom used in these animals. It is marketed both to the veterinary profession for clinical use and directly to farmers who use it to control fighting when mixing litters in intensive units.

Azaperone must be given by deep intramuscular injection, the neck muscles behind the ear usually proving to be the most convenient and best site. Subcutaneous injection is ineffective and intravenous injection results in a phase of violent excitement. The doses used depend on the effects sought and range from 1–8 mg/kg, but it is recommended that a dose of 1 mg/kg is not exceeded for adult boars as higher doses cause protrusion of the penis with the risk of subsequent damage to that organ. Following an intramuscular injection of 1–8 mg/kg of azaperone, the pig should be left undisturbed for 20 minutes, as interference before this time may provoke an excitement reaction. Excitement may occur during this induction phase even in the absence of stimulation, but it is usually mild and rarely of clinical significance. After the induction period of some 20 minutes, the pig is deeply sedated and handling for the administration of other drugs or minor procedures is greatly facilitated.

Azaperone causes vasodilatation resulting in a small fall in arterial blood pressure, and some slight respiratory stimulation. The vasodilatation of cutaneous vessels makes the sedated pig particularly likely to develop hypothermia in a cold environment so warm surroundings are essential, but the dilated ear veins are easy to enter for the intravenous injection of drugs.

Droperidol

The butyrophenone compound, droperidol, has been used in pigs and doses of 0.1–0.4 mg/kg give similar sedation to that produced by azaperone. The fentanyl with droperidol produced better sedation than droperidol alone.

More recently at the Cambridge Veterinary School it has been found that a combination of droperidol (0.5 mg/kg) with midazolam (0.3 mg/kg) given separately or, where appropriate, from the same syringe, into the gluteal or biceps femoris muscles, produces ideal sedation for radiography, lancing of abscesses, etc.

Dependable sedation of approximately 15 minutes follows some 10 minutes from the time of injection, but it is important to leave the pig undisturbed whilst the effects are developing. As with ketamine, sudden awakening without prior warning may occur.

Acepromazine

Pigs are easily restrained for intravenous injection if acepromazine (0.03–0.1 mg/kg) is given by intramuscular injection before venepuncture is attempted. Under the influence of acepromazine they do not squeal when handled and are much less likely to dislodge the venepuncture needle by head shaking (Fig. 22.1). Acepromazine may itself be given intravenously but may cause thrombosis of the vein unless very dilute solutions are used. When given by intravenous injection the drug should be allowed 10–20 minutes to produce its full effects. Intravenous injection may be followed by hyperpnoea which lasts for about 15 minutes, but the reason for this is unknown.

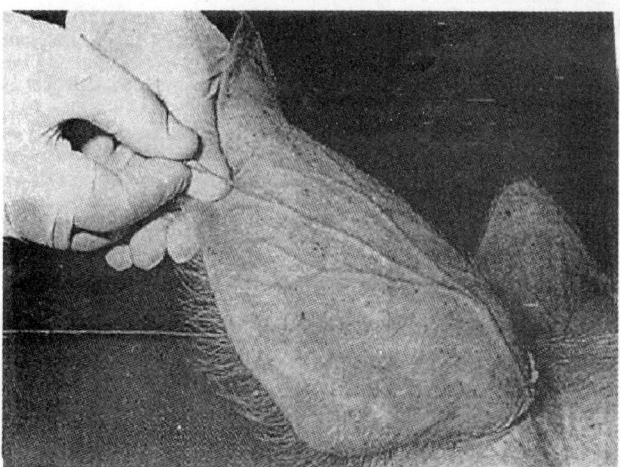

Fig. 22.1: Distension of the ear veins by the application of an elastic band around the base of the ear

PREPARATION FOR GENERAL ANAESTHESIA

In pigs, 6–8 hours' fasting and 2 hours' deprivation of water is usually adequate to ensure that the stomach is empty. Vomiting at induction is rare in pigs (although it used to be seen regularly during recovery from cyclopropane anaesthesia) but a full stomach exerts pressure on the diaphragm and reduces respiratory efficiency. The majority of surgery carried out in pigs, whether clinical or experimental, is elective and fluid deficits are seldom present before anaesthesia. An intravenous infusion may be needed, however, before anaesthesia for the correction of a strangulated hernia. Details of existing drug therapy such as antibiotic food additives, or anthelmintics, should be noted — especially if muscle relaxants whose action they may lengthen are to be used in the anaesthetic technique.

PREMEDICATION

During general anaesthesia salivation, even if not excessive, may cause respiratory obstruction. Atropine, intramuscularly or intravenously, in doses of 0.3–2.4 mg, or glycopyrrolate (0.2–2.0 mg), depending on the size of the pig, will usually control this salivation.

The degree of sedation required depends on the anaesthetic technique which is to follow. Some anaesthetists prefer to dispense with sedation at this stage, while others use it to facilitate the administration of the anaesthetic and to reduce the squealing which would otherwise occur at induction. Only rarely is there any need for analgesics to be included in the premedication but if required they may be employed in slightly larger doses than are used in dogs. It is probable that azaperone is the most widely used medicant drug for porcine anaesthesia. As already mentioned, it is given by intramuscular injection in doses of 1–8 mg/kg according to the degree of sedation required.

INTRAVENOUS TECHNIQUE

Intravenous injections are best made into one of the auricular veins on the external aspect of the ear-flap. Small pigs are restrained on their side on a table. One assistant leans on the neck and trunk, at the same time gripping the legs, whilst the second assistant holds the uppermost ear at the base of the conchal cartilage and applies pressure to the vein as near to the base of the ear as possible. If a second assistant is not available, a rubber band is applied around the base of the ear-flap. In large pigs, a noose is applied around the upper jaw behind the tusks as previously described. As in small pigs, the ear veins are distended by the application of pressure as near to the base of the ear-flap as possible.

Once the ear-flap has been cleaned, the veins are usually easily visible, but if necessary they can be made more obvious by gentle slapping and brisk rubbing of the ear-flap with an alcohol-soaked gauze swab. Venepuncture is then carried out using a needle about 2.5 cm long and, depending on the calibre of the vessel, 21–23 gauge (0.8–0.65 mm). In large pigs blood can be aspirated into an attached syringe once the needle has been inserted into the vein but in small pigs the amount of blood in the vein between the points of pressure and insertion of the needle may be so small that it is impossible to withdraw any into the syringe. In such cases injection must be attempted and if the needle is not in the lumen of the vein a subcutaneous bleb will develop. When it is certain that the needle is in the vein the pressure is released (if a rubber band has been applied to the base of the ear-flap the band must be cut with scissors) and the injection made. It will be noticed that the solution injected washes the blood out of the vein and this affords further evidence that the needle is correctly placed in the lumen of the vessel.

Introduction of a catheter into an ear vein is not difficult but these veins are not very suitable for the administration of large quantities of fluid. Fortunately such treatment is seldom needed, but if it is necessary it is usually best to implant surgically a catheter into the jugular vein of the anaesthetized pig, as the subcutaneous fat makes percutaneous puncture of this vein difficult. Some workers prefer to catheterize the anterior vena cava by a blind technique. Small pigs are restrained on their backs in a V-shaped trough with the neck fully extended and the head hanging down. The forelegs are drawn back and a 5–7.5 cm long, 16 s.w.g. (1.65 mm) needle is pushed through the skin in the depression which can be palpated just lateral to the anterior point of the sternum and formed by the angle between the first rib and trachea. The needle is directed towards an imaginary point midway between the scapulae and advanced until blood can be freely aspirated when a syringe is attached to it. A fine plastic catheter is then threaded through the needle into the anterior vena cava and after its position has been verified by the aspiration of blood through it, or by radiography, the needle is completely withdrawn and the catheter secured in position with a skin suture. In large animals the procedure is carried out with the animal standing and hanging back on a nose snare. It is always important to ensure that the head does not deviate from the midline and that the neck is well extended (Fig. 22.2).

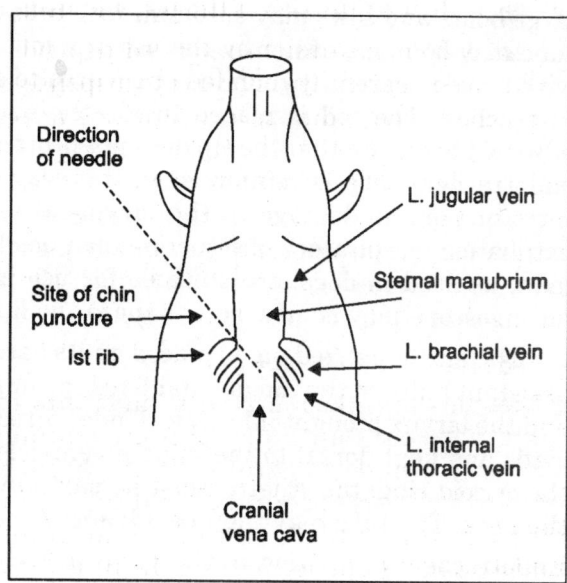

Fig. 22.2: Site for the introduction of a needle to penetrate the anterior vena cava. The needle tip is advanced towards an imaginary point midway between the scapulae

INTRAPERITONEAL INJECTION

This method of administration of anaesthetic drugs is sometimes employed by the less skilled veterinarian, but it is far from ideal. Response is variable, and accidental injection into the liver, kidney or gut lumen may occur. The injection of irritant solutions may lead to the subsequent formation of intraperitoneal adhesions. However, if for any reason intravenous injection is impossible, this route of administration may have to be used. Preferably, pigs should be starved for 24 hours to reduce the gut volume before the injection is made. The animal is then restrained on its back, or by its hind legs, and an area of skin in the region of the umbilicus is clipped and cleaned. A needle is inserted 2–5 cm from the midline at the level of the umbilicus and the injection made. A complete absence of resistance to pressure on the plunger of the syringe indicates that the solution is being injected into the peritoneal cavity or, possibly into the lumen of the gut.

Endotracheal intubation in the pig is not easy. The shape and size of the head and mouth make the use of a laryngoscope difficult. The rima glottis is extremely small, and the larynx is set at an angle to the trachea, causing difficulty in passing the tube beyond the cricoid ring. Laryngeal spasm is easily provoked so that intubation must be carried out under deep general anaesthesia or with the aid of a relaxant.

The sizes of endotracheal tubes suitable for pigs are unexpectedly small when compared with those used in dogs of similar body weight. A 6 mm tube may be the largest which can be passed in a pig weighing about 25 kg; a 9 mm tube is suitable for a 50 kg animal, and large boars and sows may accommodate tubes of 14–16 mm diameter. Introduction of the tube may be made easier by the use of a metal stilette. The ideal stilette is a copper rod with one end carefully rounded or covered to prevent damage to the mucosa of the larynx or trachea. The rod is placed inside the endotracheal tube, and a moveable side-arm adjusted to ensure that the tip does not protrude beyond the end of the tube. Whenever an endotracheal tube is reinforced in this way care must be taken not to use force in its introduction, as damage to the laryngeal mucosa with subsequent oedema and, after extubation, respiratory obstruction, can easily occur. Laryngoscopes designed for use in man, as used in dogs, are suitable for use in small pigs, but in large ones the Rowson laryngoscope may be needed to expose the larynx to view.

The anaesthetized pig is placed on its back with the neck and head fully extended. An assistant pulls on the tongue and fixes the upper jaw while the laryngoscope is introduced and the larynx brought into view. Under direct vision the tube is passed between the vocal cords and kept dorsal to the middle ventricle of the larynx. If its progress is arrested at the cricoid ring, the stilette must be partially withdrawn and the head flexed slightly on the neck. The tube may then be advanced into the trachea.

Endotracheal intubation in the pig is greatly facilitated by the use of muscle relaxants, such as suxamethonium, which relax the jaw muscles and prevent the larynx from going into a spasm. The anaesthetized pig is given oxygen to breathe through a face-mask and the relaxant is administered intravenously. The pig is intubated as soon as the jaw muscles relax and IPPV is carried out until spontaneous respiration is resumed. If suxamethonium is the relaxant used, spontaneous respiration will begin within 1–2 minutes from the time of its injection. Should one attempt at. This time, there will be a larymgospasm.

Bibliography

1. Bustad L.K., McClellan, *Swine in Biomedical Research*, p. 679, 1966.
2. Kirk R.W., *Current Veterinary Therapy*, Small Practice, Vol. 3, 1968.
3. Soma L.R., *Textbook of Veterinary Anaesthesia*, 1971.

23

Anaesthesia of the Dog

ANALGESIA

Opioid Analgesics

Opioid analgesics selected for use in dogs to provide analgesia before, during and after surgery are those usually of medium potency and duration of action, such as morphine, pethidine, methadone and papaveretum, but buprenorphine and butorphanol appear to be an acceptable alternative to these and are not 'controlled' drugs. It must be remembered that all are potent respiratory depressants, particularly when combined with barbiturates, so that subsequent anaesthesia should be administered with this in mind. Potent short-acting analgesics such as fentanyl may be used during surgery to obtain an increased analgesic effect and this and similar drugs are components of 'neurolept analgesic' mixtures. For postoperative analgesia any of these drugs may be used but its long duration of action may make buprenorphine particularly useful at this time provided its bell-shaped dose response curve is remembered. Suitable dose rates and the durations of the action in dogs are given in Table 23.1 and for premedication the lower dose rates should be selected unless preoperative pain is severe. Morphine frequently causes ambulatory dogs to vomit and defecate. This side-effect also occurs following the use of other narcotic analgesics (except pethidine) but it is much less likely to occur if the animal is in pain when the drug is administered. When given intravenously to dogs pethidine causes a severe but usually short-lived hypotension which is thought to be due to histamine release. It is, therefore, best given by other routes. The other drugs of this group may be given by the intravenous or intramuscular routes depending on the need for rapidity of action, but intramuscular injection is to be preferred for both premedication and postoperative analgesia because it tends to produce a more level, prolonged effect.

Pentazocine and butorphanol have the advantage of being subject to less stringent statutory controls, and both have the added advantage that they may be given by the oral route (although much higher doses are needed). Butorphanol has proved a useful analgesic in experimental trials and is said to be a satisfactory premedicant but in clinical use it has sometimes proved disappointing. To avoid dysphoric reactions with pentazocine it is important not to overdose. There is no question that the best analgesia is provided by the pure μ agonists.

Table 23.1: Opiate analgesics used in the dog

	Dose (mg/kg)	Approximate duration of action	Route of administration effect	Main uses
Morphine and postoperative	0.1–0.2	4 hours	i.m.	Premedication
Pethidine and postoperative	1–2	2–4 hours	i.m.	Premedication
Methadone and postoperative	0.1	4 hours	i.m. or i.v.	Premedication
Fentanyl	0.001–0.007	20–30 minutes	i.v.	During surgery and Postoperative
Buprenorphine	0.006	6–8 hours	i.m. or i.v.	Postoperative

Non-steroidal Anti-inflammatory Drugs (NSAIDs)

Flunixin meglumine, a potent analgesic with anti-inflammatory, antipyretic and antiendotoxic properties is indicated for the alleviation of inflammation and acute pain in musculoskeletal disorders and as an adjuvant in the treatment of endotoxic or septic shock. In dogs it is important not to exceed a maximum of three doses because the drug can have serious gastrointestinal effects. The recommended dose is 1 mg/kg by slow intravenous or subcutaneous (not intramuscular) injection every 12 hours and this can produce dramatic pain relief following surgery involving the musculoskeletal system.

SEDATION

Many nervous, 'highly strung' dogs do not tolerate minor procedures such as clipping, grooming or bathing without vigorous protest, and handling at these times is greatly facilitated by the use of suitable sedation. The genuinely vicious animal is, fortunately, not often encountered but when it is, it may need to be heavily sedated for the safety of the veterinarian, nursing staff and, not infrequently, the owner during even a simple physical examination. Heavy sedation is usually necessary to preserve an aseptic routine when operations are performed under epidural or other nerve block. Owners often seek advice about the prevention of travel sickness and although in some cases specific antiemetics may be necessary, for many dogs a simple sedative given in good time before the journey commences is all that is required to solve the problem.

Phenothiazine Derivatives

The action of acepromazine is primarily of an anxiolytic nature. In nervous animals its sedative effects are often marked, but in the fortunately rarely encountered genuinely vicious animal it is usually ineffective. Because of the nature of the dose-response curve, increasing the dose in these vicious animals will not increase sedation, although ataxia and a reduced speed of response may make them slightly easier to handle.

Doses of 0.03–0.05 mg/kg, preferably by intramuscular injection, are usually quite adequate for the production of sedation and are certainly adequate when the drug is used for premedication. These are lower doses than those recommended on the product data sheets, but increasing the dose rarely increases the sedative effect of the drug and merely prolongs its action. Acepromazine and atropine solutions may be mixed in the same syringe, and if time is short the intravenous route may be employed (at 0.03 mg/kg), but the drug may still take up to 20 minutes to produce its full effects. Acepromazine is said by some to be poorly absorbed from subcutaneous sites but has, in fact, been used satisfactorily by this route in dogs. Oral administration is much less reliable and doses of 1–3 mg/kg are needed at least 1 hour prior to induction of anaesthesia.

Other phenothiazine derivatives which are used include propionyl promazine, promazine, promethazine, trimeprazine and chlorpromazine. The side effects produced by them and the provisions of use are similar to those of acepromazine but metho-trimeprazine, which is used as part of the neurolept analgesic mixture. Small animal (immobilon), is said to have the added advantage of possessing analgesic properties.

α_2-Adrenoceptor Agonists
Xylazine

Xylazine was the first α_2-adrenoceptor agonist to be widely used in veterinary medicine. Given by intramuscular injection in doses of 1–3 mg/kg it will produce good sedation and even hypnosis in dogs. As the drug is classified as a sedative/hypnotic, as might be expected, increasing the dose leads to greater sedation as well as increased duration of action. Although high doses will apparently produce unconsciousness (absence of response to external stimuli) this is associated with very severe cardiovascular effects and prolonged recovery, so that high doses cannot be recommended. The major side effect of xylazine in dogs is vomiting or severe retching as sedation develops. Although on occasion this vomiting is useful for emptying the stomach of a dog which has been fed, it appears to be distressing to the dog as well as being unpleasant for the staff who have to clear up the vomited material.

In dogs, xylazine often causes a rise in arterial blood pressure which is followed by hypotension with severe bradycardia and dose-related respiratory depression. Although atropine may be given to prevent bradycardia its effect is variable, sometimes being apparently ineffective while in other cases its administration results in tachycardia accompanied by severe arterial hypertension.

Even if sedation is not marked, the doses of induction agents which are needed after xylazine premedication are greatly reduced, and any agent which is given subsequently must be used with great care. Xylazine slows the circulation, so there is a long delay between the intravenous injection of an anaesthetic drug and its effects becoming apparent; unless due allowance is made for this, intravenous anaesthetic agents will be overdosed.

Medetomidine

Medetomidine is a recently introduced α_2-adrenoceptor agonist for use in dogs and cats. It is a very potent, selective drug which produces a dose-dependent decrease in the release and turnover of noradrenaline in the central nervous system which is manifested as sedation, analgesia and bradycardia. In the periphery, medetomidine causes vasoconstriction by activation of postsynaptic receptors in the vascular smooth muscle. Thus, as with xylazine, there is an initial increase in arterial pressure due to an increase in systemic vascular resistance. However, when used by the intramuscular route at doses which produce moderately deep sedation (40 µg/kg) the rise is minimal and arterial blood pressure rapidly falls to slightly below the normal resting level. Following medetomidine administration dogs often breathe in an irregular manner, periods of up to 45 seconds of apnoea being followed by several rapid breaths. Although the mucous membranes sometimes appear cyanotic, P_aO_2 is only slightly depressed.

α_2-Adrenoceptor Antagonists

In recent years the use of antagonists to terminate prolonged sedation induced by the α_2-adrenoceptor agonists has become more common.

Atipamezole is a new, specific α_2-adrenoceptor antagonist and in dogs arousal occurs within minutes of its intramuscular injection at five times the dose of medetomidine, the respiratory rate also returning to normal. Although, this dose of atipamezole increases the heart rate this does not return to presedation levels. For this, a dose of 10 times the original medetomidine dose must be given or the sedation allowed to wane before the antidote is administered. After large doses of atipamezole dogs have been described as over alert' but convulsions have not been encountered. Although atipamezole is marketed specifically for use as an antidote to medetomidine, in the authors experience intramuscular doses of 200 µg/kg are equally effective in reversing the sedation induced by 3 mg/kg of xylazine in the dog.

Starvation for about 12 hours usually ensures a dog will have an empty stomach but gastric emptying is delayed in the parturient bitch and in dogs which have been involved in accidents or fights. If the stomach is not empty before anaesthesia dogs often vomit during the induction or recovery periods and inhalation of this vomit may be fatal. Dogs appear to have very weak protective laryngeal reflexes and have been known to inhale vomit even after they have regained their feet following anaesthesia. Water need not be withheld until premedication is given or until about 2 hours prior to anaesthesia and, indeed, further deprivation can cause renal failure in dogs which have compensated chronic kidney disease.

When a dog is obviously fluid depleted, or when blood loss during surgery is likely to be unavoidably great, an intravenous infusion should be set up before anaesthesia is induced. Percutaneous venepuncture may prove to be almost impossible if left until circulatory failure is established. Ideally, fluid deficits should be replaced before anaesthesia but if this is impracticable, then at least an adequate circulatory volume should be ensured by infusion of blood, plasma or plasma substitute.

PREMEDICATION

Premedication in the dog usually involves the administration of anticholinergic, sedative and analgesic drugs, the combination chosen depending on the circumstances and the anaesthetic technique which is to follow.

Anticholinergic Drugs

Atropine sulphate is the anticholinergic drug frequently used in dogs, and may be given by the intramuscular, subcutaneous or intravenous routes. Dose rates commonly range from 0.02–0.1 mg/kg (about 0.25 mg to a puppy and up to 1.8 mg for a large dog when the 0.6 mg/ml solution is used). The dose rate is not critical as atropine is very rapidly removed from the bloodstream of a dog, and overdose is very rare. When it does occur, it results in convulsions which, if the dose is high enough, maybe followed by coma and death.

Other anticholinergic drugs are sometimes used as part of neuroleptanalgesic mixtures. Hyoscine is combined with papaveretum in omnopon-scopolamine and diphenylpiperidinoethylacetamide in combelen/polamivet and when such mixtures are used atropine is not required. Glycopyrrolate has also been used in dogs at a dose rate of 0.01 mg/kg. It appears to have no clear advantages in this species of animal over atropine except that it does not readily cross the blood-brain barrier and is less likely to produce central nervous stimulation.

Sedative and Analgesic Premedication

Premedication with sedative and opioid drugs contributes to a smooth induction of anaesthesia by reducing stress and allowing easy handling of the dog. It also reduces the dose of subsequent anaesthetics and helps to provide a calm and pain-free recovery from anaesthesia. Thus, it becomes an integral part of the anaesthetic procedure. It is, therefore, particularly important to allow sufficient time to elapse for the maximal effects of premedication to develop before anaesthesia is induced, as failure to do this may result in overdosage of induction agents. The influence of high doses of premedicant drugs on subsequent induction doses of anaesthetics can be dramatic (Table 23.2) and the decision to use high or low doses is influenced by the personal preferences of the anaesthetist.

Table 23.2: Effects of premedication on the subsequent dose of induction agent

Premedicant drug and dose	Induction agent
No premedication	Thiopentone 10 mg/kg
Acepromazine 0.03–0.05	Thiopentone 7–8 mg/kg mg/kg i.m.
Medetomidine 5 n.g/kg i.m.	Thiopentone 7–8 mg/kg
Medetomidine 10 μg/kg i.m.	Thiopentone 6–7 mg/kg
Alfentanil 5 μg/kg i.v.	Thiopentone 3–5 mg/kg
No premedication	Propofol 6–7 mg/kg
Acepromazine 0.03–0.05 mg/kg i.m.	Propofol 4 mg/kg
Medetomidine 40 μg/kg i.m.	Propofol 1–1.5 mg/kg
Alfentanil 5 μg/kg i.v.	Propofol 3–4 mg/kg
Alfentanil 10 μg/kg	Propofol 1–2 mg/kg

The examples in this table refer to the situation in fit, healthy dogs. Sick animals may require considerably less while individual dogs may require more or less of the induction agent following premedication.

INTRAVENOUS ANAESTHESIA

In dogs, as in other animals, intravenous agents may be used either to induce anaesthesia which is then maintained by inhalation methods, or as sole anaesthetic agents. Despite their dangers and disadvantages when used as sole anaesthetic agents, this use is increasing because of fears over the effects of pollution of the atmosphere by volatile inhalation anaesthetics.

The use of intravenous drugs as sole anaesthetics does not mean that anaesthetic machines are unnecessary. All the measures normally taken to maintain proper respiratory function during anaesthesia must still be employed. The intravenous agents commonly produce respiratory depression and endotracheal intubation, the administration of oxygen, and even IPPV, may be necessary if hypoxaemia and hypercapnia are to be avoided.

Some intravenous agents may also be given by subcutaneous or intramuscular injection but these routes of administration always suffer from the disadvantages of variable absorption leading to a sometimes stormy induction, and the difficulty of gauging the dose.

Intravenous Technique

If the vein on the right foreleg is to be punctured an assistant stands on the left side of the animal, passes his or her left arm around the animal's neck and raises its head. The assistant's right hand grips the animal's right foreleg so that the middle, third and fourth fingers are immediately behind the olecranon and the thumb is round the front side of the limb. The limb is extended by pushing on the olecranon and the vein is raised by applying pressure with the thumb. Venepuncture must, of course, be carried out with the usual aseptic precautions, so the hair over the vein is clipped and the skin is disinfected.

Suitable needle sizes depend to some extent on the size of the dog and the quantity and viscosity of the fluid to be injected. For most purposes a needle 2.5 cm long and 23 gauge (0.6 mm bore) is quite satisfactory. The points of the needle should not be cut too acutely, the so called 'short bevel' or 'dental cut' being preferred.

Two methods of stabilizing the vein prior to needle puncture are employed. In one, the skin over the vein is kept taut by the thumb and forefinger of the anaesthetist's left hand which grasps the animal's forearm immediately below the site of puncture. In this position it is easy for the anaesthetist to grip the syringe between the left thumb and forefinger once the vein has been entered. The skin should be pierced immediately over the vein to avoid the branches of the radial nerve which run on either side of the vein in the region of the limb.

In the second method, the anaesthetist's left thumb is placed just alongside the vein, and the skin is not tensed. The vein is stabilized between the needle and the thumb as the needle is advanced through the skin into the vein. With this method there is a greater tendency to make contact between the needle point and the branch of the radial nerve running alongside the vein.

In Dachshunds and dogs with similar short, bent forelimbs venepuncture is best attempted in the angle where the veins join to form the cephalic vein just cranial to the carpus (Fig. 23.1) become occluded. Failure to aspirate blood into the syringe is also encountered if the vein is already thrombosed, or if peripheral perfusion is very poor as it may be after the use of α_2-adrenoceptor agonists. The recurrent tarsal vein may be used for intravenous injection at the point where it passes cranially and dorsally on the lateral aspect of the leg just cranial to the tarsus. Either hind leg may be used with the animal restrained on its side, but two assistants may be required.

The femoral vein in the middle part of the medial aspect of the thigh may also be used. It is rendered obvious by pressure applied to the inguinal region and is usually more prominent in the cranial part of the thigh. Care should be taken to ensure that injections are not made into the femoral artery which lies directly beneath the vein.

ENDOTRACHEAL INTUBATION

In dog is held in a position with its mouth field open in such a way that neither the assistant nor the anaesthetist will get bitten should the depth of anaesthesia not have been judged correctly. The assistant holds only the upper lips and the anaesthetist's finger is placed between the dog's lower incisor teeth and its tongue to prevent injury to the underside of the tongue as this is drawn forward out of the mouth. The epiglottis is clearly visible when the tongue is held in this position but its tip is usually positioned behind the soft palate.

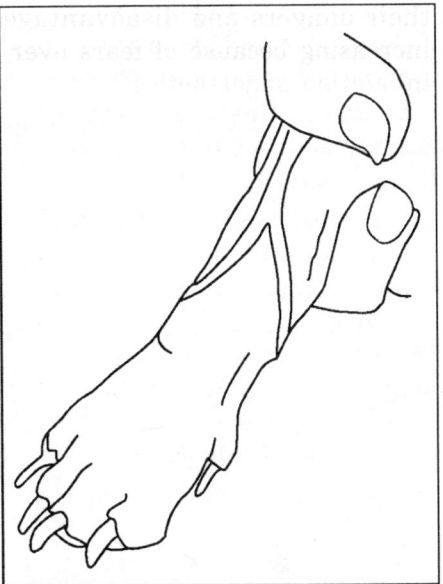

Fig. 23.1: In short-legged dogs such as Dachshunds with very mobile skins the easiest point for venepuncture is at the junction of the veins from the medial and lateral aspects of the carpus where they form the cephalic vein

The lubricated tube is introduced into the mouth and its tip used to deflect the soft palate upwards and backwards so as to bring the entire epiglottis into view. The tube is then used to depress the epiglottis anteriorly on to the base of the tongue and to keep it there whilst the tube itself is advanced in front of the arytenoid cartilages into the trachea. Should any difficulty be encountered, a laryngoscope may be used to allow vocal cords to be seen or, alternatively, a finger may be inserted into the pharynx and used to direct the tube into the glottis. Care should always be taken to avoid injury to the larynx and forceps should never be applied to the epiglottis, or to the fold of mucous membrane between the epiglottis and the tongue, in order to expose the laryngeal opening. Trauma to the larynx or to the tissues around it may give rise to oedema which can, when the tube is removed, cause complete obstruction of the airway and necessitate the performance of an emergency tracheostomy.

Standard cuffed Magill endotracheal tubes are suitable for use in all but small dogs, the tube sizes up to 11 mm internal diameter are those designed for use in man. However, man has a very small trachea in comparison with that of dogs, so that the larger tubes required for medium and big dogs are produced only for veterinary use. In very small dogs it is preferable to use uncuffed tubes because the added dimensions of the cuff-inflating tube increase the overall diameter and thus decrease the bore of the tube which can be accommodated by the trachea. When these uncuffed or plain tubes are used a pharyngeal pack of ribbon gauze will prevent inhalation of foreign material into the trachea.

The diameter of the largest tube which can be introduced into the trachea is related to both the size and breed of the dog. For example, a 16 mm tube can usually be passed into the trachea of an adult German shepherd whilst, in an Airedale of similar size, a 12 mm tube may be the largest which can be used. For their size, bulldogs and bull terriers have exceptionally small diameter tracheas and it is often preferable to use uncuffed tubes in these breeds.

All new Magill tubes should be cut to the correct length so that endobronchial intubation is impossible and dead space is reduced to a minimum. To anchor the tube in position once it has been introduced a tie should be placed tightly around the tube where it goes over the endotracheal tube connector; this tie is secured either to the jaw where the canine teeth will prevent movement or around the back of the head in case of brachycephalic dogs. It is very dangerous to place the tie half way along the tube where it cannot be tied tightly, for looseness will allow the tube to move in the mouth and possibly to slip out of the trachea during surgery.

Agents Employed

Nitrous oxide

It is generally agreed that dogs cannot be anaesthetized with unsupplemented mixtures of nitrous oxide and oxygen and thus in canine anaesthesia the gas is used only where it can be given with other agents. It is used in a non-rebreathing or low flow system either.

1. As a vehicle for the vaporization and delivery of volatile anaesthetic agents. The proportion of oxygen in the mixture, provided it is at least 30% is unimportant because the maintenance of anaesthesia does not depend on the potency of nitrous oxide, or

2. In conjunction with thiopentone, pethidine and other analgesic supplements such as fentanyl, and with muscle relaxants, for maintaining a light 'plane of anaesthesia.' In these circumstances the proportion of oxygen in the nitrous oxide/oxygen mixture delivered to the animal becomes of great importance and two factors must be considered.

Satisfactory results may be obtained when nitrous oxide/oxygen mixtures are used to maintain anaesthesia which has been induced by the intravenous injection of thiopentone sodium following well-chosen premedication. In many cases, however, the degree of surgical stimulation produced by the operative procedure is sufficiently marked as to make the animal restless when nitrous oxide and oxygen alone are employed. This restlessness often proves to be an embarrassment both to the surgeon and the anaesthetist. In these circumstances the anaesthetist is often tempted to introduce a degree of hypoxia into the administration of the anaesthetic, but this temptation should always be resisted. Better methods are available which produce smooth anaesthesia without sacrificing the benefits of nitrous oxide.

The simplest and safest method of obtaining smooth anaesthesia is to supplement the basal nitrous oxide/oxygen mixture with a volatile agent or an intravenous drug. When a volatile agent is chosen a low concentration is introduced and the concentration is steadily increased until the desired depth of unconsciousness is reached.

The technique of induction with thiopentone sodium given after rather heavy premedication of acepromazine with a narcotic analgesic, followed by nitrous oxide/oxygen (allowing at least 30% oxygen in the respired mixture) supplemented by the intravenous injection of small doses of an analgesic as required is very satisfactory. Probably the best intravenous supplements for spontaneously breathing dogs are alfentanil (25 µg/kg) and fentanyl (0.5–1 µg/kg). A muscle relaxant may be used with this technique if abdominal section is to be performed or a thorax opened. Recovery is rapid and there seems to be the minimum of postanaesthetic nausea and hangover for if their surgical condition allows it most dogs will eat a normal meal soon after regaining consciousness. The safety of α_2-adrenoceptor agonist premedication for this technique has not been established.

Chloroform

It is generally agreed that because of its toxic effects on the liver and kidneys, coupled with its ability to sensitize the heart to adrenaline-induced arrhythmias, chloroform is not a safe anaesthetic for dogs. Only on an occasion where there is no possible alternative, such as may occur unexpectedly in the field, should chloroform now be used as an anaesthetic agent for dogs.

Halothane

Because of its potency and because it is well tolerated by the respiratory tract halothane is often used alone as an anaesthetic agent for dogs. The animal is restrained and anaesthesia induced using a face mask, the halothane being vaporized and delivered to the animal by a stream of oxygen or nitrous oxide oxygen mixture. In small dogs (up to 10 kg) induction of anaesthesia is rapid and the duration of the period of narcotic excitement is brief. In larger dogs induction and the narcotic excitement stage are more prolonged and it is usually advisable to give a minimal sleep dose of an intravenous agent before halothane is used.

Halothane is potent and anaesthesia is often difficult to control, for small alterations in the concentration of the vapour being respired result in quite gross alterations in the depth of anaesthesia. No attempt should be made to produce profound muscle relaxation by increasing the depth of halothane anaesthesia for this results in a severe fall in blood pressure and marked respiratory depression. The respiratory depression is often manifested by fast shallow breathing and the inexperienced anaesthetist may mistake this as sign of too light anaesthesia. Because of the respiratory depressant properties of the drug only minimal premedication and the smallest possible quantity of thiopentone should be given prior to the use of halothane.

Halothane lends itself to supplementation of the intravenous agent/nitrous oxide/oxygen sequence, particularly when spontaneous respiration is desirable, since very small concentrations produce a good result without marked side effects. When deeper anaesthesia or more marked muscle relaxation is required it is probably better to use a muscle relaxant rather than increase the inspired concentration of halothane.

Like any other potent volatile anaesthetic agent, halothane is best administered from a calibrated vaporizer so that the concentration delivered to the animal is known. In any case it is important that the anaesthetist should be fully acquainted with the actual concentrations delivered by any vaporizer which is used.

Enflurane

In dogs, enflurane, like halothane, produces a dose-dependent depression of both respiratory and cardiovascular function. Side effects such as muscle twitching during clinical anaesthesia were not encountered, although these have been reported as occurring in experimental situations and by some other clinicians. The ability to produce rapid changes in the depth of anaesthesia and the rapid recovery suggest that this agent may be useful in dogs undergoing surgery as day-patients. However, enflurane is a poor analgesic and dogs need pain relief very early in the postoperative period to prevent restlessness or excitement and a rather stormy recovery from anaesthesia. It is possible that the inclusion of an analgesic in the premedication would avoid the problem, but this might delay recovery and thus negate the major advantage offered by the use of this anaesthetic agent.

Isoflurane

The high volatility and low blood solubility of isoflurane suggest that it might be better than enflurane for day-patient surgery in dogs. Its high cost tends to limit its use in canine anaesthesia and when it is used low-flow methods of administration are usually employed. Up to 4% isoflurane vapour may be needed to induce anaesthesia but inspired concentrations of 1.5–2% are adequate for anaesthetic maintenance. For dogs it offers no significant advantage over halothane although there are theoretical considerations for preferring it in certain situations — for example, it has properties which make it particularly suitable for use in dogs suffering from cardiac disease.

NEUROMUSCULAR BLOCKING AGENTS

The use of neuromuscular blocking agents as part of the anaesthetic procedure is a technique which has much to offer in canine surgery for the profound relaxation produced enables the surgeon to work more efficiently. Relaxants enable the anaesthetist to take full control of respiration during a thoracotomy. Laparotomies, particularly those involving dissection deep within the abdomen, are more easily performed, and dislocated joints are more easily reduced. The profound relaxation which can be produced is also helpful for laminectomies and lumbar disc fenestrations, especially in large dogs where the surgeon has to retract deep and powerful muscles to expose the surgical target. The use of neuromuscular blocking agents and their general pharmacology in relevance to canine anaesthesia are summarized in Table 23.3.

Neuromuscular blocking agents paralyse the patient and thus by abolishing respiration and preventing somatic response to impulses in afferent nerves, they suppress many of the signs used to assess the depth of unconsciousness. When these agents are used, therefore, facilities for IPPV must be available and the anaesthetist must be capable of judging the depth of anaesthesia in the absence of many of the reflex responses normally

Table 23.3: Neuromuscular blocking agents in dogs (approximate doses and effects)

	Dose (mg/kg)	Effective length of action (minutes)	Remarks
Depolarizing			
Suxamethonium	0.3–0.4	20	Initial muscle fasciculation. No reversal
Non -depolarizing			
Atracurium	0.5	15–80	Can be given by infusion
Alcuronium	0.06–0.1	30–40	Residual effects can last some hours
Gallamine	1.0	15–20	Tachycardia
Pancuronium	0.06–0.1	20–40	Further 1 or 2 doses if required. Some tachycardia
Vecuronium	0.06–0.1	15–20	'Pure' neuromuscular blocker

used. In dogs, the following signs are useful in judging the depth of unconsciousness when the animal is paralysed.

1. *Pulse:* If anaesthesia becomes too light the pulse rate may increase, or the animal may show signs of vasovagal syncope with pallor of the mucous membranes and bradycardia.
2. *Pupil:* Paralysis of the ocular muscles means that the eye is central and the pupil is easily visible. The pupil dilates if anaesthesia becomes too light, is constricted at surgical levels, and dilates again as anaesthesia becomes too deep. Atropine premedication has no significant effect on these signs.
3. *Lacrimation and salivation:* Overflow of tears, or visible production of saliva both indicate that anaesthesia is becoming too light.
4. *Tongue:* Despite the use of neuromuscular blocking agents, in dogs the tongue will be observed to twitch if anaesthesia becomes too light. This twitching is readily detected if the anaesthetist is monitoring the sublingual artery.

If any of these signs are observed it must be taken that the level of unconsciousness should be deepened.

Agents Used

The agents currently used to produce neuromuscular block in canine anaesthesia are listed in Table 23.3 but the doses shown in this table must be regarded as a guide to the initial dose to be administered.

NEONATAL ANAESTHESIA

Occasionally it is necessary to anaesthetize very young or newborn puppies. Premedication should consist of only a very small dose of an anticholinergic agent, and as such very young animals lack the enzymes necessary for the elimination of many parenterally administered drugs and the fat needed for their redistribution, it is best to induce and maintain anaesthesia with inhalation anaesthetics. Endotracheal intubation is usually unnecessary, and indeed many consider it to be actually contraindicated, for it may induce sufficient laryngeal oedema and swelling to cause respiratory obstruction when the tube is removed. Hypothermia is easily induced and must be prevented by active warming during both surgery and the anaesthetic recovery period. Particular attention must also be paid to the replacement of fluid deficits and the maintenance of fluid balance.

In general, any inhalation anaesthetic delivered through a face mask to the puppy provides anaesthesia adequate for the majority of surgical procedures which have to be performed on puppies of this age group, and is followed by a rapid recovery. Major procedures requiring other anaesthetic techniques should, whenever possible, be deferred until the pup is at least 8 weeks old.

LOCAL ANALGESIA

In the dog, the simplicity and safety of modern general anaesthesia means that local analgesia is rarely employed except for very minor procedures. However, certain techniques of local analgesia can still prove useful where poor facilities or the condition of the patient preclude the use of general anaesthesia.

Intravenous Regional Analgesia

This method provides a very safe and simple way of obtaining analgesia of the distal part of the limb and proves useful for operations such as the wiring of dislocated toes and toe amputations in tractable dogs such as greyhounds, or in sedated dogs.

The animal is restrained on its side and its systolic blood pressure measured. The appropriate limb is held as high as possible above heart level for 2–3 minutes to partially exsanguinate it while a sphygmomanometer cuff is being applied. The cuff is placed around the fore-arm cranial to the carpus, or around the tibial region cranial to the hock, and is quickly inflated to just above the systolic blood pressure. An intravenous injection of 2–3 ml of 1% lignocaine is made through a very fine needle into any superficial vein which can be identified distal to the occluding cuff. The lignocaine should not include adrenaline which may impair its diffusion. Some animals show signs of slight discomfort as the injection is made, but the onset of analgesia up to the level of the cuff is rapid. Analgesia lasts as long as the pressure within the cuff is maintained above the animal's systolic pressure. Sensation returns to the foot within a few minutes after deflation of the cuff tourniquet.

In a series of 20 greyhounds, good results were achieved in 17 cases, while in three, although the operation could be performed satisfactorily, the animal appeared to experience slight discomfort. The tourniquet was in place for 25–55 minutes and even during the longest of these operations there was no waning of analgesia. No harmful results were observed to follow the release of the lignocaine into the general circulation, but it must be noted that none of the dogs were allowed to stand up for 2–3 minutes after removal of the tourniquet.

The major difficulty in the application of this technique in canine surgery is the identification of a suitable superficial vein distal to the occluding cuff. In greyhounds and other thin-skinned dogs this presents no problems, but in thick-skinned dogs it may be necessary to introduce an indwelling needle or catheter before partial exsanguination of the limb.

The main reasons for failure with this technique are the use of a tourniquet which does not occlude the arterial blood supply to the region, or not allowing the necessary 5 minutes for analgesia to develop after injection of the local analgesic.

Brachial Plexus Block

A technique for the production of brachial block has been described by Nutt for attaining regional analgesia of the forelimb.

With the dog standing on all four legs, the triangular area bounded by the anterior border of the supraspinatus muscle, the chest wall and the dorsal border of the brachiocephalicus muscle, is clipped and prepared for injection. The animal's head is held away from the side to be injected and the depression in the centre of the clipped area is palpated and the first rib located. A 7.5 cm needle of 1.6 mm bore is inserted into the centre of the depression and guided caudally lateral to the chest wall and medial to the subscapularis muscle until its point is judged to be level with the spine of the scapula. After aspiration to confirm that the point of the needle does not lie within a blood vessel, 1–3 ml of lignocaine hydrochloride, according to the size of the dog, is injected through the needle. Onset of analgesia should be observed in most cases within 10 minutes of injection. There is a gradual loss of motor power, followed by complete relaxation and loss of sensation below and including the elbow joint as the block develops. It is possible that paraesthesia occurs soon after injection, for some animals chew at the leg.

Certain complications may occur consequent upon this procedure: a major blood vessel may be punctured by the needle and a large haematoma develop as a result of this; the local analgesic solution may be injected intravascularly; the brachial plexus may be damaged, causing neuritis or permanent paralysis; the needle may enter the thorax and admit the entry of air into the pleural cavity; infection may be introduced into the axilla. However, if due care is exercised the technique may be regarded as a relatively safe procedure, of particular value where general anaesthesia is contraindicated owing to the state of the patient when presented for surgery.

Nutt reports that fat dogs are difficult subjects on which to perform this block and says that some failures may be anticipated in these animals. However, it must be noted that he used very small volumes of a concentrated solution of lignocaine hydrochloride (3%). The use of 5–10 ml of 2–3% procaine hydrochloride solution for this block. injected into a dog's axilla, has been reported, but more certain results were obtained by the injection of 10–15 ml of a 1% lignocaine hydrochloride solution containing 1:200 000 adrenaline to delay absorption and diminish the risk of toxic reactions.

Infiltration of the Digital Nerves

The digital nerves are approached lateral and medial to the first phalanx of the digit to be rendered analgesic. A fine needle is introduced subcutaneously on each side of the digit (Fig. 23.2) and 2 ml of local analgesic solution is injected on each aspect.

Auriculopalpebral Nerve Block

The nerve runs caudal to the mandibular joint at the base of the ear and, after giving off the cranial auricular branch, proceeds as the temporal branch along the dorsal border of the zygomatic arch towards the orbit. Before reaching the orbit the nerve divides into two branches, which pass medially and laterally to supply the orbicularis muscle. The needle is introduced through the skin and fascia over the midpoint of the caudal third of the zygomatic arch (just where the arch can be felt to dip sharply medially) and 1 ml of solution is injected.

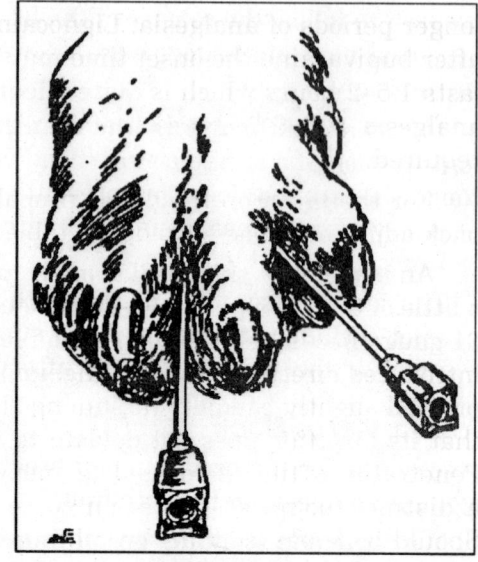

Fig. 23.2: Injection of the digital nerves

The blocking of this branch of the facial nerve does not produce any analgesia. By paralysing the orbicularis muscle it facilitates examination of, and operations on, the eyeball. It is of particular value in preventing squeezing of the eyeball after intraocular operations.

Caudal Block

In the dog, caudal nerve block may be given between the sacrum and the first coccygeal vertebra or between the first and second coccygeal vertebra. The same principles are followed as in the larger animals. The procedure is technically easy and the dose administered should not exceed 1 ml of 2% lignocaine hydrochloride solution. This block is useful for docking the tail in adult dogs and for other surgical operations upon the tail.

Epidural Block

To locate the site the iliac prominences on either side are identified. An imaginary line joining them crosses the dorsal spinous process of the last lumbar segment. The site for insertion of the needle is in the ratdline immediately caudal to this process (Fig. 23.3). The interarcual ligament lies at a depth of 2–4 cm from the skin and the approximate dimensions of the space in a 14 kg dog are: craniocaudally, 0.4 cm; laterally, 0.7 cm.

Lignocaine hydrochloride 2% with 1:200 000 adrenaline is commonly used for epidural block but bupivacaine 0.75% will produce

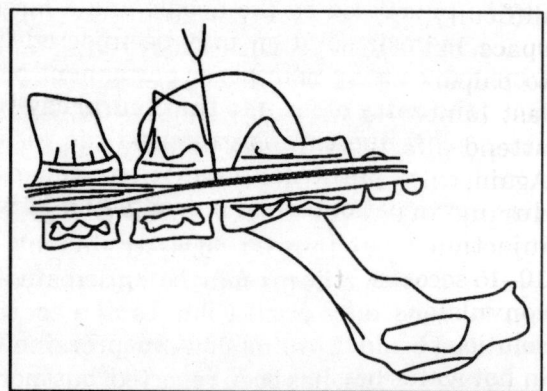

Fig. 23.3: Epidural analgesia. The site and direction for insertion of the needle

longer periods of analgesia. Lignocaine produces analgesia in about 5–10 minutes while after bupivacaine the onset time may be from 15 to 30 minutes. Lignocaine block usually lasts 1.5–2 hours which is quite adequate for most surgery but bupivacaine will produce analgesia of 5–6 hours so that this drug is to be preferred if postoperative analgesia is required.

For the injection the dog is probably best restrained firmly on its right side with its back adjacent to the edge of the table.

An insensitive skin weal is made just caudal to the last lumbar spine by the injection of a little of the local analgesic solution, using a short, fine needle. For the epidural injection a 21 gauge needle 3–5 cm long is employed. Its point should be cut at an angle of 45°. It is introduced directly in the midline, immediately caudal to the last lumbar dorsal spine, and pressed slightly caudally (assuming the animal to be in the normal position), taking care that its direction does not deviate to one side. Penetration of the interarcual ligament imparts a distinct 'popping' sensation to the finger. Should bone rather than ligament be encountered, it indicates that the direction of the needle has been wrong and that its point has struck an articular process or the roof of the first sacral segment. If this occurs the needle is slightly withdrawn and a search made for the space by redirecting it a little caudally, cranially or laterally.

Epidural 'Minipack' set, which is ideal for the introduction of catheter into a dog's epidural span, is shown in Fig. 23.4.

That the canal has been entered is indicated by the complete absence of resistance to the injection. In the majority of animals no difficulty will be experienced in locating the space, but in very fat dogs it may be impossible to palpate either the iliac tuberosities or the last lumbar spine and, in these, failure may attend efforts to induce epidural analgesia. Again, with highly nervous animals, movement during injection may cause failure. The injection must be made slowly, over some 10–15 seconds, otherwise vomiting and possible convulsions may occur. The local analgesic solution should be warmed by placing ampoules in hot water before use.

There is a rather remote possibility that the meningeal cul-de-sac will be penetrated, in

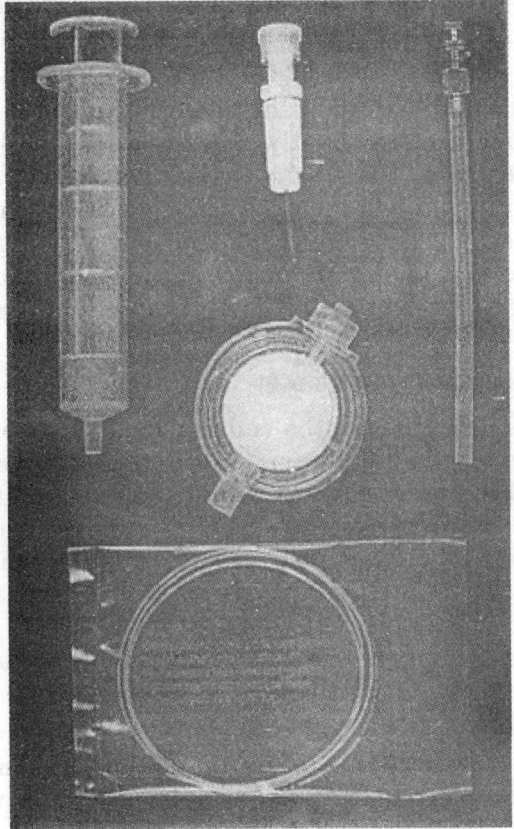

Fig. 23.4: Epidural 'Minipack' set (Portex Ltd) which is ideal for the introduction of a catheter into a dog's epidural space. The set contains a 10 ml syringe, 19 G Tuohy needle graduated 10–45 mm x 5 mm. Open-ended catheter marked at 20–100 mm x 10 mm from tip, loss-of-resistance device, flat filter and Luer lock connector

which case cerebrospinal fluid will escape from the needle. If this occurs it is probably best to withdraw the needle and abandon the attempt to produce epidural analgesia.

A catheter can be introduced easily some 2–3 cm into the epidural space through a correctly placed Tuohy needle.

In the dog interference with motor power of the hind limbs is of no consequence. To produce analgesia up to the first lumbar segment a dose of approximately 1 ml per 4.5 kg body weight is required and for cranial laparotomies where analgesia is needed to the fourth or fifth thoracic segment this dose is usually increased to about 1 ml per 3.5 kg.

The complication most likely to occur is hypotension and this is perhaps best minimized by the infusion of about 20 ml/kg of Hartmann's solution as the block develops. Certainly, a catheter should be placed in a vein before epidural block is induced so that vasopressors can be injected without delay should hypotension develop. Arterial blood pressure should be monitored by non-invasive means in every case. The dose of methoxamine, by intravenous or intramuscular injection, is up to 5 mg.

To block the thirteenth thoracic nerve a skin weal is raised at the posterior border of the dorsal spine of the twelfth thoracic vertebra, and a needle is introduced through this and directed slightly caudally and laterally to strike the caudal articular process of the vertebra. The needle is then withdrawn slightly and advanced again over this process until it meets the transverse process of the first lumbar vertebra. After withdrawing the needle point about 1 cm, 2 ml of local analgesic solution is injected. The lumbar nerves are treated in a similar manner, the landmarks sought being the caudal articular processes of the vertebrae immediately cranial to the nerves to be blocked.

POSTOPERATIVE CARE

Whether or not the endotracheal tube has been left in place, the dog must be carefully watched until it has regained its protective, reflexes, and should remain under continuous observation until it is fully conscious. Laryngeal spasm and oedema sufficient to cause respiratory obstruction is fortunately rare in the dog, but occasionally (usually in elderly dogs with a history of chronic cough) laryngeal paralysis and collapse is encountered. The arytenoid cartilages appear to collapse into the laryngeal orifice and emergency tracheostomy may be necessary to relieve obstruction from this cause. Dogs with chronic respiratory insufficiency may require the administration of oxygen in the recovery period. Initially this may be given through a face mask, but later on a nasal catheter delivering oxygen into the pharynx is usually better tolerated.

Hypothermia is better prevented than treated as energetic, rapid rewarming of the patient results in cutaneous vasodilatation which can be responsible for serious hypotension in animals which have a depleted blood volume after surgery. The rectal temperature, as measured by a mercury-in-glass clinical thermometer, is often extremely low in the postoperative period.

Excitement in the recovery period is always undesirable and the animal may even thrash about to the extent of causing itself injury, although fortunately this is uncommon. Excitement or restlessness is more common after barbiturate anaesthesia than after the use of inhalation agents and can often be prevented from occurring by adequate suitable premedication.

Intravenous infusion has been given during anaesthesia and the animal has not been catheterized, distension of the bladder can cause very great discomfort and it should also be remembered that many dogs will not urinate in a kennel. Evidence of bladder distension should always be sought whenever a dog is restless in the postoperative period and the condition should always be relieved by emptying the bladder, if necessary by catheterization. The administration of analgesics to these animals may make distension of the bladder more tolerable.

Even when its presence is recognized, pain is often treated inadequately for fear of causing respiratory or circulatory depression with the pain-relieving drugs. Surgical pain is usually severe for only the first 1 or 2 days; in this period it can usually only be relieved effectively by the narcotic analgesics, but after this non-steroidal anti-inflammatory drugs often provide adequate analgesia. Morphine may not be the best of the powerful analgesics available for use in dogs.

A dog's fluid intake should be restored as soon as possible following surgery. Oral intake is best, and if there are no surgical contraindications, the dog may be allowed access to small amounts of water as soon as it is fully conscious. Should it be impossible to provide an adequate intake by mouth, fluids must be given intravenously. This is particularly important in elderly dogs where fluid deprivation may lead to renal failure.

Bibliography

1. Grahm Jones O., *Small Animal Anaesthesia*, p. 59, 1964.
2. Kirk R.W. *Current Veterinary Therapy*, Vol. 3, Small Practice, 1968.
3. Soma L.R., *Textbook of Veterinary Anaesthesia*, 1971.

24

Anaesthesia of the Cat

SEDATIVE/OPIOID COMBINATIONS

Neuroleptanalgesic techniques employ large doses of opiate analgesics to which the cat may respond with violent excitement. They are, therefore, contraindicated for use in cats or, indeed, in all other Felidae.

Low doses of opioids such as pethidine (1–2 mg/kg) may be used together with acepromazine but the improvement in sedation over that provided by acepromazine is usually minimal.

PREANAESTHETIC PREPARATION

Preanaesthetic examination should be carried out in a manner similar to that described in Chapter 14 and any pathological conditions found, together with any pre-existing drug therapy, taken into account during the subsequent anaesthetic. In clinical practice it is common to find that cats have been exposed to organophosphorus insecticides from flea collars or sprays and this may increase the length of action of suxamethonium given for intubation. Corticosteroids are frequently used in cats to control allergies to external parasites and corticosteroid cover should be given over the anaesthetic and operating periods if the cat has received such therapy in the 2 months preceding anaesthesia.

About 12 hours of fasting will usually ensure that the cat has an empty stomach and water need only be withheld for 2 hours prior to anaesthesia, or the water bowl removed at the time premedication is given. If surgery is to be carried out on the day of admission, enquiry should be made as to whether the cat was closely confined throughout the previous night for a roaming, hunting cat may have filled its stomach by eating its prey.

ANAESTHETIC TECHNIQUES

Intravenous Infection

The minimum enforceable restraint should be used to enable intravenous injection to be carried out. Cats object strongly to restraint and respond to its imposition by trying to escape from it, thus inviting more forcible measures which only too often result in scratched and bitten assistants and a very frightened excited cat. Such stormy conditions during the induction of anaesthesia can lead to the cat dying from ventricular fibrillation.

In the conscious cat, intravenous injections are best made into the cephalic vein (Fig. 24.1). The animal is placed in a sitting position on a table of convenient height and for injection into the right cephalic vein the assistant stands to the cat's left side, raising and supporting its head between the thumb and fingers of the left hand. In this position the assistant can usually help to keep the cat

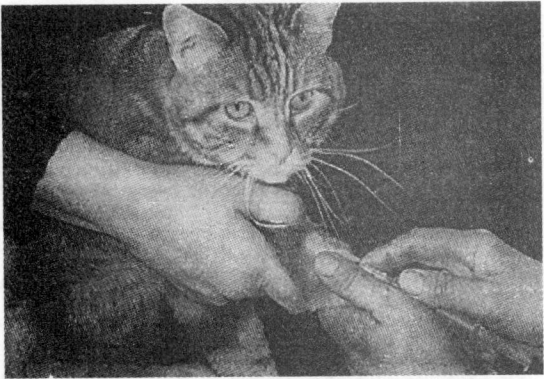

Fig. 24.1: Injection of cephalic vein

calm by tickling it below the ears. The assistant's right hand is placed so that the middle, third and fourth fingers are behind the olecranon, and the thumb is around the front of the right forelimb. The limb is extended by pushing on the olecranon and the vein is raised by applying gentle pressure with the thumb. The limb must not be held in a vice-like grip because this cuts off the arterial blood supply and distresses the cat. Venepuncture is carried out. Most friendly household cats will allow venepuncture to be carried out easily as long as the needle is sharp and no thrust is made with the needle. The needle must be introduced steadily and gently through the skin and into the lumen of the vein without stabbing. Should it become obvious that more restraint is needed, the assistant can provide this rapidly by holding the cat between his or her body and right arm while preventing movement from the hind limbs by pressing the cat firmly on to the surface of the table. The cat's head can easily be controlled when held firmly in the left hand as described. If it is clear that greater restraint than this is needed, it is probably preferable to abandon attempts at intravenous injection until an appropriate premedication has had time to take effect, or to induce anaesthesia by other means. A short needle with a fine bore is suitable for injections into the cephalic vein and, in general, a 25 gauge needle (0.5 mm external diameter), 15 mm long is ideal.

In moribund or anaesthetized animals, the jugular vein can be used. The cat is placed in lateral recumbency with its neck over a small pad or sandbag, its forelimbs are stretched backwards towards its tail, and the uppermost jugular vein occluded in the jugular groove near to the sternal inlet by the assistant's thumb. Venepuncture is then carried out as described for the dog. The jugular vein route is a particularly useful one for the administration of intravenous fluid therapy and when relatively large blood samples are required for diagnostic or other purposes the jugular vein is the only practicable source.

Endotracheal Intubation

In cats, laryngeal spasm is easily provoked, and after induction of anaesthesia a traumatic intubation can only be carried out by adopting one of the following methods.

The laryngeal mucous membrane of the anaesthetized cat can be desensitized by spraying it with a solution of a local analgesic drug, such as 4% lignocaine hydrochloride. The larynx usually goes into a spasm when the spray is applied and attempts of intubation should be delayed for about 30 seconds until it is seen to relax again. Following intubation by this method it must be remembered that the larynx will be insensitive, and the normal protective reflexes absent, until the effects of the local analgesic have worn off. Spraying the larynx has been shown to produce tissue oedema and the amount of local analgesic used is critical. Heavner has shown that lignocaine is capable of causing neurogenically mediated ventricular arrhythmias.

The anaesthetized cat may be paralysed by the administration of a relaxant drug after inhaling pure oxygen from a face mask for 30–60 seconds to prevent hypoxia during the subsequent intubation procedure. Paralysis is usually produced rapidly by the intravenous injection of 3–5 mg of suxamethonium (for an adult cat), and oxygen administration is continued during the fasciculations caused by the initial depolarizing action of this agent. When relaxation is complete the cat is intubated through completely flaccid vocal cords. Artificial ventilation of the lungs is continued through the endotracheal tube until spontaneous respiration returns some 5 minutes later. Should intubation prove difficult the cat is prevented from becoming hypoxic whilst further attempts are made by manual ventilation of the lungs using a face mask. The mask is applied and the lungs inflated several times with pure oxygen as the colour is restored to a normal pink by the lung inflation.

Manual ventilation of the lungs through a face mask is not difficult. Cats' faces are reasonably uniform in shape and it is easy to get a gas-tight seal between a properly designed mask and the face. The lower jaw must be pushed forward to ensure the airway is clear and only gentle pressure applied to the bag to ventilate the lungs or gas will be forced down the oesophagus into the stomach. It is possible to ventilate almost all unconscious cats with pure oxygen at any time and the well-oxygenated cat can be intubated under the influence of a muscle relaxant such as suxamethonium without need for haste.

Ventilation of the lungs through a face mask is only impossible in cats with upper respiratory obstruction (usually an abscess or tumour) and in these a tracheostomy may be the only way in which patency of the airway can be assured. Particular care should be taken to exert only minimal pressure on the bag in cats with ruptured diaphragms, for in them it is very easy to inflate the stomach.

The head and neck of the supine cat are extended by placing a small sandbag under the neck, or by an assistant supporting the head with a hand placed beneath the neck, and the tongue is pulled out of the mouth, taking care not to injure it on the teeth. A standard laryngoscope with an infant-sized blade is introduced and the tip of the blade placed so that it is over the dorsum of the tongue and resting just in front of the epiglottis. The laryngoscope blade is then lifted to expose the glottic opening and giving a good view of the vocal cords. The endotracheal tube may then be passed between the cords without any difficulty. If a laryngoscope is not available, a lighted tongue depressor can be used in much the same way but these tongue depressors are not so easy to control and it may be found easier to expose the larynx if the cat is lying on its side as described for the dog .

A 5 or 5.5 mm uncuffed endotracheal tube is suitable for most adult cats. A tight seal, such as may be needed to prevent inhalation of foreign materials, can be ensured by a pharyngeal pack of moistened ribbon gauze. Endotracheal tubes should be long enough to pass well beyond the larynx but not so long that they will enter the main bronchus. The correct length may be assessed as being from the nostrils to the point of the shoulder of the cat, and all new tubes should be cut to this measurement before use (Fig. 24.2).

An excess of tube between the mouth and breathing circuit should not be tolerated because this, in small animals, adds significantly to the respiratory dead space. A tape tied tightly around the tube over the endotracheal connector can be secured behind the cat's ears to anchor the tube in position once it has been introduced.

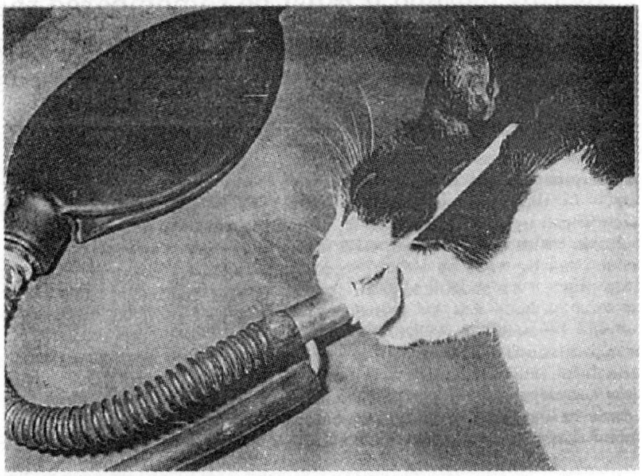

Fig. 24.2: An intubated cat with no excess length of tube protruding from the mouth and the tube securely anchored

PREMEDICATION

Anticholinergic drugs should generally be included in the premedication given to cats, both to prevent saliva and bronchial secretions from obstructing the small diameter airway, and to block vagal reflexes. The only contraindications to their use are the general ones of pre-existing tachycardia or glaucoma and they should be given whenever it is proposed to use suxamethonium for endotracheal intubation. Analgesics should be given whenever it is necessary to relieve pain. The use of sedatives is governed by the temperament of the cat and by the anaesthetic technique to follow. Phenothiazincs do little to calm a wild cat, but are useful in quieter animals to counteract excitement caused by some drugs and to improve the quality of recovery. Xylazine and medetomidine markedly reduce the dose of all other drugs used for anaesthesia and should be used with very great care.

Anticholinergic Agents

Atropine, at a total dose of 0.3 mg for an adult cat, may be given by the intramuscular or subcutaneous route. Atropine interferes with vision and cats which have received this drug should be handled particularly carefully to avoid inducing panic reactions. Glycopyrrolate, in doses of about 0.01 mg/kg by intramuscular injection, or at half this dose by the intravenous route, is probably a better anticholinergic for cats. It does not cause as marked increase in heart rate nor does it readily cross the blood-brain barrier.

Intravenous injection is relatively easy in dogs but in cats problems of restraint may make intravenous injections more difficult or even impossible, so that agents which can be given by other routes tend to have a greater role to play in feline than in canine anaesthesia. The disadvantages of such administration, e.g. slow induction, variable absorption, variable results, often prolonged recovery, and inability to dose to effect, must be weighed against the temperament of the cat and the likelihood of being able to carry out a controlled intravenous injection.

Thiopentone Sodium

Thiopentone may only be given intravenously and in cats it should be used as a 1.25% or even more dilute solution. It may be used for induction of anaesthesia at doses of up to 10 mg/kg, and if the cat has not been given a sedative premedication it is probable that the full dose will be required. Very small doses will be needed after premedication with the α_2-adrenoceptor agonists. If thiopentone is to be used as the sole agent, incremental doses up to a total dose of 20 mg/kg may be used but, at these high doses, saturation of the fat depots may mean that recovery will take several hours and effects may still be observed the next day. If recovery is prolonged, the cat must be kept warm, for development of hypothermia will delay recovery still more.

Methohexitone Sodium

Methohexitone may be given only by intravenous injection, and is used at a concentration of 0.5% for feline anaesthesia. Although it can be used for induction of anaesthesia at a dose of about 5 mg/kg, and given in incremental doses to maintain anaesthesia, in cats its tendency for causing excitement means that recovery is often far from uneventful. The use of sedative premedication helps to reduce the incidence of excitatory phenomena but, in general, methohexitone is only employed in cats when very rapid recovery is essential (e.g. after caesarean section).

Pentobarbitone Sodium

Until about 20 years ago pentobarbitone was widely used in general practice and experimental laboratories as an anaesthetic for cats. Doses of 25 mg/kg by intravenous injection, half given fast to avoid induction excitement and the rest given slowly over.

Alphaxolone and Alphadolone (Saffan)

Since its introduction into clinical feline anaesthesia this steroid mixture has become an extremely popular agent, especially in general practice.

The two steroids in Saffan are dissolved with Cremophor EL to give a total steroid concentration of 12 mg/ml and in veterinary practice it has become customary to express doses in terms of milligrams of this total steroid content. The solution is non-irritant and is given to cats intravenously or intramuscularly. In the unsedated cat, doses of 3 mg/kg by intravenous injection produced unconsciousness for a few minutes, whilst doses of 9 mg/kg give 10–15 minutes of anaesthesia with very little increase in the initial depth of unconsciousness or respiratory depression. The increased duration of action with initial dose increase reaches a plateau at about 18 mg/kg and giving higher doses is pointless and may be dangerous. If it is necessary to prolong anaesthesia further, increments of Saffan may be given later on, or an inhalation agent employed. Saffan is rapidly metabolized in the liver so that the incremental dose regimen does not result in undue delay in recovery and cats are usually completely conscious 2 hours after the last dose has been given. The rapid breakdown of the steroids, coupled with the minimal cardiovascular effects, undoubtedly make it a safe drug.

The fact that ketamine can be administered by intramuscular or subcutaneous injection makes it a very useful agent for the induction of anaesthesia in cats which are difficult or impossible to handle. The volume of solution which has to be injected is small and the injection can be made by a dart projectile fired from a blowpipe. If it is possible to give it from a syringe, the small volume can be injected very rapidly. It should be noted, however, that intramuscular or subcutaneous injection of ketamine appears to be painful, in that it is very often violently resented by the animal, and that for all but the most minor of procedures it is necessary to supplement its action with an inhalation agent, as the marked muscle tone limits the surgery possible. When given by intravenous injection there is a delay of 1–2 minutes before its effects become apparent but this is the best route for administration. Application to the mucous membrane of the mouth (squirting from a syringe) can be an effective route of administration in cats which are difficult to handle.

A wide range of sedative agents have been used for premedication, or in combination with ketamine, in order to reduce the side effects, in particular those of emergence phenomena and increased muscle tone. Where the use of such premedication allows a reduction in the dose of ketamine, speed of recovery may be enhanced. Acepromazine (0.1 mg/kg by intramuscular injection) although widely used is not totally effective in reducing the unwanted side effects and has little influence on the dose of ketamine subsequently required. Intramuscular diazepam in doses of 1 mg/kg has also often proved disappointing. However, midazolam (0.2 mg/kg) mixed in the syringe with ketamine (10 mg/kg) and administered intramuscularly provides deep sedation suitable for radiotherapy; useful sedation lasts about 30 minutes (some cats become cyanosed when breathing air) and recovery is usually complete within 2–3 hours. Xylazine has been the most commonly used sedative for cats receiving ketamine. Xylazine is extremely effective in preventing emergence excitement and increased muscle tone and it permits reduction in the ketamine dose, but its use is also associated with the side effects of bradycardia (unless anticholinergic have been used for premedication) and vomiting.

Zolazepam/Tilctamine

Zolazepam is a member of the benzodiazepine group of drugs, while tilctamine is a drug of the phencyclidine family. Their combination in equal proportions has been used intravenously and intramuscularly to produce deep sedation or even anaesthesia in cats and dogs. Intravenous doses of 15 mg/kg of the mixture produce unconsciousness in one injection site/brain circulation time and after intramuscular injection full effects are seen in 2–5 minutes. Anticholinergic premedication should be given to limit excess salivation which is a feature of the anaesthetic state. Anaesthesia or sedation may be prolonged by the injection of one-third to one-half of the initial dose. After one dose the duration of surgical anaesthesia is of the order of 20–60 minutes and recovery is prolonged, frequently taking 6 or more hours or even longer. If more than the one initial dose has been administered recovery can be very prolonged.

INHALATION ANAESTHESIA

Anaesthesia using a face mask in a restrained cat, the animal is usually placed in lateral recumbency with all four legs held by an assistant while the anaesthetist controls the head with one hand and uses the other to apply the face mask.

Cats seldom object to breathing a nitrous oxide/oxygen mixture via a face mask and Magill system and the volatile agents may be added to this in gradually increasing concentrations. The normal rule is to increase the concentration of the volatile agent after every three breaths until the safe maximum is obtained. This technique avoids the prolonged breath holding which occurs if the animal is suddenly introduced to high induction concentrations of the volatile anaesthetic agent. If the cat struggles it usually breathes rapidly and deeply so the induction of anaesthesia is more rapid; if breath holding is encountered care must be taken not to release the cat as it may be at the stage of narcotic excitement. This method of induction can be traumatic for both the cat and the anaesthetist and adrenaline release in the frightened animal may occasionally result in ventricular fibrillation and death unless acepromazine, which seems to exert some protective effect, has been given for premedication. However, it has been applied quite safely for many years and the rapid postoperative recovery which results from not having given the cat any parenteral agents may often out-weigh the disadvantages of the induction procedure. In heavily premedicated or very sick cats, induction of anaesthesia by volatile agents given by a face mask can usually be carried out without invoking excitement or struggling, and is often the method of choice. Smooth induction can usually be anticipated with halothane or isoflurane in a nitrous oxide/oxygen, but even if they are very carefully introduced into nitrous oxide/oxygen, coughing, sneezing and breath holding may be encountered in vigorous, healthy cats.

Breathing Circuits

Any breathing circuit used to administer inhalation anaesthetics to cats must have a very low resistance and small dead space. In practice, this limits the possible circuits to non-rebreathing systems as the soda lime canister of rebreathing systems creates too much resistance to respiration.

The Ayre's T-piece system

This is the circuit of choice when the cat is intubated but it may also be used with a face mask. It has minimal resistance and dead space and IPPV can be carried out very efficiently by squeezing the partially filled bag of the Jackson-Rees modification of the T-piece system. Fresh gas flow rates of twice the minute volume of respiration (Table 24.1) are sufficient to prevent rebreathing.

Table 24.1: Average respiratory and cardiovascular data for anaesthetized normal adult cats

Respiratory rate	24–28 breaths/min
Tidal volume	12–24 ml
Minute volume	280–670 ml/min
Heart rate	160 beats/min
Arterial blood pressure	120–140 mmHg (16–18.7 kPa) systolic
	70–80 mmHg (9.3–11 kPa) diastolic
Arterial blood pH	7.34
PaO_2	90–104 mmHg (12–13.9 kPa)
$PaCO_2$	35 mmHg (4.7 kPa)

Coaxial Circuits

In practice the Bain circuit does not behave like a T-piece system and appears to offer too much resistance for animals breathing spontaneously, but it seems that the performance of the modified Bain circuit is improved if the 'tail' of the bag is cut. The Lack system behaves rather like a Magill system but the tubing is much stiffer and bulkier so that it tends to drag the face mask away from the face or the endotracheal tube out of the trachea. The expiratory valve needs to be removed from the Lack circuit. The parallel circuits in these configurations offer no advantage in feline anaesthesia.

The Magill system

Although the expiratory valve of the Magill system creates rather too much resistance for cats, the system is frequently used with a face mask to administer inhalation anaesthetics to these animals. If the mask is tightly applied to the cat's face most anaesthetists lift the valve plate off its setting by introducing a pin or needle beneath the plate. Other anaesthetists use a large face mask which is not applied tightly to the cat's face so that free expiration can take place between the face and the mask.

Inhalation Agents Used

All the inhalation anaesthetics may be used in cats in a similar way to that in which they are used in dogs.

Nitrous oxide

Nitrous oxide/oxygen mixtures (3/2) are useful after anaesthesia has been induced with saffan, especially when it has been given by intramuscular injection, as they seem to suppress the muscle twitching often seen when the effects of saffan are waning. However, nitrous oxide/oxygen mixtures are usually used in feline anaesthesia simply as the vehicle for the delivery of the volatile agents.

Ether

For well over 100 years ether has proved to be a particularly safe anaesthetic for cats. Today, however, it is being discarded in most of the developed countries in favour of more recently introduced agents. Nevertheless, although induction is slower, the margin for error is much greater than it is for more potent agents such as halothane. Many thousands of cats have been anaesthetized with ether and the number of deaths which can be attributed to its proper use is small. In man, anaesthetization with ether is often followed by nausea and this may occur in cats for many are reluctant to eat for the first 12–24 hours after operation. However, this is a small price to pay for the safety of the patient and the only real objection which can be made to the use of ether in feline anaesthesia is the risk of fires or explosions when it is mixed with air or oxygen. Anticholinergics are essential to reduce the copious secretions induced by the irritant nature of its vapour.

Halothane

Cardiac arrhythmias occur quite frequently in cats under halothane anaesthesia. When they occur they can usually be abolished and normal rhythm restored by the performance of artificial respiration (IPPV) to increase the gaseous exchange in the lungs. It appears that the respiratory depressant activity of halothane allows carbon dioxide to accumulate in the body and once the concentration of this gas exceeds a certain threshold value arrhythmias appear. Lowering the $PaCO_2$ by IPPV is followed by a prompt return to normal cardiac rhythm. Very satisfactory anaesthesia results when an accurately calibrated vaporizer is used and halothane is administered in oxygen or a nitrous oxide/oxygen mixture through a non-rebreathing T-piece system. For cats the total fresh gas flow rate to the T-piece system need not exceed 1.5–2 1/min, little halothane is used and, consequently, the method is not expensive so, provided ducting of waste gases from the open end of the T-piece is practised, there is no justification for attempting to use closed methods of administration.

Enflurane

The enflurane can has been used quite successfully to produce anaesthesia with short induction and recovery periods. It may be volatilized, preferably from a calibrated vaporizer in a stream of oxygen or nitrous oxide/oxygen and delivered to the cat by any of the methods usually employed in feline anaesthesia. Evidence of central nervous irritation has not been observed, but myotonia is common during recovery.

Isoflurane

Isoflurane may eventually find a role in feline anaesthesia. Such limited trials as have been carried out in cats with isoflurane have shown it to be an apparently quite satisfactory agent although in cats not undergoing surgery respiratory depression is marked. Theoretically, for use in cats with cardiac disease isoflurane may have advantages over halothane but, in practice, this is not very obvious when halothane is given with care.

INTERMITTENT POSITIVE-PRESSURE VENTILATION (IPPV)

In the intubated cat, IPPV can be carried out by manual compression of the reservoir bag of the Jackson-Rees modification of the T-piece system, as described for small dogs. It is perfectly possible to apply IPPV when an uncuffed endotracheal tube is in place and indeed the absence of a cuff acts as a safety device by preventing the application of too high a positive pressure and overinflation of the lungs. When the cat is not intubated, IPPV can be applied through a tightly fitting face mask attached to either an Ayre's T-piece or Magill system, but care must be taken to ensure that the airway is clear and that too much pressure is not applied or the stomach will be inflated. A clear airway is produced by avoiding overflexion or extension of the head and applying forward pressure behind the vertical ramus of the mandible as the face is pushed into the mask. The Magill system is only used for emergencies because when IPPV is performed it gives rise to almost total rebreathing so that the mask has to be removed from the patient's face every few breaths to allow exhalation to the atmosphere and the mask to refill with fresh gas.

Most mechanical ventilators used in canine surgery produce tidal volumes which are too large for cats and if they are used in these animals a controlled leak has to be introduced into the circuit. Human paediatric ventilators are available which are quite suitable for use in feline anaesthesia but they are likely to be needed too infrequently to justify their purchase.

NEUROMUSCULAR BLOCKING AGENTS

In cats there is seldom any indication for the use of competitive neuromuscular blocking agents as muscle tone is insufficient to interfere with most feline surgery. However, when they arc indicated they may be used at the same dose rates, and their action antagonized in the same way, as described for dogs. The depolarizing agent suxamethonium is used to aid endotracheal intubation or endoscopy, and in adult cats doses of 3–5 mg by intravenous injection will, after the initial muscle fasciculation, give complete relaxation for some 4–6 minutes, depending on the anaesthetic agents in use. During the period of apnoea IPPV is of course, necessary, and no difficulty is experienced in continuing this IPPV for much longer than the paralysis due to the relaxant lasts.

NEONATAL ANAESTHESIA

The small size of neonatal kittens make them particularly prone to develop hypothermia and to respiratory obstruction. Kittens should always be premedicated with an anticholinergic (0.005 mg of atropine is sufficient) and anaesthesia is best induced and maintained with volatile anaesthetics. Endotracheal intubation should be avoided unless absolutely essential — as it is if IPPV is needed. Very careful attention should be given to the maintenance of body temperature and to the replacement of blood or fluid losses.

POSTOPERATIVE CARE

Endotraeheal tubes should be removed from cats when anaesthesia is still reasonably deep as their removal during light anaesthesia can give rise to troublesome laryngeal spasm. The quality of recovery in the cat depends to a great extent on the anaesthetic agents which have been employed. It is usually smooth and uneventful following the use of inhalation anaesthesia, but cats may be hypersensitive to noise and other stimulation after treatment with propofol (saffan) or ketamine use of this agent be restricted to preoperative use. In the authors' experience, pethidine in doses of 10–25 mg (depending on the size of the cat) given by intramuscular injection at 3–4 hourly intervals produced excellent pain relief in the postoperative period for the majority of animals. Buprenorphine (0.006 mg/kg) can also be effective.

Cats may always be encouraged to eat and drink, provided that there are no surgical contraindications, as soon as they have fully regained consciousness.

LOCAL ANALGESIA

Local analgesia is seldom used in cats because of the problems involved in adequate restraint of the animal, but it can be valuable in very sick or moribund animals or when the animal is controlled by deep sedation or light anaesthesia. Whatever method of local analgesia is employed care must be taken that the total dose of the agent does not constitute a toxic dose. Extrapolating from the levels considered to be toxic in other species of animal, a dose of about 0.12 g, i.e. 12 ml, of 1% lignocaine should be the maximum employed in a 4 kg adult cat. In cats local analgesia usually involves local infiltration of the operation site, but techniques such as intravenous regional analgesia or specific nerve blocks can be employed if restraint is adequate.

Epidural Analgesia

The use of epidural analgesia in cats has been described. The technique is identical to that used in dogs and, using 2% lignocaine, doses of 1 ml/4.5 kg given at the lumbosacral space block.

Bibliography

1. Healy E.G., In Gahm Jones O., ed. *Small Animal Anaesthesia,* p. 59, 1964.
2. McDonell W., *Modern Veterinary Practice* p. 31, 53, 1972.
3. Soma L.R. *Textbook of Veterinary Anaesthesia*, p. 250–81, 1971.

25

Anaesthesia for Small Laboratory Animals

The small animals require restraint. If used, local analgesic drugs should be diluted and care taken not to overdose. General anaesthesia is preferred for most purposes and may be induced and maintained with volatile agents, induced with injectable drugs and maintained with volatile agents or maintained with injectable drugs alone.

ANAESTHESIA WITH VOLATILE AGENTS

The safest method of anaesthesia for the veterinarian who is inexperienced in anaesthetizing small mammals is that of induction and maintenance with volatile anaesthetics. The most popular agents are methoxyflurane, halothane and isoflurane. Ether, often used in the past, is not recommended as the excessive bronchial secretions it provokes may cause respiratory obstruction even if an anticholinergic premedication has been given. Methoxyflurane has the advantage of a high safety margin due to its low volatility while halothane and isoflurane allow for faster induction and recovery, but are easier to overdose.

Mask induction can lead to handling stress and the use of an induction chamber is to be preferred. Several such chambers are commercially available but they are very easy to construct and there is now little reason to use the much more dangerous method of simply putting the agent on cotton wool into a jar with the animal. This can result in very high concentrations of the anaesthetic agent in the animal. If this dangerous method has to be used it is safest with methoxyflurane, and the animal should be removed from the jar as soon as it becomes recumbent and care should be taken not to allow direct contact between the animal and the soaked cotton wool.

Once induced, anaesthesia should be maintained by volatilizing the agent in a stream of oxygen and administering the mixture through a T-piece or similar low-resistance breathing circuit. Suitable face masks for small mammals can be made from syringes and should not be a tight fit around the muzzle, for allowing gas to escape in this way reduces the resistance to breathing. Such a leak of gas does, however, cause problems of atmospheric pollution and some form of active scavenging should be used.

ANAESTHESIA WITH INJECTABLE DRUGS

Theoretically, any injectable anaesthetic can be used in small mammals and usually the necessary doses are well known from the original development work in laboratory animals carried out by the drug company. However, practical limitations are set by the possible methods of administration. In some animals with easily accessible veins (e.g. rabbits) drugs such as propofol or thiopentone can be used in doses similar to those used in cats and dogs (although the duration of effect may be shorter). Where intravenous injection is more difficult, drugs which can be given by intraperitoneal, intramuscular or subcutaneous injection are generally used. The most popular combinations of drugs are the neuroleptanalgesics or incorporate ketamine. There are marked differences between species responses and even within one species of animal actions may be unreliable, a given drug producing deep anaesthesia in one animal whilst only providing some sedation in another.

Ketamine has the advantage that it is effective no matter what the route of administration. Doses required and efficacy vary greatly between the various species of animal (Table 25.1). Lower doses may be used for sedation and immobilization for non-surgical procedures. As in other species of animal, ketamine is used in combination with sedative drugs such as the benzodiazepines (diazepam or midazolam) and/or α_2-adrenoceptor agonists (xylazine or medetomidine) in order to reduce the dose of ketamine, improve muscle relaxation and to increase the effectiveness of the dissociative agent as an anaesthetic. It is worth noting that the formulations of ketamine at lower concentrations, which are available for use in children, can prove more convenient for use in very small animals than the standard veterinary preparation which needs to be diluted before use. Although most commercially available neuroleptanalgesic combinations can be used, the mixture of fentanyl and fluanisone (Hypnorm) has proved to be most popular in the UK and this again can be administered by any route.

Alphaxalone/alphadolone (**Saffan**) has proved useful in some species of animal when given intravenously (Table 25.1) and may also be given intramuscularly. Propofol and thiopentone should only be given intravenously. Pentobarbitone may be used by intra-peritoneal injection in some animals but gives prolonged sedation and respiratory depression so that it cannot be recommended for clinical use.

Postoperative analgesia should not be neglected. Some suitable opioid drugs are listed in Table 25.1 and oilier methods utilizing such agents as the local analgesics should be considered. It is regrettable that the rat, which has probably contributed more than most animals to advances in medical and veterinary sciences, still seems to be neglected when postoperative analgesia is indicated.

Rabbits

Rabbits *(Oryctolagus ainwuhis)* and hares *(Lepus europaeus)* need to be handled carefully; they tend to panic if placed on slippery surfaces and are best held for injection wrapped in a towel in the arms of an assistant or placed in a restraining box. A rabbit' struggling against forcible restraint may fracture a vertebra, especially if restraint is applied to the neck, so any anaesthetic technique used should entail only the minimum of physical restraint. Intramuscular injections are made into the quadriceps or triceps muscles and intravenous injections are given into the marginal vein of the ear.

Although any intravenous anaesthetic agent may be used to induce anaesthesia in rabbits, they are not good subjects in which to maintain anaesthesia with injectable agents,

Table 25.1: Recommended doses of injectable anaesthetics and analgesics for small mammals

	Rabbits	Guinea pigs	Hamsters	Gerbils	Rats	Mice	Ferrets
Ketamine combinations	Ketamine 25 mg/kg i.m. (sedation only) (sedation only) Xylazine 3 mg/kg i.v. followed by 10 mins later by ketamine 3 mg/kg i.v. Ketamine 20 mg/kg Mcdctomidine 300 µg/kg Diazepam 0.75–1.5 mg/kg[4]	Not effective on its own (sedation only) Ketamine 40 mg/kg\ Xylazine 5 mg/kg s.c. (restraint only)[l]	Not very effective	Always unreliable, not effective on its own Ketamine 50 mg/kg Xylazine 2 mg/kg (still unreliable)	Ketamine 60 mg/ kg i.m. (sedation) Ketamine 25 mg/kg \ Diazepam 2 mg/kg i.m. (anaesthesia)	Ketamine 100 mg/kg	Ketamine 20–30 mg/kg i.m.
"Hypnorm' combinations 1 ml Hypnorm contains fentanyl 0.315 mg + fluanisone 10 mg. Reversal of Fentanyl if necessary with Naloxone 0.1 mg/kg	Hypnorm 0.3 ml/kg Diazepam 1–2 mg/kg[l] Hypnorm 0.3 ml/kg Midazolam mg/kg	Hypnorm 1 ml/kg- i.m. Diazepam 2.5 mg/kg Diazepam 5 mg/kg 5 mg/kg i.p. or i.p. or Midazolam mg/kg Hypnorm		Hypnorm 1 ml/kg Diazepam 5 mg/kg 0.3 ml/kg 5 mg/kg i.m. or i.p.	Hypnorm 1 ml/kg Midazolam or Midazolam 5 mg/kg i.p. Diazepam 5 mg/kg [P-D]	Hypnorm 0.3 ml/kg Diazepam	Hypnorm 0.01 ml/30 g
Alphaxalone/alphadolone	6–9 mg/kg i.v. (best used only for induction) 12 mg/kg i.m. (sedation only)						10–15 mg/kg i.v.
Postoperative analgesia Buprenorphine	0.02–0.05 mg/kg s.c 8–12 hours	0.05 mg/kg s.c. 8–12 hours			1.0–0.2 mg/kg s.c. 8–12 hours	2 mg/kg s.c. 12 hours	
Pethidine	10 mg/kg s.c. or i.m. 2–3 hours	20 mg/kg s.c. or i.m. 2–3 hours		20 mg/kg	20 mg kg s.c. 2–3 hours	20 mg/kg s.c. 2–3 hours	

even very small incremental doses causing death through respiratory arrest. Similarly, unexpected deaths may occur following ketamine.

Induction with thiopentone (10–12 mg/kg), methohexitone (5–10 mg/kg) or saffan (2–8 mg/kg), given intravenously to effect, is satisfactory, but it is doubtful whether methohexitone or saffan have any real advantages over thiopentone. These agents are best given through a 0.8 mm (21 s.w.g.) butterfly needle strapped into the ear vein and may be followed with halothane/oxygen or isoflurane/oxygen to produce satisfactory anaesthesia for several hours should this prove necessary.

For an inhalation induction a 1:1 mixture of nitrous oxide/oxygen should be administered through a face mask from a T-piece system at a flow rate of about 21 min for 1–2 minutes before halothane or isoflurane is cautiously added in small step concentrations up to 2-3%. Induction of anaesthesia is usually quiet when the volatile agents are vaporized in a nitrous oxide oxygen mixture in this way and once anaesthetized the rabbit may be intubated with a 3–3.5 mm uncuffed endotracheal tube under direct vision using a laryngoscope with a small paediatric blade. An alternative method which is probably better if nitrous oxide is not available is to place the rabbit in a box and introduce a stream of halothane or isoffurane volatilized in oxygen into the box until the animal is unconscious. Anaesthesia is usually maintained with 1.5–2% halothane or 2–3% isofurane vapour given by lace-mask or through an endotracheal tube.

Judgement of the depth of anaesthesia is assessed by tickling the inside of the ear pinnae, since with many anaesthetic methods the pedal withdrawal reflex may remain strong until the animal is very close to death.

There are very many ways of anaesthetizing rats and mice but simple halothane or isoflurane anaesthesia is very satisfactory for all clinical purposes. Anaesthesia may be induced in a box used as an induction chamber, or by a face mask, with the agent volatilized in a stream of oxygen.

Ketamine is generally unsatisfactory in rats and mice (Table 25.1) and although a neuroleptic combination, given by subcutaneous injection, may be used, in experienced hands inhalation anaesthesia is safer.

It is most important to keep the rats and mice warm whilst they are anaesthetized and in the recovery period.

Guinea pigs are not good subjects for anaesthesia with injectable agents whether given by intravenous injection or by parenteral routes. Visible veins are fragile and venepuncture is often difficult, while the use of other routes necessitates an accurate estimation of body weight for computation of the dose. Since the gastrointestinal tract can contribute anything from 20–40% of the total weight of the animal, depending on its content of ingesta, it is not surprising that variable results follow from intraperitoneal or intramuscular injections of computed doses of injectable drugs. Moreover, respiratory disease is common. Fortunately, halothane or isoflurane anaesthesia meets most of the needs of clinical practice. A mixture of the volatile agent with oxygen is supplied to an induction chamber (box) or to a face mask at 1–2 l/min, starting with a minimal concentration of the vapour and gradually increasing it until the animal loses consciousness. Anaesthesia is usually produced in about 2–3 minutes and can be maintained with concentrations of halothane

(0.5–1.5%)) or isoflurane (1–2%), given through a face mask from a T-piece system. Full recovery follows in less than 20–30 minutes after termination of anaesthesia.

Maintenance of a clear airway is not always easy in guinea pigs since nasal and oropharyngeal secretions tend to become viscid during anaesthesia and are liable to give rise to obstruction. The risk may be countered by frequent aspiration of the mouth and oropharynx using a line rubber catheter attached to a 60 ml syringe. Endotracheal intubation is virtually impossible in these animals. As with all small mammals, conservation of body heal is important and a warm environment should be provided.

Ketamine, whether used alone or in combination with α_2-adrenoceptor agonists, immobilizes and produces anaesthesia in these animals.

Hamsters and gerbils are best anaesthetized by inhalation methods. They should be placed in an induction chamber such as a small cardboard box with a perforated lid and anaesthetized with isoflurane, halothane or methoxyflurane. These volatile agents can be introduced into the box in a stream of oxygen. The animal is removed from the box as soon as it becomes unconscious and anaesthesia is maintained using a face mask. If injectable agents are obligatory, neurolept analgesic techniques appear to give the most reliable results. Ketamine is again very variable in effect.

Mink are not domestic animals — they are nervous, fast and vicious. All mink are best anaesthetized in a mink carrying box with a volatile anaesthetic such as isoflurane, halothane or methoxyflurane. If necessary, the box may be covered with transparent plastic sheeting to make it more gas tight, and the animal is not removed from the box until it is unconscious.

Ferrets and *skunks* can be anaesthetized with isoflurane or halothane vapour passed into an induction box until they are unconscious and then through a face mask from a T-piece circuit. Inhalation anaesthesia presents no special features in these animals.

Stoats and *weasels* can be dealt with in a similar manner, but it should be remembered that they are much more vicious than ferrets or skunks.

The preferred injectable agents are ketamine with xylazine or a benzodiazepine or saffan (Table 25.1).

Tortoise

In tortoises, terrapins and turtles anaesthetic problems are posed by the very low metabolic rate which varies with environmental temperature, and the ability to retract the head into the protective shell. Some species present further problems due to their adaption to a semi-aquatic or aquatic mode of life. It should be remembered that some species of soft-shelled aquatic turtles can move quickly and handlers can be bitten or scratched.

The lungs are well developed and the respiratory movements are produced chiefly by muscles at each leg pocket beneath the viscera. Although these muscles have been described as diaphragms, they are too weak to drive gases around any anaesthetic system. Most chelonians have the ability to survive on a single ventilatory movement per hour, making attempts to induce anaesthesia with inhalation agents rather unsuccessful. Ketamine is probably the anaesthetic agent of choice although it does not produce muscle relaxation.

It may be given in doses of 60–80 mg/kg into gluteal muscles and if the sedation produced is not adequate for surgery it may be deepened by the administration of isoflurane or halothane because the head will protrude from the shell and breathing will be reasonably rapid. Saffan may be used instead in doses of 12–18 mg/kg. Loss of muscle tone in the neck and limb muscles is the best guide to the depth of central nervous depression. Chelonia are easily intubated.

Recovery from a dose of 60 mg/kg of ketamine takes up to 24 hours. Tortoises should be allowed to recover at normal room temperature, preferably in a strawfilled box. Terrapins and turtles should be kept at a slightly lower environmental temperature and have their bodies kept damp by the application of cold water at fairly frequent intervals.

Snakes

Snakes are difficult subjects for the anaesthetist. They have a low basal metabolic rate which is directly related to the environmental temperature so that if parenteral agents are used the induction and recovery times are very variable. Moreover, they are relatively resistant to hypoxia and can hold their breath for several minutes so that the induction of inhalation anaesthesia may be very prolonged.

Snakes also have peculiar anatomical features. The absence of an epiglottis and the position of the glottis makes it possible to intubate non-venomous snakes under simple physical restraint and inhalation anaesthesia may then be induced by the use of IPPV. (Even so, non-venomous snakes can still inflict bite wounds which often become septic!) Most snakes have only one functional lung which consists of a thin-walled hollow tube terminating in an air sac extending to the level of the cloaca, the trachea being open along one side within the lung. There is no diaphragm and the three-chambered heart yields a slushing noise instead of the clear 'lub-dup' of the mammalian heart on ausculatation.

Rabbits are also subject to respiratory infections, and animals showing signs of such infection should not be used.

Rabbits very seldom can be included to bite but will attempt to scratch strongly with their hind claws when picked-up. They can be safely handled by grasping the scruff of the neck firmly behind the ears and taking care to avoid the hind legs. A rabbit placed on a slippery surface (tile floor or formica countertop) can be easily managed by one person when giving injections or wrapping in a sheet or towel.

Two methods of anesthesia are acceptable when working with the rabbit. Procedures which require placing the rabbit in a prone position (ear flap) may utilize gas anesthesia with a vaporizer. Those which place the rabbit in a supine position (oviductal anastomosis) are best managed with injectable anesthetics.

Gas anesthesia: The rabbit should be securely wrapped in a small sheet, leaving only its head free. (Rabbits have a bundling reflex and when tightly wrapped tend to remain still.) Set the Fluotec vaporizer to deliver 5% Fluothane and 2 L O_2/min, and place the nose cone securely over the rabbit's nose.

Expect most rabbits to hold their breath as long as they can. When the corneal reflex is absent, set the vaporizer back to 3% for maintenance anesthesia. If respiratory depression occurs administer doxapram.

With animal clippers, shave the rabbit's ears and the top of its head. The interscapular area is also shaved to accommodate a cautery ground.

Place the rabbit in the restraining box and pass the ears through the central hole in the earpiece, giving rompun 5–7 mg kg IM in paraspinal muscles or in the large muscles of the hip. The rabbit will become drowsy in 10–15 minutes and will then be more easily handled.

Induction proceeds with a 12–15 mg kg IM injection in either of the afore mentioned sites followed by atropine 0.16 mg. IM.

A maintenance dose of ketamine 12–15 mg; kg IM is given every 30–90 minutes and rompun 20 mg IM is given at 3–4 hours. This anesthetic regimen should be adequate for 5 or 6 hours of anesthesia with the rabbit in a supine position.

The following suggestions may prove helpful in selecting rats and preparing them for surgery.

Rats weighing over 250 gms will usually have femoral vessels approximately 1 mm in external diameter, which is practical size for microvascular surgery.

Rats are subject to mycoplasmal infections. An animal showing signs of such infection (i.e. cough, wheezing, or a watery discharge from eyes or nose) is likely to develop respiratory distress and die when anesthetized.

After weighing the rat, determine the appropriate dosage of pentobarbital and draw it up in a syringe with a 3 8" needle. Place the rat on the lid of his cage, or some other surface to which he can cling with his front feet. Hold the syringe in one hand, and with the other hand lift the rat's tail and hind legs off the cage lid, thus exposing the lower abdomen. Aiming cephalad, penetrate the lower abdomen with a quick jab and inject the pentobarbital intraperitoneally.

Rats may also be immobilized for injection by using a commercially available restraining cage, or by grasping the animal firmly around the neck and shoulder girdle with a leathergloved hand, or by wrapping the animal loosely in a towel or soft cloth.

If the rat does not move when placed on its back, it is ready to be prepped. Use clippers to remove the hair from the lower abdomen, hind legs, and scrotum (you may wish to use a depilatory agent in addition). Wash the shaved area to help remove extraneous and annoying bits of hair.

Place the rat supine on the dissecting board and secure its hind-legs with tape or rubber bands. Test periodically for depth of anesthesia by pinching the base of the tail or the interdigital webs of the forepaws with a pair of toothed forceps. A maintenance dose of 0.1 cc of pentobarbital solution may be given as needed.

When the rat is restrained in the supine position, mucous will often collect in the trachea and cause respiratory obstruction. This is usually heralded by noisy breathing and retraction of the diaphragm. To remove the mucous, retract the tongue and suction the trachea with a piece of small bore plastic tubing attached to a 10 cc syringe. To keep the tubing from becoming plugged with tissue, move it back and forth while aspirating. Repeat this procedure until the obstruction is removed. If respiratory depression occurs, doxapram may be given IM as a stimulant.

The agents described below are those used in laboratory.

Anesthetic Agents
Rats

Sodium pentobarbital (Nembutal Veterinary) is supplied in 100 cc vials containing 60 mg cc. For ease of administration, portions of this solution are diluted 1:1 with physiologic saline. For induction of anaesthesia, a dose of 6 mg (0.2 cc)/100 gm body weight is injected intraperitoneally. For maintenance, an additional 3–6 mg (0.1–0.2 cc) is given every one to two hours as needed.

Rabbits

Two methods of obtaining anesthesia are recommended.

The safest and most efficient gas anesthetic agent for rabbits is halothane (fluothane). Induction is accomplished using a Fluotec Vaporizer set at 5% halothen, with oxygen flow at 2 L/minute. After induction. The halothane concentration is decreased to a maintenance level (3–4%).

A combination of IM injectable rompun 5–7 mg kg (available from veterinary supply companies or a local veterinarian) followed by ketamine 12–15 mg kg and atropine 0.16 mg will provide anesthesia and a dose of ketamine 12–15 mg kg every 30–90 minutes and rompun 5–7 mg/kg every 4–5 hours will maintain it for 5–6 hours.

Respiratory Stimulant

Doxapram (dopram) is a direct stimulant to the central respiratory center (not a specific narcotic antagonist). It is supplied in 20 cc vials containing 20 mg cc. In the event of respiratory depression, the rat is given 4 mg (0.2cc) IM; the rabbit 5 mg (0.25 cc) IV.

Anticoagulant
Rats

Heparin sodium is supplied in 10 cc vials containing 100 μ/cc. Approximately 100 μ/100 gm body weight will give adequate anticoagulation. A solution of 1000 μ/1000 cc physiologic saline is used for irrigation (rats are relatively hypercoagulable. An anticoagulant may be necessary to prevent thrombosis of venous anastomoses).

Rabbits

No anticoagulation is necessary for the rabbit.

Vasodilating Agent

Lidocaine (Xylocaine) 1% is the vasodilating agent we prefer for both rats and rabbits. It is applied (undiluted) directly to the vessel, and allowed to remain for 3–5 minutes.

Sacrificing Agent

20% KCl is a convenient solution to use for sacrificing fully anesthetised animals. Three to five ml (administered IV) rapidly causes cardiac arrest in rats; 10 cc usually suffices for rabbit.

Handling of Rats during Anaesthesia

Rats are widely preferred for microvascular practice work. They have the advantages of being hardy inexpensive, and easy to obtain in addition they withstand prolonged anesthesia veil. Rat vessels have thinner walls than human vessels and in this respect, they are more difficult to work on. In addition, the femoral vessels are smaller than almost any vessels that will be encountered clinically. These factors will give you a certain theoretical margin of competence when you make the transition to wonting on human vessels. However, experience with the rat fails to simulate the difficulties of access, exposure, and control of unwanted movement which are often encountered in clinical work.

Laboratory rats are clean creatures and generally docile. They become nervous and aggressive if kept alone in a cage and also if they hear loud, sudden noises. Rats dislike open spaces and are peaceful only if they are in close contact with things.

Do not use a rat that makes wet, snuffly noises when it breathes or that has blood-stained nasal discharge. These are signs of mycoplasma infection, and such rats are unfit for anesthesia.

ANNEXTURE

Rat Groin: External Features

The anatomy of the rat groin is roughly analogous to that of the human. One important difference is that when the hind limb is extended (i.e. when it is immobilized on the rat board) it joins the long axis of the body at a 135° angle. The inguinal fold makes a 45° angle with the long axis and corresponds to the location and course of the underlying inguinal ligament.

Skin and Subcutaneous Tissue

The skin is quite lax and mobile. There is a thin layer of muscle and fat. The panniculus carnosus which is loosely connected to the dermis. A pronounced inguinal fat pad overlies the entire femoral triangle and extends over the lower quadrant of the abdomen, where it gradually thins out.

Femoral Triangle

The femoral triangle is bounded superiorly by the inguinal ligament, laterally by the extensor muscles and the adductor muscles of the thigh. It is covered by a very thin but definite, superficial fascia. Beneath this fascia, and contained within the femoral sheath, run the femoral vessels and the femoral nerve (Fig. 25.1).

The femoral artery (0.6–1 mm external diameter), vein (1–2 mm external diameter) and nerve enter the left; through the femoral canal which passes beneath the mid point of the inguinal ligament. There is a fairly dense femoral sheath which envelops the femoral vein (medial), femoral artery (lateral to the vein), and femoral nerve (lateral to the artery), and forms septae between these structures. The femoral artery and vein give off deep branches about midway in their course through the femoral triangle, but otherwise are devoid of major branches. The deep branches (profunda femoris artery and vein) are usually single large vessels which dive into the underlying muscle; however, there may be two or more of each of these branches.

As the femoral vessels leave the femoral triangle they give off the superficial epigastric artery and vein. Accompanied by a branch of the femoral nerve, these branches ascend superficially into the inguinal fat pad and curve superiorly and medially to supply the skin and subcutaneous tissues of the groin and lower two thirds of the abdomen. Where these branches arise several other muscular branches are seen.

Rat Sciatic Region

The sciatic nerve arises from the lumbosacral plexus at the caudal end of the spinal cord. It exits from the dorsal pelvis and crosses the posterior thigh overlying the adductor femoris and subjacent to the biceps femoris. As it enters the popliteal space, it gives rise to the peroneal, tibial, and sural nerves which are monofase-

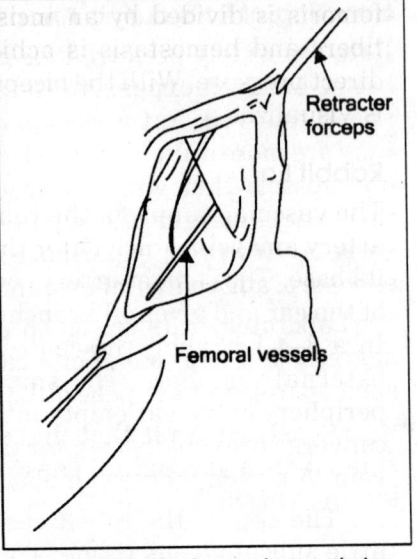

Fig. 25.1: Rat femoral vessels in femoral triangle

icular. A tiny fourth branch to the biceps femoris is often present and is usually transacted when the nerve is mobilized. For oviductal anastomoses, position the animal supine and shave the lower abdomen. Apply adhesive tape to remove loose hairs and prep with alcohol. After the animal is anesthetized as previously outlined and prepped a midline incision is made in the lower abdomen with dissection continued down through the subcutaneous tissue, incising the fascia in the midline and entering the peritoneal cavity (Fig. 25.2). Retraction exposes the abdominal viscera. A rubber sheet should be prepared that will cover the animals' abdominal wall. A slit is made in this rubber sheet measuring two to three cms in length. The uterine horn and oviduct from one side is then manually elevated and placed through the slit in the rubber sheet to isolate it from the other abdominal contents. Oviductal approximating clamps can be utilized if desired to maintain the oviducts on the rubber drapes. The uterine tubal junction is then identified by inspection and palpation. The oviduct is much more narrow and less firm than the uterus itself. The gross dissection is done with the aid of ocular loupes. When the exposure is complete the operating microscope is positioned over the operating field.

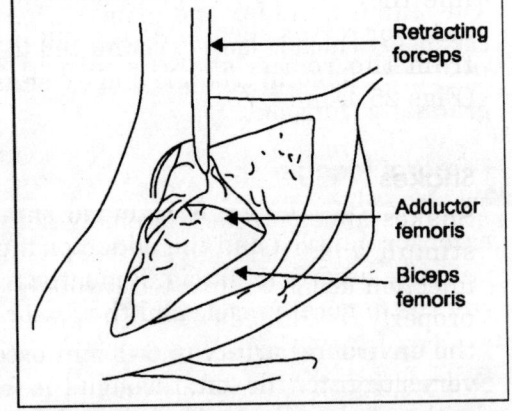

Fig. 25.2: Sciatic region showing muscles

The animal is anesthetized and the dorsal hindquarters are shaved. After stabilization on the dissecting board a transverse incision is made with a scalpel or scissors and the skin is blunt dissected from the underlying muscles. With the skin retracted, the biceps femoris is divided by an incision running parallel to its fibers and hemostasis is achieved with hot cautery and direct pressure. With the biceps retracted, the sciatic nerve is visualized.

Rabbit Ear

The vascular supply of the rabbit ear consists of a central artery and vein which enter the dorsal aspect of the ear at its base. The central artery courses along the central axis of the ear and gives off branches in a herringbone pattern. In a 3–4 kg rabbit the central artery is 0.75–1.0 mm in external diameter. The small venous branches at the periphery of the ear empty into two marginal veins which converge proximally to enter the main trunk of the central vein. A central nerve can also be identified (Fig. 25.3)

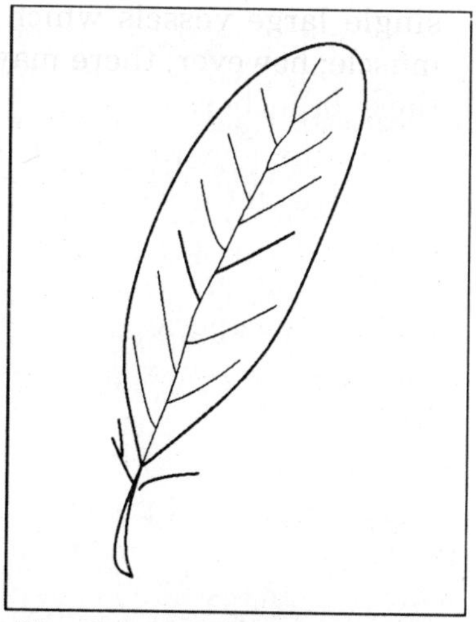

Fig. 25.3: Rabbit ear with central vessels

The skin of the rabbit ear is quite thin and has very little subcutaneous tissue. The vessels are distributed on the deep surface of the dermis, and when dissecting a skin flap in this model care must be exercised in order to avoid damage to these vessels. The skin is more or less tightly adherent to the underlying cartilage.

Rabbit Abdomen and Pelvis

The anatomy of the rabbit abdomen and pelvis is similar to that in most mammals. In the lower abdomen the external oblique and internal oblique are separate and distinct muscles. As they approach the midline they form an aponeurosis which becomes the anterior rectus sheath. At the midline contributions from the rectus sheaths join at the linea alba (Figs 25.4 and 25.5).

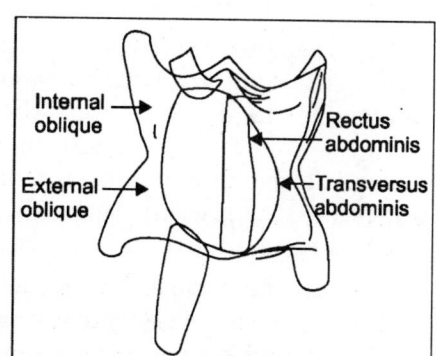

Fig. 25.4: Rabbit abdomen muscles

Snakes

Snakes appear to be extremely sensitive to painful stimuli and strike or contract violently when an injection needle is inserted through the skin. It is, therefore, essential to have the snake properly restrained before attempting any injection. A simple aid to handling is to reduce the environmental temperature to below 10°C for this makes the poikilothermic snake very sluggish. If injectable agents are to be used only the lightest level of narcosis compatible with safe handling should be used, for deeper levels which require larger doses of drug may be followed by a recovery period extending over several days. Of the injectable central nervous depressants only ketamine is really useful and initial intramuscular doses of the order of 50 mg/kg produce moderate sedation which facilitates handling but muscle relaxation is poor and serpentine movements may occur. Ketamine anaesthesia can be supplemented by infiltration of the surgical site with 0.5–1% lignocaine, or by the administration of isoflurane or halothane after endotracheal intubation.

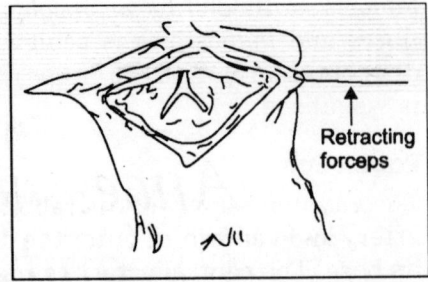

Snakes may also be anaesthetized with inhalation anaesthetics when a rapid recovery is important. Induction is best achieved by placing the snake in a clear plastic box, plastic bag or an aquarium tank into which 7–10% halothane or isoflurane vapour in oxygen or nitrous oxide/oxygen is piped. Induction may take as long as 15 minutes and the creature should not be removed until agitation or turning of the container

Fig. 25.5: Lower abdomen dissection of rabbit

demonstrates that the righting reflexes have been lost. It is then removed, intubated and anaesthesia maintained with about 3% of halothane or 4% of isoflurane vapour. Even when the anaesthetic is delivered through a T-piece system the expiratory movements of the snake will be too weak to expel gases and the lung must be ventilated artificially. Gases may be introduced into the lung by occlusion of the open limb of the T-piece and expelled by massaging the snake from the cloacal region towards the head. Induction of anaesthesia in a tank has the advantage that venomous snakes can be anaesthetized with the minimum of handling, but because the vapours are heavier than air they sink towards the bottom of the tank and snakes can raise their heads above the anaesthetic layer and delay the onset of anaesthesia so it is always wise to ascertain that the righting reflexes really have been abolished before removing the snake from the tank.

Most snakes exhibit a short period of excitement or agitation when first placed in a tank containing anaesthetic vapour but they quieten down and it is not always easy to determine the depth of anaesthesia. The first indication that the snake can be safely removed from the tank is certainly the loss of the righting reflexes but the tail withdrawal reflex is also valuable. Absence of response to pricking of the tail indicates that surgical anaesthesia is present. If the tip of the tongue is gently grasped with forceps there is a marked resistance to its withdrawal until the stage of surgical anaesthesia is reached.

When inhalation anaesthesia is employed it is important to ventilate at the respiratory rate observed in the previously conscious individual, and fluid balance should be maintained by giving 5 ml/kg of isotonic saline subcutaneously every 1–2 hours. Most snakes may be kept at normal ambient temperatures of around 20°C unless it is wished to cool them for the purpose of restraint.

Bibliography

1. Grahm O., *Small Animal Anaesthesia,* p. 50–106, 1964.
2. Soma L. R., *Textbook of Veterinary Anaesthesia,* p. 150, 1971.
3. *Occupational Safety and Health Administration.* New Publication of National Institute of Occupational Safety and Health (NIOSH) Washington DC. US Govt. Printing Office, 1992.

26

Anaesthesia for Fish, Birds and Wild Animals

FISH

Fish are usually anaesthetized by allowing them to swim in a solution of the anaesthetic agent. The solution should be made up in some of the aerated water in which they normally swim and various drugs are used.

1. Carbon dioxide may be used at a concentration of 200 ppm.
2. Diethyl ether 10–15 ml per litre of water is usual but 50 ml per litre has been used for large fish. In goldfish anaesthesia is induced in about 3–5 minutes; recovery takes 5–15 minutes.
3. Tricaine methanesulphonate is probably the best agent. It is a white powder which dissolves in both fresh- and sea water. Concentrations of 25–300 mg/l are employed, the more concentrated solutions being used for larger fish. Anaesthesia is induced in 1–2 minutes and fish recover in about 15 minutes.

When a fish is immersed in the anaesthetic solution there is initial excitement followed by erratic swimming. The fish then becomes inactive, sinking to the bottom of the tank to rest on its back. For surgery, the fish is removed from the tank and placed on a moist cloth. Complete recovery from the effects of the anaesthetic ensues when the fish is immersed in clean, aerated water.

BIRDS

In recent years interest in conservation of wild life appears to have led to an increased demand for anaesthesia for surgical purposes in wild or semi-wild birds as well as the more domesticated chicken, duck or goose. Cage birds have also become popular as companions, especially for elderly people living in urban districts, and as a result of these trends it is now commonplace for the veterinary anaesthetist to be confronted with avian patients requiring anaesthesia for a wide variety of conditions.

It is well known that birds do not react in the same way as mammals to stimuli which in man cause pain. For example, after a slight reaction to the skin incision, conscious birds do not show any response to the manipulations involved in caponization. Many operations on hens, such as the suturing of a torn crop or the removal of superficial neoplasm, cause little response and the heart rate, which might be expected to increase if pain was experienced, remains normal. In spite of these differences humane considerations seem to dictate that anaesthesia should be used for birds as it is for mammals.

The special problems presented by birds, especially wild ones, are related to their physiological, anatomical and metabolic differences from mammals. The problems of handling wild birds are often greatly exaggerated. Provided they are handled quietly and that the normal precautions are taken (such as the wearing of gauntlets when dealing with birds of prey), few difficulties or dangers are encountered.

The high metabolic rate has several implications for the anaesthetist. It implies a higher rate of utilization of foods so that starvation of 6–8 hours is often sufficient to produce fatal hypoglycaemia and ketosis. Metabolism of parenterally administered agents is also rapid.

The high avian body temperature means that excessive cooling occurs when the bird is exposed to a cool environment during or after anaesthesia, especially if many feathers are plucked around an operation site. Small birds such as budgerigars have very high, labile heart rates and heart failure is frequently encountered when these birds are frightened by handling. The blood volume of birds is such that small surgical haemorrhages may be sufficient to induce shock.

The avian respiratory tract is very different from that of mammals, one obvious difference being that inspiration in birds is normally passive whilst expiration is active. The respiratory system is constructed around a central 'core' of relatively fixed lung volume. The trachea divides into two mesobronchi which in turn divide to give secondary bronchi, one group of which, the ventrobronchi, communicates with the cranial air sacs (cervical and interclavicular). The dorsal and lateral secondary bronchi arise from each mesobronchus before these terminate in caudal air sacs (abdominal and posterior thoracic air sacs). The dorsal and ventral bronchi are joined by narrow tubes, the parabronchi, which form the analogue to the mammalian lungs and are where gaseous exchange takes place between the air and the blood. Air passing through the parabronchi moves in only one direction during both inspiration and expiration; blood flows across the direction of gas flow. Thus, the gas composition must change from the inspiratory to the expiratory ends of the parabronchi so that the capillary blood must equilibrate with parabronchial gas at widely differing oxygen and carbon dioxide tensions. The arrangement is such that gas exchange takes place during both inspiration and expiration and its efficiency is dependent on an uninterrupted flow of air through the lungs. Tidal exchange is generated through the air sacs and fluid such as blood or injected solutions in these sacs will interfere with ventilation. Even short periods of apnoea are serious and will produce marked hypoxia. Anaesthetic gases and vapours are rapidly absorbed into the blood stream so that induction is rapid when inhalation anaesthesia is used and, equally, recovery is also rapid. Most inhalation anaesthetics are less soluble in avian than in mammalian blood so that brain tensions equilibrate more rapidly with lung tensions and the clinical anaesthetist will often find induction and recovery disconcertingly abrupt.

After anaesthesia birds must be kept warm in a darkened, padded box and they should be supported in sternal recumbency. During recovery, vigorous flapping of the wings may occur and this should be prevented by wrapping the bird in a towel because a wing bone may be fractured if the wing beats against the cage or box wall.

Local Analgesia

Because birds such as budgerigars are so small it is very easy to give a gross overdose of a local analgesic agent, but in larger birds local analgesia can be used without difficulties. Even so, in large birds it is wise to watch the total dose which is administered and to use very dilute solutions (e.g. 0.25–0.5% lignocaine) for injection because there is some evidence that birds are more sensitive to local analgesics than are mammals of the same body weight. Many workers consider that local analgesia has no place in avian anaesthesia because even when it is correctly used the bird still requires restraint and this may produce undue distress.

Injectable Agents

Whenever possible birds should be weighed before any drug is given by injection. This is usually possible if the subject can be confined to a plastic box. Physical restraint should be kept to a minimum because small birds such as budgerigars and canaries are prone to become very distressed and large birds may fracture bones whilst trying to escape. Poultry should be grasped so that the wings are held along the thorax, turned on their backs and stroked on the abdomen to quieten them. Hawks usually present no problem after being hooded and parrots may be gripped around the neck and wings with a hand wrapped in thick towelling.

Intramuscular injection is made into the pectoral muscles on either side of the cariniform sternum or into the thigh muscles. Intravenous injections are made into the brachial vein where it passes over the ventral aspect of the elbow joint.

Although very many injectable agents have been used in birds of all kinds it is probable that ketamine is the one of choice in every case. When an injectable agent has to be used ketamine may be given intramuscularly in doses of 15 mg/kg. The bird should be confined in a warm, darkened box as soon as the injection has been made and the depth of anaesthesia produced is assessed by noting the response to pinching the wattle or the skin of the neck and although the eyelids often close the corneal reflex should persist throughout. Increments can be given to produce the desired degree of unconsciousness. There is a wide safety margin and doses of 25 mg/kg of ketamine may be safely given to all species of birds, although recovery may sometimes be prolonged.

Inhalation Anaesthesia

Whenever possible anaesthesia should be induced and maintained with an inhalation agent. Birds may be restrained so that anaesthesia can be induced using a face mask or they can be confined in a box made of transparent plastic material while anaesthetic gases or vapours are introduced into the box. Probably the best method is to induce anaesthesia by passing halothane and oxygen into the box in which the bird is confined and then to maintain anaesthesia by administering the same agent through a face mask or endotracheal tube.

Endotracheal intubation is not difficult in birds and suitable tubes may be constructed from silicone rubber or PVC tubing. The tube should be long enough to reach the syrinx but dead space must be kept to a minimum and the end should be cut at a bevel to facilitate passage into the trachea. Airway secretions may block the flow of gas in both intubated and non-inlubated birds so it is always wise to have suction available for their removal by aspiration. Adequate suction can be provided from a 60 ml syringe tilted with a short length of fine catheter.

Most birds can be anaesthetized with 0.5–1% halothane vapour in oxygen delivered to the endotracheal tube or face mask through an Ayre's T-piece but if it is available isollurane should be used, for induction and recovery are more rapid and the safety margin appears greater. The air sacs should be flushed at about 5-minute intervals by occlusions of the open arm of the T-piece system, their overdistension being prevented by escape of gas around the loose-fitting endotracheal tube or by partial lifting of the face mask. Total gas flow rates should be about two to three times the estimated minute volume of respiration of the bird, an adult domestic hen has a minute volume of about 750 ml, a pigeon of about 250 ml and a budgerigar of about 25 ml.

Inhalation anaesthetics may also be administered through a needle introduced directly into an air sac, but this, has little to commend it.

Recovery from anaesthesia is accelerated by administering oxygen and flushing the air sacs from time to time until the bird has regained its righting reflexes. Unless this is done the anaesthetic which passes into the air sacs may not be cleared by the depressed respiratory activity so that it will be taken up again by the parabronchiai capillary blood and recovery will be prolonged.

Combination of Inhalation and Injectable Agents

Very satisfactory results are obtained by the combination of injectable and inhalation agents. Although many combinations have been used, the induction of unconsciousness with ketamine (10–15 mg/kg) followed by the inhalation of isoflurane/oxygen or halothane/oxygen is probably the simplest and the safest.

Measurement of the dose of ketamine for small birds such as canaries and budgerigars which may weigh from 30–60 g is not easy and these birds may be dosed with 1–2 mg per bird. The standard solution of ketamine for veterinary use contains 100 mg/ml and if 0.1 ml is diluted to 1 ml birds may be given 0.1–0.2 ml of the diluted solution by intramuscular injection into the pectoral muscles. The larger dose (0.2 ml of the diluted solution) will usually produce light anaesthesia in 2–3 minutes from the time of injection.

Saffan can be used in place of ketamine for most birds but when given by intramuscular injection it produces more variable results, probably due to the difficulty of ensuring that the dose is correctly administered into a muscle mass.

The aim should always be to give just enough of the injectable agent to make the bird unconscious and to use only as much isoflurane or halothane as is necessary for the maintenance of anaesthesia.

ANAESTHESIA OF WILD ANIMALS

Difficulty in getting close to the subject, either because of its timidity or aversion to mankind, and the obvious need to avoid being attacked, have led to two approaches to the problems of anaesthetizing wild animals. The first is the use of squeeze cages, the animal being enticed into the cage then squeezed between a fixed and movable wall so that it cannot turn around or move very far whilst being given an injection of a sedative or anaesthetic agent. These cages should be standard equipment at zoos, some research centres and similar establishments, and they have a role in the capture of farm deer, but they are unlikely to be available to the veterinarian in general practice. The second, which is, perhaps, more generally applicable, is the administration of agents from projectile syringes. These syringes may be projected from rifles, pistols, crossbows or blowpipes so that the administrator can remain a safe distance from the subject. They were originally developed for the capture of wild game animals but they are now finding a use in ordinary veterinary practice where, for example, current methods of farming.

The projectile syringe is designed to inject its contents after the needle has penetrated the skin of the animal and its impact with the tissues can result in serious bruising. They should empty within seconds of penetration and the force of the injection should be adequate to push the plunger fully home even if the needle is partially obstructed by a skin-plug. To minimize tissue damage the syringe should strike the beast towards the end of the firing trajectory, although obviously this is less important when the projectile is propelled from a blowpipe. When fired from a gun or crossbow at too close range the syringe may enter the abdominal or thoracic cavities, and often when striking too hard, syringes bounce off without penetrating effectively in spite of barbs and collars on the needles. Extensive and fatal trauma may be caused by injection into the thoracic or abdominal cavities.

In all cases the shortest needle commensurate with penetration of the skin should be used and large-bore needles should terminate in a cone, with holes on the side of the shaft, for the ordinary open-ended needle may block with a core of skin. Collared needles are seldom satisfactory and tend to allow fluid to flow back out of the hole caused by penetration of the collar. To remove a barbed needle a small incision is made over the site of the barb.

Irritant solutions may not be used since their administration under the non-sterile conditions associated with the use of dart-guns may produce an abscess, but when simple precautions are routinely observed, untoward reactions at the site of injection are surprisingly rare. Valuable animals may be given a precautionary dose of antibiotic and in summer the wounds should be treated with fly repellants.

There are now many patterns of projectile syringe designed for use with rifles, pistols and crossbows but, in general, they usually inject their contents through the agency of an explosive cap and striker mechanism, or by gas evolved from a chemical reaction initiated in a capsule by a similar striker mechanism, incorporated behind the plunger. The projectiles used with blowpipes have needles with side holes which are covered with a short plastic sleeve and displacement of this sleeve as the needle penetrates the skin allows the pressure of air or gas previously injected behind the plunger to inject the syringe contents. Detonation of an explosive cap produces such a force that the ejected fluid penetrates far into the tissues and haematoma formation is common, so that the slower injection due to gas propulsion is usually to be preferred.

Projectile syringes usually have a capacity of up to 4 ml so that only relatively soluble drugs can be administered. If they are to be used on common land or in dense undergrowth any temptation to use immobilon or etorphine should be resisted, for should the projectile bounce off the animals or the animal be missed completely, these projectiles are surprisingly difficult to locate in spite of their bright silver barrels and coloured flights, and their subsequent discovery by a child or even an adult could have fatal consequences for that individual. It must be appreciated that projection is very far from accurate. The weight of the projectile varies according to its capacity and degree of filling, and the wind velocity has a great influence at all but the shortest of ranges which can, in any case, only be estimated. Experience has shown that best results are obtained by getting as close to the animal as is possible or safe, and aiming for the neck or shoulder region.

It is always advisable to use doses of injectable agents which do no more than permit the animal to be approached with safety and so allow general anaesthesia to be produced with intravenous or inhalation agents.

Although a quick recovery is essential in the wild, as partially sedated animals are at risk from predators, it is not so important in captive animals. To date, the techniques most frequently used for immobilizing a wide variety of species have been based on the use of potent opioids such as etorphine or carfentanil coupled with sedatives, anaesthesia being terminated with antagonists such as diprenorphine. For felidae, ketamine has long been the drug of choice, usually in combination with the α_2-adrenoceptor agonist xylazine or more recently with medetomidine. With the recent development of potent and effective α_2-adrenoceptor antagonists, such as idazoxan, RX82100A and atipamezole, the use of ketamine/α_2-adrenoceptor agonist combinations has become more popular in a wide range of species of animals since, providing low doses of ketamine are employed, immobilization can now be countered. A major advantage of ketamine-based combinations in ruminants is that regurgitation occurs less frequently than after the etorphine-based combination Immobilon has been used. The use of antagonists is not totally without risk, however. Often there is residual sedation from the non-reversed component of the drug combination (e.g. from ketamine or acepromazine).

The doses of drugs required by the various species of animal and the breeds within a species varies enormously so that an extensive literature on the subjects is now available.

Deer

There can be little doubt the xylazine/ketamine or medetomidine/ketamine mixtures are the drugs of choice for use in deer at the following doses, the smaller animals requiring proportionately larger amounts.

Maximum effect is obtained in about 10 minutes from the time of injection and recovery usually follows in about 2 hours unless antagonists are given. More recently, medetomidine/ketamine has been used successfully.

Immobilon has been used successfully in sika, fallow and red deer, for short periods of immobilization needed for blood sampling, faeces sampling and dosing for worms. Fallow deer seem to be particularly difficult and perhaps the safest combination for these is fentanyl (0.3–0.6 mg/kg) with xylazine (0.5–1.25 mg/kg).

All these agents are usually administered intramuscularly by projectile syringe and if the dose given does not produce surgical anaesthesia an inhalation agent should be administered as needed.

Wild Cats

Large zoological felidae can usually be trapped in squeeze or transport cages and when properly placed in a squeeze cage, a limb can usually be roped and pulled through the bars so that an intravenous injection can be made without much difficulty. They may then be treated as large domestic cats and the procedures are not as difficult or hazardous as might be anticipated. If thiopentone is used the dose should be kept to a minimum since recovery from its effects can take up to 2 days in the larger animals such as lions and tigers. Many lions and tigers in zoological collections and circuses can be enticed up to the bars to have their backs scratched and, although some caution is needed, subcutaneous injections can often be made while they are apparently enjoying the scratching.

If the animal cannot be approached closely, xylazine/ketamine or medetomidine/ketamine can be administered intramuscularly by projectile syringe.

Bears

Bears do not have retractile claws and even a playful blow from a paw can inflict a severe injury; their faces are curiously expressionless and it is difficult to detect their mood. Grizzly and polar bears may deliberately attack human beings.

In zoos and circuses, bears can be confined in squeeze cages or airtight boxes where a number of drugs can be administered but if these facilities are not available, ketamine can be administered by a projectile syringe. The dose is not well established but various doses from 15 to 25 mg/kg have been administered with atropine to control salivation.

Venepuncture is not easy, even in sedated bears, because the limb veins are small and embedded in fat so that if sedation produced by ketamine does not allow surgery an inhalation agent such as isoflurane or halothane should be given. Endotracheal intubation is not difficult in the unconscious animal.

Non-human Primates

Not only can monkeys inflict bites and scratches, they are also carriers of viruses which are extremely pathogenic to man as well as diseases such as tuberculosis, salmonellosis and shigellosis. For these reasons it is always undesirable to handle conscious monkeys and even domestic pets should be viewed with suspicion. Handling of the domestic pet monkey should be left to its owner.

An intravenous injection of an anaesthetic such as thiopentone or alphaxalone and alphadolone (saffan) into the recurrent tarsal vein on the dorsal surface of the gastrocnemius muscle. Caution is necessary for these monkeys often weigh much less than is estimated and it is seldom necessary to exceed 5 mg/kg of thiopentone or 2 mg/ kg of saffan. Once unconscious the monkey may be given a small dose of suxamethonium (i.e. 1 mg/kg) and intubated with an uncuffed tube. Anaesthesia may then be maintained by the administration of isoflurane or halothane in nitrous oxide/oxygen, or oxygen alone, from a T-piece system. When suxamethonium is to be given it is wise to inject atropine (0.15–0.3 mg) intravenously as soon as the induction agent has been given.

Alternatively, if the owner or an assistant can hold the monkey, again with its arms held behind its back, an inhalation agent can be used both for the induction and maintenance of anaesthesia. The use of nitrous oxide is a distinct advantage in these circumstances and halothane is probably the volatile agent of choice for, isoflurane often provokes breath holding. A suitable face mask is held over, but not touching, the face and nitrous oxide/oxygen (3/1) is administered at a flow rate of 4 l/min for 1–2 minutes. Halothane is then introduced into the gas mixture, increasing the concentration of the vapour every 3–4 breaths to a maximum of about 3%.

The mask is applied to the face as soon as it is judged that the monkey is unconscious and induction is usually free from excitement and struggling. Anaesthesia is maintained with a 1.2–1.5% of halothane vapour in the nitrous oxide/oxygen mixture.

Larger or less cooperative monkeys may need sedating by intramuscular injection before an attempt is made to induce anaesthesia. The use of projectile syringes is not to be recommended for monkeys are adept at dodging or even deflecting the projectile with their hands, and they usually pull the needle out before the injection is complete even when a hit is obtained! In the case of the smaller varieties it is usually possible to catch the monkey's arm and draw it out through the bars of the cage so that injection can be made into the deltoid muscle, but a squeeze cage may be needed for the larger, strong animals such as adult chimpanzees.

Ketamine is probably the agent of choice in all except squirrel monkeys and marmosets for chemical restraint or preanaesthetic sedation. At dose rates of 10–25 mg/kg, the volume of the veterinary preparation Vetalar which needs to be injected is small so that the drug can be given rapidly into the thigh muscles of even struggling animals. The peak effect is obtained 5–10 minutes after injection and the period of sedation is from 30 to 60 minutes. Recovery is complete in 1.5–4.5 hours depending on the dose and species of monkey. When the desired degree of sedation is not produced by the ketamine, further depression of the central nervous system is probably best produced by the administration of nitrous oxide/ oxygen supplemented with 0.5–1% halothane delivered through a face mask from a T-piece system.

For squirrel monkeys and marmosets saffan is the sedative of choice and this preparation is also useful in other species of non-human primates. In squirrel monkeys and marmosets doses of 15–18 mg/kg produce light general anaesthesia some 5 minutes after injection into the thigh muscles. Anaesthesia lasts about 45 minutes and is followed by recovery to full consciousness 1–3 hours later. In baboons, doses of 12–18 mg/kg make the animal safe to handle about 10 minutes after injection and recovery is much quicker than in squirrel monkeys. In all monkeys anaesthesia may be deepened by giving increments of Saffan intravenously until the desired depth is obtained. The animals can then be intubated and maintained unconscious with inhalation agents such as halothane, or sequential incremental doses of saffan can be given intravenously over several hours if need be. The main disadvantage of saffan is the large volume of solution which has to be given intramuscularly, although such injections do not appear to result in pain at the injection site.

When it is impossible to give an intramuscular injection to a large monkey or ape the simplest thing is to entice the animal into the cage which can be made airtight by covering with a sheet of plastic material so that anaesthetic gases and vapour can be piped in. The animal must be observed carefully and removed from the cage as soon as it is unconscious and relaxed.

It is important to conserve body heat and the anaesthetized monkey should be placed on a warm water blanket maintained at 38°C. If sedation or anaesthesia is to last for more than about an hour, an intravenous drip infusion of N/5 saline or Hartmann's solution (Ringer's lactate) should be started as soon as the animal is anaesthetized or sufficiently sedated. The fluid should be given at the rate of 10 ml/kg and, for the smaller monkeys, it should be warmed to 38°C by passing it through a blood warmer before it reaches the animal. The use of atropine is somewhat controversial but it is probable that it should be given as soon as the monkey becomes anaesthetized, in a dose of 0.15–1.2 mg depending on the size of the animal.

Recovery from anaesthesia should take place in a warm environment and endotracheal tubes and intravenous cannulae should be removed while it is still safe to handle the animal. Postsurgical analgesia should be provided by the intramuscular injection of a suitable analgesic (e.g. pethidine at a dose of 2 mg/kg) as late as possible in the recovery period.

Bibliography

1. Edwards G. B., Allen W. E., New Combe I.K. Equine Veterinary Journal, p. 6, 122,2, 1974.
2. Dodman N.H., Journal of Small Animal Practice, p. 20, 449, 1979.
3. Finster M., Morishima H.O., Mark L. C., Ferel J. M. , Daylom P.G. and James I.S., Anaesthesiology, p. 36; 65, 1972.

27

Veterinary Obstetrics

OBSTETRICS ANAESTHESIA IN HORSE

The insoluble inhalation anaesthetics given to the mare are readily excreted by the foal if it breathes properly after delivery. Although neuromuscular blocking drugs such as vecuronium, alracurium and pancuronium will not cross the placental barrier in significant amounts, guaiphenesin will, so for obstetrical anaesthesia it should be avoided if the foal is alive when anaesthesia is induced. Respiratory depression in the foal which results from the administration of narcotic analgesics to the mare can be antagonized by giving naloxone to the foal.

The abdominal distension of the mare will probably be the problem which gives rise to most concern because many mares have great difficulty in breathing spontaneously once they are recumbent under general anaesthesia. Due to intrapulmonary shunting of blood they may also be difficult to keep asleep with inhalation anaesthetics. In the supine position which some surgeons prefer for caesarean section in mares, the weight of the uterus and its contents will compress the vena cava and aorta, reducing venous return and causing a marked reduction in cardiac output and arterial blood pressure. Once the foal is delivered, the condition of the mare shows a dramatic improvement, pulmonary ventilation increases and the arterial blood pressure rises towards normal levels. To minimize difficulties before delivery of the foal, the mare should be positioned so that she is lying inclined towards her left side and respiration may need to be controlled. As always in equine anaesthesia, the magnitude of the problems encountered is related to size and small pony mares present only relatively minor problems. The techniques which have been successful for elective caesarian section in small experimental pony mares operated on in lateral decubitus are often inadequate for the large mares of the heavy breeds which may need emergency obstetric procedures in clinical situations.

In practice, vaginal repositioning and delivery of the foal can often be carried out in the sedated mare using one of the drug combinations discussed earlier in this book, but if general anaesthesia is needed the α_2-adrenoceptor agonist/ketamine combination, in spite of some theoretical objections, can be recommended, for it has been used without giving rise to problems. Should a longer period of anaesthesia be required small intravenous doses of a thiobarbiturate may be given to prolong the effects of this combination of drugs. Caudal epidural block is not as useful as it is in cattle because in mares there is a rather long delay between injection and the full development of analgesia.

For caesarian section, if the foal is alive, induction with an α_2-adrenoceptor agonist before thiopentone or methohexitone followed by endotracheal halothane/ oxygen seems to be satisfactory but ketamine is undoubtedly better than either of the barbiturates as the induction agent. Only the minimum amount of halothane should be used and IPPV may be necessary until the foal is delivered. Involution of the uterus is hastened when xylazine has been used and may be assisted by the intravenous injection of 2.5–10 units of oxytocin. Bleeding from the uterus is best controlled by the intravenous injection of 3–5 mg of ergometrine tartrate, but this may give rise to cardiac arrhythmias if given to a hypercapnic or hypertensive animal. If the foal is dead any technique of general anaesthesia suitable for laparotomy may be used and often vigorous supportive therapy with intravenous fluids will be necessary.

ANAESTHESIA FOR OBSTETRICS IN CATTLE

In cattle, caudal block is nearly always satisfactory for vaginal delivery of the fetus. Whenever possible sedation should be avoided but if needed to control the animal the intravenous injection of 0.05 mg/kg of xylazine will, in most cases, provide adequate maternal tranquillization to enable the block and delivery to be undertaken with minimal trouble.

Lumbar segmental epidural block may be useful for caesarian section carried out through the left flank of the standing animal but it is not easily performed and most veterinarians prefer to use paravertebral block of the thirteenth thoracic, first, second and third lumbar nerves that side.

Local infiltration techniques can be employed but they do not relax the abdominal muscles and, if the fetus is alive, the injection of large volumes of the amide-type local analgesics may result in cardiopulmonary depression in the neonate.

Caesarian section via a ventral abdominal incision is usually carried out under general anaesthesia with endotracheal intubation. Anaesthesia may be induced by the intravenous injection of minimal doses of xylazine/ketamine, thiopentone or methohexitone and, after endotracheal intubation, maintained with a halothane/oxygen mixture. Alternatively, after xylazine or detomidine has been given to produce deep sedation, the animal may be intubated and anaesthesia completed by the administration of halothane. Guaiphenesin should be avoided since it crosses the placental barrier, while ketamine, entlurane and isoflurane may be too expensive for use in all except very valuable cattle.

Involution of the uterus after delivery may be assisted by the use of ecbolic drugs provided the animal is not hypercapnic or hypertensive. All cows subjected to caesarian section under general anaesthesia should be given a subcutaneous injection of calcium borogluconate to prevent the occurrence of hypocalcaemia which is otherwise frequently seen in the postoperative period. Postoperative analgesia is also important and 0.5–1.0 g of pethidine, depending on the size of the cow, repeated at 4–6-hourly intervals for the first 24 hours has proved to provide adequate analgesia as shown by the cow looking comfortable and cudding or eating.

Removal of a dead, putrefying normal-sized calf by hysterotomy should only be attempted after resuscitation of the cow with intravenous fluids; antibiotic cover is essential.

Anaesthesia for Obstetrics in the Sheep and Goat

Sheep are seldom given any analgesia or anaesthesia for the vaginal delivery of lambs but in difficult cases requiring extensive repositioning of the lamb in the birth canal caudal block is very satisfactory. For caesarian section, which is usually carried out through the left flank, epidural or paravertebral blocks local infiltration and general anaesthesia are all suitable. The ewe is easily restrained for operation and hence techniques of local analgesia are popular. Probably the technique of choice is paravertebral block of the thirteenth thoracic, first, second and third lumbar nerves for the ewe is then able to stand and nurse her lambs immediately the operation is completed and the wound area remains analgesic for one or more hours depending on the local analgesic drug used. If local infiltration is used care must be taken to restrict the dose of any amide-type local analgesic to minimize the likelihood of depression of the lambs.

Ewes carrying dead lambs or suffering from pregnancy toxaemia are often very toxic, dehydrated and dull or collapsed. Hysterotomy, if the expense of operation can be justified, should be preceded by resuscitation with intravenous fluids.

Postoperative analgesia is all too often neglected. The ewe, like any other animal, is entitled to adequate pain relief in the postoperative period and morphine, pethidine or epidural drugs should be used as freely as may be required to keep the animal comfortable.

Anaesthesia for Obstetrics in Pigs

Anaesthesia for obstetrical procedures in sows is almost completely limited to the provision of anaesthesia for caesarian section. The general principles are similar to those in all other species of animal. It is necessary to provide adequate surgical conditions to prevent the sow from experiencing pain and to use a method which produces minimal depression of the piglets. Ideally, both the sow and piglets should recover from the effects of the anaesthetic in the minimum of time.

Caesarean section may be carried out under conditions which vary from those encountered on the farm to those provided in an operating theatre. Fortunately, the need for caesarean section to be performed on the farm is uncommon, due to the relatively small size of the piglets compared with that of the dam, making vaginal delivery relatively easy. Elective caesarean section, for the production of minimal disease herds of pigs, or gnotobiotic animals for research purposes, is much more common, but is usually performed in well-equipped operating theatres.

On the farm, caesarean section is probably best carried out under local or regional analgesia. Although paravertebral blocks are theoretically possible, they are difficult to perform because the thick layer of subcutaneous fat makes palpation of landmarks almost impossible, and infiltration of the line of incision is the method usually employed. Epidural block may also be used.

The major problem is the restraint of the sow and today sedation with azaperone is usually used for this although the drug does cross the placental barrier and the piglets are sleepy when delivered. However, respiratory depression in the offspring is minimal and if kept warm they usually survive. The sedative effects of azaperone on the sow are rather prolonged; she may not be able to suckle the piglets for some hours; if left unattended with the piglets she may suffocate some by lying on them. If the sedation produced by azaperone is inadequate, intravenous thiopentone or metomidate may be given. This does not appear to add to the depression of the piglets and is preferable to increasing the dose of azaperone. If thiopentone or metomidate is used the sow loses control of her airway, so care must be taken to see that respiratory obstruction does not develop. Local analgesia is usually still required.

Probably the most viable piglets are delivered when anaesthesia is induced and maintained with a volatile inhalation agent given with a high concentration of oxygen. In the majority of sows anaesthesia is rapidly induced with agents such as halothane or enflurane, but if the sow is very large or difficult to handle, a minimal dose of a short-acting intravenous induction agent, e.g. methohexitone or propofol, can be employed.

Satisfactory results are also achieved by the use of ketamine, usually in combination with diazepam. Premedication with diazepam (2 mg/kg intravenously) and atropine is followed by the intravenous injection of ketamine given to effect. Usually about 5–10 mg/kg of ketamine is needed to produce a peculiar state in which the sow appears to be aware of the environment yet does not react to skin incision or other surgical stimulation. Necessary nitrous oxide can be used to control any slight restlessness which may occur towards the end of the operation.

Sedative premedication with azaperone, followed by induction with intravenous or inhalation agents, has been widely used for elective caesarean section with generally satisfactory results. However, in the authors' experience, there can be no doubt that piglets delivered after the use of this sedative drug are, for some hours, sleepier than if no sedation is employed. This may be acceptable under farm conditions where equipment and assistance are not plentiful, but there seems little point in using the drug where it is not necessary.

Methods of anaesthesia involving the use of neuromuscular blocking agents result in the delivery of lively piglets and rapid recovery of the sow; they can be used whenever endotracheal intubation and IPPV can be carried out. However, it is essential to ensure that the sow is completely unconscious and it is sometimes difficult to be sure of this without having to administer large doses of anaesthetic or other drugs which will give rise to marked respiratory depression in the piglets. Techniques of this nature are, therefore, best avoided except by the experienced veterinary anaesthetist.

Involution of the uterus after delivery of the piglets may, if the animal is not hypercapnic, be helped by the intravenous injection of 2–10 units of oxytocin or, if bleeding is a problem, 1–1.5 mg of ergometrine tartrate, but this latter drug may produce cardiac arrhythmias if the $PaCO_2$ is elevated when it is given.

ANAESTHESIA FOR OBSTETRICS IN DOGS

The bitch may be fit and healthy at the time of operation or she may be exhausted from a prolonged obstructed labour and even after several hours of starvation she often has a full stomach, so vomiting at induction of anaesthesia presents a major hazard. Premedication with a low dose of morphine or paraveretum (Omnopon) will usually provoke vomiting and ensure an empty stomach but will cause some degree of respiratory depression in the pups. However, as long as only low doses of these opioids are used this respiratory depression will rarely be serious. In any case, respiratory depression in the pups which results from opioid premedication of the bitch may be overcome by giving the pups naloxone. Similarly, the use of xylazine or medetomidine premedication for its emetic properties may cause prolonged and serious respiratory depression in the offspring but this can be overcome by the administration of atipamezole. Sleepiness of the pups caused by premedication of the bitch with acepromazine cannot, however, be counteracted for there is no specific antagonist to the phenothiazine derivatives.

Pressure on the major blood vessels from the gravid uterus causes circulatory disturbances in the supine animal and pressure on the posterior vena cava can interfere with venous return to the heart.

This pressure can be avoided by the use of a wedge of plastic foam material placed under the right side of the supine bitch. Major circulatory disturbances also occur once intra-abdominal pressure has been reduced by removal of the gravid uterus or the pups and the ability of the bitch to compensate for these disturbances may have been reduced by the drugs used for general anaesthesia or the sympathetic blockade induced by some techniques of local analgesia.

Some of the agents used during anaesthesia may interfere with the involution of the uterus after delivery of the pups. In women, halothane is particularly likely to lead to severe postoperative haemorrhage after caesarean section but the difference in placental attachment makes this complication much less common in bitches. Halothane, enflurane and isoflurane can all be used for caesarean section in bitches with very satisfactory results, but methoxyflurane usually produces marked depression of the pups for some time after their delivery. Provided the bitch is not hypercapnic an ecbolic (such as oxytocin, 2–10 units, or ergometrine up to 0.5 mg intravenously, depending on the size of the bitch) may be given after delivery of the pups to promote involution of the uterus. Although there are considerable differences in the rate at which drugs cross the placenta, it is always safest to consider that any drug given to the mother will exert an influence on the pups in the post-delivery period. As long as respiratory depression is not severe, the pups will rapidly eliminate any of the less soluble inhalation agents which may have come to them from the mother but elimination of parenterally administered anaesthetic agents may be much more difficult due to the immaturity of the newborn pups' detoxicating mechanisms.

Anaesthetic-induced depression of the offspring can be avoided by the use of local analgesia. Epidural block is particularly suited to caesarean section but it should only be used in quiet bitches. If heavy sedation is needed for the performance of the operation the pups will be affected and the method will offer no advantage over a well-administered general anaesthetic.

In bitches of reasonable temperament, premedication may be limited to the use of an anticholinergic agent, but minimal doses of opioids may be used to cause vomiting and thereby ensure that the stomach is empty when anaesthesia is induced.

Induction of anaesthesia is best carried out with an inhalation agent given via a face mask, and is usually rapid and excitement free in parturient bitches. The main disadvantage of inhalation induction is that vomiting may occur before endotracheal intubation is possible, so suction apparatus should be available to enable the anaesthetist to clear the airway rapidly should this complication be encountered.

In large or bad-tempered bitches it may be necessary to use an intravenous agent for induction of anaesthesia. Methohexitone, at a maximum dose of 2.5 mg/kg, or propofol in doses of 4–6 mg/kg are probably the drugs of choice, but thiopentone can be used in doses of up to 5 mg/kg without risk of serious depression of the pups. All that is required of the intravenous induction agent is to make the bitch lie down, and if intubation is not possible at this stage, anaesthesia may be deepened with an inhalation anaesthetic administered by the mask. When intravenous agents are used it is advisable to wait a few minutes (about 15 minutes when propofol is used) before delivering the pups in order to let the blood levels of the parenterally administered agents decline.

The volatile agents used, whether for induction or maintenance, should be those which are associated with a fast recovery from anaesthesia. Enflurane might seem to be the ideal anaesthetic, for the pups are born lively and the bitch is fully awake within a few minutes of the end of the operation. Halothane has been widely and successfully used, although it may delay involution of the uterus.

Techniques involving the use of neuromuscular blocking agents can be used very satisfactorily for caesarean section, as these drugs do not cross the placenta in sufficient quantities to paralyse the muscles of the offspring. However, the administration of the anaesthetic drugs necessary to ensure that the bitch is unconscious will result in slight depression of the pups and muscle relaxation for closure of the abdomen is quite adequate after delivery of the pups and involution of the uterus, so there is apparently no real advantage to be gained from the use of relaxants.

Where apparatus for the administration of inhalation anaesthesia is not available many veterinary anaesthetists use neuroleptanalgesic mixtures, such as hypnorm. Small Animal immobilon for caesarean section — their use is associated with severe and prolonged respiratory depression of the pups and although the effects of the opioid agents may be countered with naloxone or diprenorphine, the sedative effects of the tranquillizer components cannot be antagonized so that the pups are exposed to the dangers of hypothermia and failure to feed. The neuroleptanalgesic techniques may be preferable to other methods of intravenous anaesthesia in these circumstances, but they must always be recognized as being considerably inferior to well-administered inhalation anaesthetics for the delivery of lively pups.

Enterohepatic recirculation of etorphine may result in the bitch and pups returning to a narcotized state even when diprenorphine has been used.

Postoperative pain relief for the bitch should be regarded as essential but care must be taken to ensure that any drugs used for this purpose are not excreted in the milk in concentrations which may affect the suckling pups. The provision of adequate pain relief may pose problems when opioid antagonists have been used to produce more rapid awakening of the bitch.

ANAESTHESIA FOR OBSTETRICS IN CATS

The requirements of anaesthesia for caesarean section in the cat, and the problems likely to be encountered, are similar to those already discussed above for dogs.

Although cats may vomit on induction of anesthesia, inhalation of vomit is less likely than in dogs, for cats have more active laryngeal reflexes. Nevertheless, endotracheal intubation should be carried out as soon as anaesthesia is induced and a pharyngeal pack should be introduced around the tube.

Many cats presented for caesarian section or hysterectomy are carrying dead kittens and the uterus may be infected, ideally, in such cases an intravenous drip infusion should be set up before anaesthesia but, unless the mother is exhausted or otherwise very ill, this is usually delayed until after anaesthesia has been induced.

Premedication before caesarian section is usually limited to the administration of anticholinergics, and induction with low-solubility volatile agents leads to the quickest recovery of both mother and kittens. With care, such an induction can be smooth, but many anaesthetists prefer to induce unconsciousness with small intravenous doses of thiopentone, propofol, methohexitone or saffan, before going on to the inhalation anaesthetic. Only minimal quantities of any intravenous agent should be used, and volatile anaesthetics should be employed to maintain the lightest possible levels of anaesthesia.

If facilities for the administration of inhalation agents are not available and intravenous anaesthetics have to be used for caesarean section, saffan is probably the best available agent. Although the saffan steroids cross the placenta and will affect the kittens, no noticeable respiratory depression results. If it is necessary to use saffan for this operation it is probable that it should be used in conjunction with local analgesic techniques so that the lightest level of general anaesthesia can be employed.

Neurolept analgesic methods are contraindicated in cats and after ketamine anaesthesia recovery is too prolonged for this drug to be used alone if the offspring are alive and need maternal care soon after delivery. The advent of medetomidine, however, has changed this situation in that after its use for premedication (in doses of up to 80 µg/kg) the dose of ketamine can be reduced to low levels (e.g. 2 mg/kg), while the effects of the medetomidine itself can be antagonized with atipamezole.

Epidural analgesia can provide excellent analgesia and muscle relaxation for caesarean section, but in cats the need for deep sedation to control the head end of the animal severely limits its usefulness. All sedatives in current use will depress the kittens and their condition will be no better than after well-administered general anaesthesia.

Maternal postoperative analgesia may be provided by the use of small doses of morphine or pethidine, any suckling kittens being carefully watched for signs of undue sleepiness that indicate high drug levels in the milk.

Bibliography

1. Edwards G.B., Allen W.E. and Newcombe, J.K. *Equine Veterinary Journal*, p. 6. 122. 2, 1974.
2. Dodman, N. H. *Journal of Small Animal Practice*, p. 20, 449, 1979.
3. Finster M. Morishima H. O., Mark L.C. Perel, J.M. Daylon P.G. and James S. *Anesthesiology*, p. 36, 155, 1972.

28

Complications During Veterinary Anaesthesia

PNEUMOTHORAX

The anaesthetic management of the pneumothorax created by the wide opening of the chest wall and/or diaphragm for surgical access to the contents of the thoracic cavity involves 'controlled respiration' or IPPV. Although in veterinary practice ventilation of the lungs by manual squeezing of the reservoir of the anaesthetic breathing circuit is still carried out in centres where little intrathoracic surgery is undertaken, the use of mechanical ventilators is becoming widespread. Surgeons find it easier to work with the regular movement produced by these machines and their use makes it possible to stabilize the tidal and minute volumes of respiration, the airway pressures and the duration of the inspiratory and expiratory periods in a way which cannot be achieved by manual 'bag squeezing'. Apart from the fact that IPPV is obligatory while the pleural cavity is open, the actual anaesthetic methods employed for intrathoracic surgery are largely governed by the personal preferences and experience of the anaesthetist. The main anaesthetic problems centre around the elimination of any pneumothorax remaining after closure of the thoracotomy incision and here close cooperation between the surgeon and anaesthetist is essential if they are to be satisfactorily resolved.

CLOSURE OF THE CHEST

The anaesthetic technique used while the chest is being closed varies with the nature of the operation but should always include drainage of the pleural cavity. In the past, after a limited operation not involving injury to the lung the chest was often closed without drainage. An attempt was made to achieve full reexpansion of any collapsed area of the lung tissue and to maintain full control of the breathing until the chest was airtight. However, the methods employed never succeeded in removing all the residual air from the pleural cavity, portions of the lung remained collapsed and often became a focus of infection. The air trapped in the pleural cavity caused movements of the chest wall to be transmitted to the lung by negative intrapleural pressure and pleural exudation occurred as a result of this. Proper drainage of the pleural cavity with removal of all the residual air overcomes all of these problems but if, on occasion, the chest has to be closed without drainage the amount of air trapped in the pleural cavity can be minimized by inserting a catheter through an intercostal space and applying suction after the chest wall is closed.

269

The catheter is then pulled out with a sharp tug. Alternatively, when the thoracotomy wound has been closed a large-bore catheter connected to a suction apparatus is inserted into the pleural cavity and suction applied until there is a negative pressure present in the system. The catheter may become blocked by the lung and the method is therefore not very satisfactory. It is, however, commonly used in cats where after closure of the thorax a large (13 s.w.g.) intravenous catheter may be introduced into the pleural cavity, the needle part being withdrawn after penetration of the skin and the blunt plastic catheter forced through the intercostal muscles and parietal pleura.

When there is an injury to the lung which could cause an air leak, or there is any likelihood of continuing haemorrhage into the pleural cavity, the chest must be drained. Underwater drainage is undoubtedly the most reliable and informative procedure and for this the drain tube is connected to a bottle containing water or a weak aqueous solution of chlorhexidine. This acts as a non-return valve and allows air or fluid to be expelled from the pleural cavity but prevents the indrawing of air during inspiration. The drain tube dips about 2.5 cm below the surface of the water and should have an internal diameter of about 0.5 cm. The bottle must have an internal diameter of not less than 15 cm.

Causes of Respiratory Obstruction

In the non-intubated animal respiratory obstruction is usually due to the base of the tongue or the epiglottis coming into contact with the posterior wall of the pharynx. This type of obstruction may be overcome by extending the head and drawing the tongue forwards out of the mouth. In pigs overextension of the head will also cause respiratory obstruction and in these animals care should be taken to keep the head in a normal position in relation to the neck. Brachycephalic dogs may develop respiratory obstruction due to the ventral border of the soft palate coming into contact with the base of the tongue, for many of these animals are almost unable to breathe through their nostrils. This type of obstruction can only be overcome by endotracheal intubation. The main problem in these breeds occurs during recovery, from the time when the dog will no longer tolerate the endotracheal tube until it is fully conscious and able to maintain its airway. Ideally, anaesthetic agents which ensure a very rapid return to consciousness should be used to reduce this danger time, but spraying of the larynx with local analgesic at the end of the anaesthetic may enable the endotracheal tube to be tolerated for an adequate period.

Large blood clots may accumulate in the pharynx after tonsillectomy, tooth extraction or endotracheal intubation when the tube has been passed through the nostril. These blood clots must be found and removed at the end of the operation. Animals unconscious after mouth, nose and throat operations should be placed in a position of lateral decubitus during the recovery period and kept under observation until fully conscious.

The fact that an endotracheal tube is in the trachea does not necessarily mean that the airway is clear. Endotracheal tubes may kink (particularly if the head is flexed). They may become blocked with mucous and in the case of cuffed tubes a faulty cuff may actually occlude the end of the tube, or its pressure obliterate the lumen of the tube. An overlong endotracheal tube may pass down one bronchus (usually the right), effectively obstructing the airway to the other lung. Obstruction may also be caused by the animal biting on the tube.

An uncommon but serious cause of respiratory obstruction is impaction of the epiglottis in the glottic opening. This may occur during 'blind' intubation in young horses and sheep, when a soft, flexible epiglottis is forced backwards into the laryngeal opening by the forcible passage of an endotracheal tube. Unless the epiglottis is dislodged by the withdrawal of the tube at the end of anaesthesia, it can give rise to serious respiratory obstruction in the recovery period until either coughing occurs, or the cause of the obstruction is diagnosed and overcome by the anaesthetist hooking the epiglottis out of the airway.

In horses, oedema of the upper respiratory passages develops during general anaesthesia if the head is in a dependent position or if the jugular veins are partially occluded for any length of time. This can result in serious respiratory obstruction in the recovery period that can only be relieved by endotracheal intubation, preferably with a tube passed through one nostril.

Animals suffering from laryngeal paralysis or tracheal collapse may obstruct during the recovery period when the increased effort of breathing tends to draw the sides of the larynx and/or the trachea together. As with the brachycephalic breeds, it may be necessary to leave an endotracheal tube in place for longer than would otherwise be done.

Laryngeal and Bronchial Spasm

Laryngeal spasm appears to be seen more commonly than bronchial spasm, but both conditions can occur together during general anaesthesia. Laryngeal spasm can occur in all kinds of animals but it is perhaps most frequently encountered in cats when attempts are made to force them to breathe high concentrations of an inhalation agent before the protective laryngeal reflexes have been subdued. Another common complication of anaesthesia in cats is laryngeal 'crowing', the crowing noise being caused by a partial spasm of the vocal cords due to irritation by a blob of mucous, saliva, blood or vomit.

When laryngeal spasm is troublesome the best treatment is to administer a relaxant, in order to relax the spasm, and then to intubate with an endotracheal tube. Attempts at intubation without the aid of relaxants will usually be unsuccessful and will prolong the spasm. Forcible intubation through a closed glottis may result in oedema of the mucous membrane of the larynx and necessitate tracheotomy.

Constriction of the bronchioles or bronchial spasm' is uncommon but occasionally seen in all kinds of animal. Ruminants appear to be particularly liable to develop this complication of general anaesthesia. This may well be due to unsuspected regurgitation and inhalation of fluid from the rumen. Bronchial spasm may also be initiated reflexly during light anaesthesia by stimuli from the site of operation and there is some evidence which suggests that the passage through the brain of blood deficient in oxygen and rich in carbon dioxide causes bronchoconstriction.

The first warning sign that bronchial spasm is imminent is a bout of coughing and if an endotracheal tube is not in use the larynx closes. Complete respiratory arrest follows. The chest is rigid and the lungs cannot be inflated by pressure on a rebreathing bag, nor can they be deflated by pressure applied to the chest wall. Cyanosis sets in and is soon replaced by a grey pallor. If ill, the animal may die, but usually the severe hypoxia releases the spasm and the animal gasps. The gasp is followed by normal spontaneous respiration and the animal recovers. Unfortunately bronchial spasm may recur if the stimulus responsible for the first attack is still present. In all cases where bronchial spasm occurs the anaesthetist must ensure that the upper airway is clear and that whenever possible the first gasp of the animal will be of an oxygen-enriched atmosphere.

Vomiting is an active process which occurs in light anaesthesia either during induction or recovery. It is often preceded by swallowing or 'gagging' movements.

When vomiting occurs, the protective mechanisms of laryngeal closure, coughing and breath holding are present, and the accident should not have serious consequences. All that is necessary is for the anaesthetist to clear the pharynx of the vomited material, by swabbing or suction, and to allow the animal to cough vigorously before proceeding with further administration of the anaesthetic. The dog, however, has very weak protective reflexes and in a few cases, particularly where vomiting occurs during the recovery period and the dog is still sleepy, these reflexes fail and the food material is inhaled. In such a case it may even prove necessary to reanaesthetize the animal in order to use vigorous suction to clear the tracheobronchial tree.

It is obvious that if anaesthetics are not given to animals whose stomachs might contain food then aspiration is unlikely to occur, but this is counsel of perfection which cannot, always be realized in veterinary practice. Clearly it can never be achieved in ruminants and in simple stomached animals the stomach may contain material many hours after the eating of a meal, particularly if an accident has occurred in the meanwhile or if the animal has gone into labour.

Passive regurgitation is most commonly seen in ruminant animals but it also occurs in horses, pigs, dogs and cats. It usually happens when the animal is in a head-down position, or lying horizontally on its side, and relaxation is induced by deep anaesthesia or the use of relaxant drugs. In these circumstances the protective reflexes are not active and aspiration occurs all too readily. In deeply anaesthetized ruminants any increase in intra-abdominal pressure will force fluid ingesta up the oesophagus into the pharynx, and this regurgitation is frequently seen in adult cattle when anaesthesia is induced with a small, rapidly injected dose of thiopentone sodium. To prevent regurgitation in cases of equine surgical colic the stomach should be decompressed by the passage of a stomach tube prior to the induction of anaesthesia. It is almost impossible to pass a tube into the stomach of an anaesthetized horse.

In cases of oesophageal dilation or obstruction there may be an accumulation of fluid on the oesophagus, while the stomach may contain fluid material if there is an obstruction of the pylorus or small intestine.

The most certain practical way of preventing the aspiration of material from the oesophagus and stomach is to perform endotracheal intubation with a cuffed tube immediately after anaesthesia has been induced. In the case of small animals, keeping the head raised after induction of anaesthesia until the trachea is intubated and the cuff inflated will completely prevent the danger of inhalation from passive regurgitation, but this is obviously not practicable in the ruminant.

Often, the first sign that aspiration has occurred is the unexpected appearance of cyanosis, dyspnoea and tachycardia. Obviously the severity of the condition depends on the quantity of fluid aspirated and the extent of the lung area involved.

Immediate treatment consists of thorough aspiration of the tracheobronchial tree—although this is more easily advised than performed. Oxygen should be administered and attention directed towards the relief of bronchiolar spasm. If, after operation, the animal develops bronchopneumonia the appropriate treatment must be instituted (antibiotics, etc.).

Emergency Tracheostomy

The obvious treatment of respiratory obstruction is to locate the obstruction and remove it, but this is not always possible and occasionally an emergency tracheostomy is required to save the animal's life. In a cat, a 14 gauge needle or catheter, disposable trachcostomy tube placed, percutaneously directly into the trachea, provides an adequate airway in the short term, and 10 gauge catheters may be used in a similar manner in dogs up to medium size. In all but small dogs the size of such an airway is totally inadequate for any length of time, but may be sufficient to sustain life whilst a tracheostomy is carried out. This type of tube is suitable for dogs, cats, sheep, goats and small calves. Curved plastic tracheostomy tubes or cannulae are available in sizes suitable for most dogs, and are inserted through the cricothyroid membrane, between two tracheal rings, or by slitting a tracheal ring longitudinally. Once such a tracheostomy tube is in place in a dog, the patient should be under constant observation as the tube may become dislodged or blocked by folds of skin, secretions, or the dog flexing its neck.

In the horse, tracheostomy is much easier to carry out, and if necessary can provide a safe airway for a long period of time. In emergency, or for short-term use, narrow curved tubes are used. On superficial examination these tubes appear to provide far too small an airway, but they are fully effective in such situations.

For more prolonged use a tracheostomy tube which can be removed and cleaned is employed.

It must be pointed out that the need for an emergency tracheostomy is rare. In the cat it is required because of severe, persistent laryngeal spasm, but in most other species it is made necessary by pathological obstructions of the airway which prevent endotracheal intubation. In many cases, therefore, the requirement can be foreseen and equipment for tracheostomy kept readily available.

BREATHING

Respiratory Insufficiency and Arrest

Apnoea during anaesthesia is very common, and its successful treatment depends on the original cause. Although respiratory arrest is obvious, it is often preceded by respiratory insufficiency, which is much more difficult to assess. In either case, the immediate requirement is that oxygenation of the tissues should be maintained, so that as soon as the problem is noted the anaesthetist should carry out the following routine.

1. Check the airway and, if necessary, take steps to clear it.
2. Apply artificial respiration (ensuring there is no anaesthetic in the inspired gas).
3. Check the pulse.

Assuming that the circulation is adequate, in the majority of cases these measures should prevent further hypoxia and hypercarbia, and give the anaesthesia.

Methods of Ventilation

The efficiency of artificial ventilation in emergency situations depends on the apparatus available and the size of the patient. Where anaesthetic circuits utilizing reservoir bags are being employed it is possible to ventilate by squeezing the bag, but otherwise resuscitation is more difficult. Self-filling bag/valve units such as the Ambu bag.

Where respiratory depression is due to opioid drugs such as morphine, it may be reversed by the use of specific antagonists. Diprenorphinc (Revivon) is the specific antagonist to etorphine, whilst naloxone (Narcan) is the drug in current use to reverse the effect of the other opioid agonists. Naloxone is a pure antagonist, and should have no effects of its own on the animal. The dose required depends on the depth of narcosis to be reversed, and as naloxone is very short acting further doses may be required. Naloxone is most effective against the pure opioid agonists, and is less effective against partial agonists such as buprenorphine.

Doxapram hydrochloride has replaced most of the earlier analeptic drugs. It increases the respiratory minute volume by acting on the respiratory centre and, in general, doses considerably larger than those used clinically must be used before general stimulation results in convulsions. There are reports of its safe and successful use at intravenous doses of 2 mg/kg in a wide range of species. For clinical purposes an initial intravenous dose of 1 mg/ kg is usually employed and further doses given if required. Doxapram may also be used by the sublingual route to stimulate respiration in the newborn. Despite the claims as to the specificity of the action on the respiratory centre, in practice, clinical doses are usually found to decrease the levels of unconsciousness of the anaesthetized animal. Whilst this is useful if apnoea is due to central depression, this drug must be used with care in large animals such as horses, where the awakening may be violent.

Normal levels of carbon dioxide in the blood are necessary to maintain spontaneous respiration. However, the role of carbon dioxide in resuscitation in veterinary anaesthesia has been grossly abused. Although a slight increase in carbon dioxide stimulates respiration in the conscious animal, this reflex is considerably reduced under anaesthesia. Further increases in carbon dioxide tension in the blood causing increasing central nervous depression, which will itself eventually result in apnoea. Hypercapnia also sensitizes the heart to arrhythmias and may precipitate cardiac arrest. In the majority of cases apnoea is preceded by respiratory insufficiency and by the time that respiration ceases, hypercapnia already exists. The only circumstances where carbon dioxide is required to stimulate respiration is following hyperventilation, usually after vigorous IPPV. If carbon dioxide is required to correct hypocapnia it is best added to the inspired gas either from cylinders on the anaesthetic machine, or by increasing the dead space of the patient circuit, as in this way it is possible to continue ventilation and prevent hypoxia from occurring. Artificial ventilation should never be stopped to allow accumulation of carbon dioxide.

Failure to reverse the effects of muscle relaxants used during the anaesthetic technique will result in respiratory failure. Treatment consists of the continuation of artificial ventilation until the relaxant's effects have worn off or been adequately antagonized. Pain, particularly involving the thorax and abdominal regions, may cause hypoventilation in the post-operative period. If opioid analgesics in limited doses are used in such circumstances, the increased ventilation through pain relief is usually greater than any respiratory depression as a direct result of the drug. Other causes of inadequate ventilation include pathological changes in the lung which prevent its aeration, such as space-occupying lesions of the lung or pleural cavity, and bleeding into the substance of the lung. Normal carbon dioxide tensions are essential for the maintenance of normal tissue perfusion and hypocapnia leads to a decrease in cerebral blood flow. However, severe hypocapnia does not occur in spontaneously breathing animals and the cerebral circulation is only likely to be affected when IPPV is carried out in such a way as to remove excessive amounts of carbon dioxide.

Hypoxaemia

Hypoxaemia can be very difficult to detect as cyanosis, usually considered the commonest sign, may be masked by pigmentation of the skin and mucous membranes, and may not be seen at all in anaemic or shocked animals. Hypoxaemia may result from any of the airway or breathing problems already discussed, or through problems preventing oxygen transfer into the blood. However, assuming ventilation to be adequate, the commonest cause in anaesthesia is an inadequate level of oxygen in the inspired gas as the result of apparatus failure (sometimes to an empty cylinder), an inadequate oxygen input, an accumulation of nitrogen or nitrous oxide in a low-flow circuit, or faulty valves preventing the correct gas circulation around a circle absorber system. Such accidents occur far too commonly, and should be suspected if an animal becomes cyanotic despite an adequate respiratory minute volume and an apparently adequate circulation. Treatment consists of the administration of oxygen, preferably utilizing a simple non-rebreathing patient circuit. However, as long as the animal is breathing spontaneously, simply disconnecting it from the machine and allowing it to breathe room air will usually provide adequate oxygen whilst the fault in the apparatus is located.

Respiratory Acidosis

Serious consequences are seen when the minute volume of respiration is decreased since this causes a diminished excretion of carbon dioxide from the lungs and therefore results in the development of respiratory acidosis. This state is commonly seen when the total gas flow rate in a non-rebreathing circuit is too low, or when the soda lime in an absorber is exhausted. It also occurs when the airway is obstructed, or when the respiratory movements are hampered by the position of the animal's body on the bed or operating table. Usually this disturbance of the acid-base balance of the blood results in very little harm when the duration of anaesthesia is short, but it may have serious effects if the anaesthetic period is prolonged. Death occurs when the pH of the blood falls below about 6.7.

The signs of respiratory acidosis are not always obvious. Hypoxaemia may have been avoided by an increase in the inspired oxygen tension so that the animal's mucous membranes remain pink and its pulse slow and of good volume. It is important to note that, although in the normal animal an increase in the alveolar carbon dioxide tension causes a frank increase in the tidal volume, in the anaesthetized animal this may not be seen. The blood pressure first rises, then returns to normal and finally falls. Circulatory failure, when it occurs, is rapid and is due to heart failure. When respiratory acidosis has developed, the animal may collapse at the end of the operation, for the excess carbon dioxide is rapidly excreted as respiratory depression decreases and the circulatory reflexes are not active enough to compensate for the sudden change in the acid-base status of the blood. The condition may be diagnosed as shock, but unlike shock, is characterized by a slow pulse and, in otherwise fit animals, by rapid spontaneous recovery.

Inadequacy of the Circulating Fluid Volume

Inadequacy of the circulating fluid volume to fill the existing vascular bed may be due to an absolute reduction in blood or body fluid volumes, or to an increase in the vascular space as a result of peripheral vasodilatation. In either case the immediate treatment is to ensure that the animal is lying flat out or in a head-down position to improve venous return and the cerebral circulation, and to administer fluids intravenously as rapidly as possible.

A common cause of circulatory failure under anaesthesia is surgical haemorrhage. There may be a sudden effusion of blood or, more commonly, an almost imperceptible loss over the course of a long operation. Unless blood loss is actually measured by swab weighing or some other technique, it is very difficult to estimate the amount of haemorrhage occurring, and most surgeons tend to underestimate grossly the blood loss they cause. Many of the drugs used in anaesthesia abolish the normal physiological response to haemorrhage, and cardiovascular collapse can occur following even moderate blood loss. For practical clinical purposes an animal can be considered to have a blood volume of 88 ml/kg and when a loss of 10% of this (i.e. 8–9 ml/kg) has occurred infusion of fluid should be commenced.

Where blood loss is not too severe, infusion of crystalloid solutions (in four times the volume needed for a solution which is retained within the circulation) may be adequate until the homeostatic mechanisms come into effect, but when gross and/or rapid loss occurs, compatible whole blood, plasma or a plasma substitute such as one of the gelatine solutions should be given; the quantity and speed of replacement are the factors which determine the fate of the patient. Dextran solutions which are often used in veterinary practice as plasma substitutes should always be used with caution, because the infusion of large quantities of dextran results in failure of the blood-clotting mechanism, and bleeding may be increased.

Fluid deficits which may have arisen in the pre-operative period may lead to circulatory failure under anaesthesia. When the fluid loss is primarily an electrolyte loss, such as seen in vomiting dogs or equine colic cases, circulatory changes are severe and the animal appears shocked. However, in cases where the depletion is primarily of water, the deficit is more difficult to recognize and assess but unless this is done such animals will develop cardiovascular failure following the administration of vasodilator anaesthetic drugs, or following an apparently small blood loss. Also, elderly animals often do not tolerate haemorrhage well. In all these cases deficits should, whenever possible, be corrected before anaesthesia is induced, the only exceptions being cases of intestinal obstruction where it is sufficient to restore only the circulating fluid volume prior to anaesthesia.

Peripheral vasodilatation due to drugs administered during anaesthesia or, more serious, due to endotoxins may lead to circulatory failure but in their absence major changes in the peripheral circulation and the volume of the vascular bed can occur in response to autonomic reflex activity. For example, a sudden fall in blood pressure during an operation sometimes occurs without warning in an animal whose cardiovascular system is apparently healthy and where there has been little loss of blood. The pulse becomes imperceptible, respiration ceases and the veins (noticeably in the tongue) are dilated. The pupils remain normal in size and this may be the only indication that the heart has not stopped beating. This rather alarming reaction appears to be initiated by certain surgical manipulations. For example, it may be seen during caesarean hysterotomies in cattle and sheep when traction is exerted on the mesovarium or on the broad ligament of the uterus. It may also be seen in dogs and cats when swabs or retractors are allowed to press upon the coeliac plexus, or when the stomach and liver are handled by the surgeon. When it arises the surgeon should stop and not recommence operating until recovery has occurred. The reaction may be avoided by gentle surgery and the anaesthetist should note that gentle surgery is only possible when the patient's muscles are adequately relaxed.

Shock

Shock is a caricature of the physiological responses to haemorrhage; the outline of the defensive features remains recognizable but it is exaggerated and distorted to a degree which becomes both absurd and damaging. The major factors in its initiation and maintenance are decreased cardiac output, increased vascular resistance and decreased effective circulating blood volume. Each of these feeds back, either directly or through the sympathetic nervous system, to perpetuate the condition of shock. Reduction in cardiac output leads to increased sympathoadrenal activity which leads in turn to a selective reduction of blood flow in the splanchnic and cutaneous circulations, thereby producing the clinical signs of shock. Hypotension is not a primary manifestation or feature, and only occurs when the increased sympathoadrenal activity fails to compensate for losses in effective circulating blood volume and decreased myocardial contractile force.

The most common and dramatic cause of shock is sudden external haemorrhage, but a similar state can arise if blood is lost internally or if large quantities of electrolytes and water are lost to the body through vomiting and diarrhoea or intestinal obstruction. Nearly all cases of surgical or traumatic shock respond to prompt transfusion and a fatal outcome is usually due to undiagnosed complications such as pneumothorax, fulminating cerebral fat embolism, cardiac tamponade, bilateral adrenal haemorrhage, air embolism or preexisting cardiac, pulmonary or other diseases, such as diabetes mellitus.

Sometimes, however, shock is unresponsive to treatment and the condition is said to be 'irreversible'. This state is not uncommon in animals suffering from systemic bacterial infection or peritonitis. It can also arise from undertransfusion or too long a delay before replacing fluid losses. Dogs bleed until they have become severely hypotensive recover if the blood is replaced within a certain time but after a delay of 2–4 hours transfusion has little or no effect. The animals die and their intestinal mucosa, especially in the ileum, is found to be haemorrhagic and haemorrhages are found under the endocardium and elsewhere.

The processes which lead to irreversibility are complex and difficult to unravel, but if peripheral circulatory failure is the mechanism, then the final common pathway should be found in the microcirculation. It has been suggested that irreversibility begins when ischaemic anoxia changes to stagnant anoxia in certain tissues, and prolonged vasoconstriction is thought to be a key factor. After severe haemorrhage, sympathetic activity and catecholamine secretion produce vasoconstriction and ischaemia anoxia in the splanchnic bed, liver and kidneys. This regional vasoconstriction enables the circulation to be maintained through the unconstricted cerebral and coronary vessels in spite of any reduction in cardiac output. Transfusion at this stage improves cardiac output, relieves hypotension and much of the vasoconstriction, allowing tissue perfusion to be restored. If transfusion is delayed, the constricted arterioles become less and less responsive to adrenaline, apparently due to accumulation of metabolites in the tissues. Eventually the capillaries become engorged and flow stagnates because it is suggested that venules remain constricted. The reason for the persistence of venular spasm when the arterioles become paralysed is not at all clear, however. Capillary engorgement then raises the hydrostatic pressure so that fluid exudes from the capillary beds and oligaemia becomes more severe. Anoxic changes become serious, local haemorrhages appear and the cycle to death begins. Transfusion is now of no avail, because it merely engorges further the stagnant capillary bed. The venous return and the cardiac output continue to fall and the heart stops or fibrillates as the coronary flow is reduced.

Changes in the abdominal viscera and sympathetic activity are of importance in irreversibility as is the endotoxin of Gram-negative bacilli. This toxin is absorbed from the damaged (anoxic) bowel, acts on the nervous system, produces a relentless abdominal sympathetic induced vasoconstriction, and then cannot be detoxicated because of failure of a reticuloendothelial enzyme in the hypoxic spleen and liver. Endotoxin action certainly has an important adrenergic component; its lethal effect is counter acted by adrenolytic compounds and it potentiates the pressor responses to catecholamines.

Vasopressors are much more likely to be harmful than beneficial in shocked animals. The only measures which consistently reduce mortality are those which increase blood volume or reduce vasoconstriction and this leads to the inference that vasodilators may have a place in the treatment of shock. Although not to be used when the blood volume is already reduced and no substitute for correct fluid therapy, there are some encouraging reports that antiadrenergic drugs and other methods of inhibiting sympathetic activity improve survival after haemorrhage or trauma, provided further transfusion is also given to cover the increased capacity of the vascular system. It is extremely doubtful if the adrenal cortex plays any part although hydrocortisone (itself a vasodilator) given in massive doses of 50 mg/kg has been used. Such massive doses are impracticable for large animals, but phenylbutazone, in doses of 15 mg/kg, were as effective as corticosteroids in the treatment of endotoxic shock. Unfortunately, the best results are only obtained when these drugs are given before shock actually develops. Flunixin (1 mg/kg, intravenously) is claimed to have a beneficial effect by countering endotoxaemia in equine colic cases. During shock the endogenous opioid β-endorphine is released from the pituitary and it has been suggested that it may contribute to hypotension since this is alleviated by the administration of naloxone. Although the use of naloxone may be efficacious it might also restore pain sensitivity which is usually reduced in shock.

Currently, there are indications that the infusion of small volumes of *hypertonic saline* may be beneficial in shocked animals. This approach is quite distinct from volume replacement therapy and may be useful in veterinary practice since it necessitates the use of only small volumes of solution. More research is needed to evaluate its real worth.

Much work has been done to establish the best methods of estimating the state of the circulation. Undoubtedly the most useful determinations are measurement of the arterial blood pressure, the central venous pressure and the urinary output. Capillary refilling time and the state of distension of the peripheral veins may also be of assistance.

Obviously, the best treatment for shock is to prevent it from occurring. Early transfusion to restore the blood volume and expeditious operation to arrest bleeding, remove damaged tissue and, if necessary, fix broken bones, will prevent shock from becoming irreversible.

Disturbance of Cardiac Rhythm

Tachycardia is usual in young animals, but in adults the pulse rate increases in shock or after the administration of anticholinergics. It must be emphasized, too, that in cases where relaxants are being used tachycardia may indicate an insufficient depth of anaesthesia.

Cardiac arrhythmias are common in all kinds of animal under all forms of anaesthesia but they are frequently unrecognized since unless the ECG is continuously displayed the anaesthetist is unlikely to become aware of them.

The origin of these disturbances of cardiac rhythm is still uncertain. If the anaesthetic agent is known to depress the functional capacity of the heart muscle it is natural to assume that the direct action of the drug on the myocardium is the cause, but it is more probable that serious arrhythmias are caused by the action of autonomic nerves to the heart. The nervous system is often hyperactive immediately before operation, especially if the animal is frightened, and stimulation of sympathetic nerves to the heart may cause ventricular ectopic beats or even ventricular fibrillation if the heart muscle is sensitized by anaesthetic agents. Carbon dioxide may accumulate in the body, and mild degrees of hypoxia may cause stimulation of the sympathetic nervous system, so arrhythmias are common when respiration is depressed or obstructed.

Treatment of cardiac arrhythmias will depend on their cause and an accurate diagnosis can only be made when an electrocardiograph is available. The use of drugs for the treatment of cardiac irregularities is not justified in the absence of an accurate diagnosis. However, during general anaesthesia most cardiac arrhythmias disappear once an adequate respiratory exchange has been established. An unobstructed airway must be ensured and pulmonary ventilation assisted by IPPV whenever respiratory depression is encountered.

Heart Failure

There are two distinct types of heart failure: the first is ventricular fibrillation, the second is ventricular asystole, frequently termed 'arrest of the heart'.

The causes of heart failure are numerous and in any one case it is likely that several factors may be implicated but in the majority of cases hypoxia and hypercapnia contribute significantly to its occurrence. Fibrillation is more common under conditions of oxygen lack (e.g. in shocked or anaemic animals). Cardiac arrest or asystole is the type of heart failure associated with overdosage of anaesthetic agents. Gross overdosage is probably rare, but relative overdosage is more frequent (e.g. the use of normal doses or concentrations of anaesthetic agents in old or debilitated animals).

Cardiac arrest of neurogenic origin, usually stimulation of the vagus nerves, is the exception to the general rule of multiple causation. Where the surgeon stimulates the vagus nerve, either directly or by initiating a reflex such as the oculocardiac, the heart may stop with no prior warning. Such a cardiac arrest can only be detected by continuous palpation of the pulse, or with an electrocardiograph, as the suddenness of the cessation of circulation means that the tissues are initially well oxygenated, the mucous membranes remain pink, and spontaneous respiration may continue for 2–3 minutes until the respiratory centres become anoxic. By the time respiration has ceased and the pupil has dilated, cerebral hypoxia makes successful resuscitation much more difficult. The horse and the cat are the species of animal most sensitive to vagal arrest of the heart and they should be protected by the administration of anticholinergics prior to surgery in the head and neck regions.

If counter measures are to be successful, diagnosis of heart failure must be rapid. Where, as may happen during anaesthesia, circulatory arrest has been preceded by respiratory or circulatory insufficiency, the brain may already be hypoxic when the crisis occurs and in these circumstances even less time is available in which to restore an effective cerebral circulation.

Diagnosis of Circulatory Arrest

Diagnosis of circulatory arrest is based on the absence of a peripheral pulse, absence of heart sounds, and ashencoloured mucous membranes. The surgeon will notice an absence of bleeding from the wound but the anaesthetist should have diagnosed the condition before this is obvious. These signs are closely followed by wide dilatation of the pupil and either agonal gasping or apnoea. It must be remembered that respiration does not cease immediately the circulation fails, but continues until the respiratory centres become anoxic.

Treatment

Conservative treatment is not only useless but also wastes valuable time. The only way of restoring an effective circulation is the immediate institution of resuscitative measures. Once an effective circulation has been produced, the immediate danger is over.

There are two ways of attempting to provide an effective circulation to the brain and myocardium. One, and the first that should be tried, is chest compression; the second is direct compression of the surgically exposed heart. The use of cardiac stimulant drugs should not be considered until the myocardium is once more well oxygenated and, therefore, they have no place in the initial treatment.

The veterinary anaesthetist should have a simple, set routine for the treatment of circulatory arrest, which is known to all those working in the theatre or recovery unit. Table 28.1 sets out such a routine.

Table 28.1: Cardiac resuscitation routine

Stage 1: *Establishment of an artificial circulation*
1. Notify surgeon and note time
2. Clear and maintain airway
3. Ventilate (if possible with O_2)
4. External compression; if ineffective, internal massage
5. Where possible, maintain in head down position

Stage 2: (this is sometimes left until after Stage 3). Infuse fluid to restore or maintain circulating volume

Stage 3: *Restoration of normal cardiac rhythm*

Heart in

Ventricular fibrillation	Adrenaline, Lignocaine, i.v
Asystole	Electric defibrillation

Stage 4: *Post-resuscitation*
1. Continue pulmonary ventilation
2. Counteract acidosis — hyperventilate or give sodium bicarbonate
3. Prevent cerebral oedema — corticosteroids, diuretics
4. Circulatory support as needed — adrenaline
    dopexamine
    dopamine
    dobutamine

As soon as circulatory arrest is detected, the anaesthetist should inform the surgeon and stop the administration of any anaesthetic; a clear airway must be ensured and IPPV instituted, preferably with oxygen. At the same time external chest compression (see below) should be commenced in order to improve the venous return to the heart; whenever possible the animal should be placed in a headdown position. The effectiveness of chest compression may be judged by the presence of a palpable carotid pulse caused by each compression and a reduction in the diameter of the pupil. If chest compression does not prove to be effective, then direct cardiac compression via a thoracotomy must be considered.

Effective external chest compression is possible in most animals although it is probable that except in cats and other small animals this will not compress the heart itself. In cats and small dogs the chest walls over the region of the heart are compressed between the fingers and the thumb of one hand. Larger animals are quickly placed on their side on a hard, unyielding surface. The upper chest wall over the region of the heart is then forced inward and allowed to recoil outwards, movement of the lower chest wall being restricted by the hard surface on which the animal is lying. It is an advantage if the lower chest wall can be supported. In dogs and other small animals pressure on the uppermost chest wall with the hand is adequate, but in adult horses and cattle the knee or foot is used. The rate of compression should be about 60 compressions/min in dogs, or 30 compressions/min in adult horses and cattle. A remarkably effective circulation can be maintained in this way. Regular respiratory movements may return, although they are usually inadequate to provide proper gaseous exchange and it is inadvisable to cease IPPV. The size of the pupils should decrease and the level of unconsciousness should lighten. The authors have seen a horse start to recover consciousness and to move its limbs while thoracic compression was being performed.

The way in which external chest compression produces blood flow in the body is somewhat debatable. It was initially thought that when the chest was compressed the heart was squeezed, so ejecting blood into the aorta. This may be so in small animals, particularly in cats and narrow-chested dogs where it is usually possible to feel the resistance to compression of the ventricles through the compliant chest wall but it is unlikely to occur in larger animals. Recent evidence suggests that blood flow is induced by intrathoracic pressure changes, pushing blood in a retrograde and forward fashion, but due to the presence of the valves and the collapse of veins, retrograde flow is stopped early on and blood is allowed to flow into the aorta. The flow of blood through the lungs is thought to be due to a cascade effect between the right and left sides of the heart but emptying of the lungs is also augmented by pulmonary ventilation.

Several techniques have been advocated for improving the pulmonary pump mechanism. The first is to bind the abdomen with an Esmarch bandage to limit the caudal displacement of the diaphragm and hence increase the intrathoracic pressure during chest compression. The second is to alternate compression of the chest and abdomen but this gives rise to risk of damage to abdominal viscera such as the liver. A third technique is to limit the collapse of the lungs during compression by ventilating as the compression is applied. None of these techniques have been shown to improve survival in veterinary clinical practice.

Fibrillation may be present when circulatory arrest occurs or may be precipitated in an asystolic heart by the effects of drugs or even chest compression. The best and most specific treatment is to pass an electric shock through the myocardium so that when the contraction which this causes passes off the whole muscle remains in a relaxed state of asystole. Then, it is hoped, normal contractions will start spontaneously. Electrical defibrillation attempts will do no harm to a heart that is in asystole and may even induce it to start beating, so applying a shock, or shocks, is now regarded as one of the first measures to be undertaken in cases of cardiac failure during anaesthesia and time should not be wasted in applying ECG leads for diagnostic purposes.

Electrical defibrillation should, however, only be attempted with properly constructed apparatus.

Bibliography

1. Healy E.G., In Graham Jones O., ed. *Small Animal Anaesthesia,* p. 59, 1964.
2. Mc Donell W., *Modern Veterinary Practice,* p. 53, 31, 1972.
3. Occupational Safety and Health Administration, New Publication of National Institute of Occupational Safety and Health (NIOSH), Washington DC, US Govt. Printing Office, 1992.

with the hand is adequate, but in adult horses and cattle the knee or foot is used. The rate of compression should be about 60 compressions/min in dogs, or 30 compressions/min i

Index

❑❑❑

CBS Veterinary Science Texts

Veterinary Andrology & Artificial Insemination..Saxena M.S.
Microbiology and Infectious Diseases of Domestic Animals, 8/e ....Hagan & Bruner's
Veterinary Bacteriology and Virology ....Merchant / Packer
Veterinary Surgery...Dollar's
Veterinary Surgery...Frank E.R.
Feeds and Feeding..Frank B. Morrison
Veterinary Obstetrics and Genital Diseases, 2/e...Roberts S. J.
Ruminant Surgery...Jit Singh / Tyagi R. P. S.
Veterinary Radiology...Jit Singh / A. Singh
Veterinary Pathology, 7/e..Ganti A. Sastry
Veterinary Clinical Pathology, 3/e...Ganti A. Sastry
Veterinary Clinical Diagnostic Technology ....Prasad B.
Veterinary Pharmaceuticals, 4/e...Prasad B.
Poultry Production..Das
Poultry Meat and Egg Production..Parkhurst / Mountney
Physiology of Reproduction & Artificial Insemination of Cattle, 2/e ....Salisbury et al.
Physiology of Domestic Animals, 9/e..Duke's
A Handbook of Practical and Clinical Immunology (in 2 Vols.)...Talwar G.P.
Veterinary Practitioner's Manual...Saxena / Dabas
Handbook of Histological, Histochemical Techniques ....David S.K.
The Invertebrates (in 6 vols.)..Hyman L.H.
Animal Feed Formulation ....Pesti / Miller
Veterinary Systemic Bacteriology and Pathogenic Fungi...Rao V.P.
Dogs (Breeding, Nutrition, Diagnosis, Health Management)...Sharma et al.
Veterinary Dictionary...Sood M.S.
Oxford Concise Veterinary Dictionary...Oxford
Veterinary Toxicology ....Garg S.K.
Animal Physiology, 2/e ....Eckert / Randal
Clinical Book of Veterinary Medicine, 2/e (Hindi)...Parihar M.L.
Wonderful World of Dogs, 2/e (Hindi)...Parihar M.L.
Guidebook of Pet Owners and Practitioners: Dogs & Cats ....Prasad D.
Breeds and Health Management of Dogs..Sharma/Pathak
Blood Groups of Indian Livestock ....Sharma M.C.
Handbook of Veterinary Clinical Pathology ....Mouddin S.M.
Veterinary Parasitology..Levine Norman D.
Special Veterinary Pathology ....Thomson
Veterinary Radiological Interpretation...Douglas
Modern Veterinary Laboratory Techniques in Clinical Diagnosis ....Vihan V.S.
A Textbook of Veterinary Anaesthesia...Pramod Kumar
MCQs & Short Answer Questions in Veterinary Bacteriology and Mycology, 2/e ....Malik B.S.
MCQs and Short Answer Questions in Veterinary Virology, 2/e ....Malik B.S.
Laboratory Manual of Veterinary Microbiology (in 4 Vols.) ....Malik B.S.

Vol. I   : General Bacteriology   Vol. II : Immunology and Serology
Vol. III : Pathogenic Bacteriology, Mycology   Vol. IV : Virology

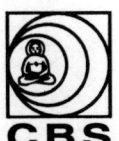

CBS PUBLISHERS & DISTRIBUTORS PVT. LTD.

4819/XI, 24 Ansari Road, Daryaganj, New Delhi - 110 002 (India)
e-mail: cbspubs@vsnl.com; delhi@cbspd.com • www.cbspd.com

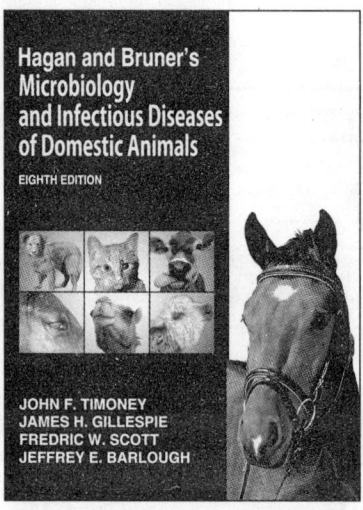

Hagan and Bruner's
Microbiology
and Infectious Diseases
of Domestic Animals

EIGHTH EDITION

JOHN F. TIMONEY
JAMES H. GILLESPIE
FREDRIC W. SCOTT
JEFFREY E. BARLOUGH

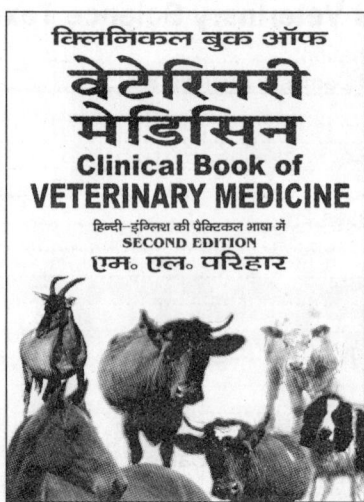

क्लिनिकल बुक ऑफ
वेटेरिनरी
मेडिसिन
Clinical Book of
VETERINARY MEDICINE
हिन्दी-इंग्लिश की प्रैक्टिकल भाषा में
SECOND EDITION
एम॰ एल॰ परिहार

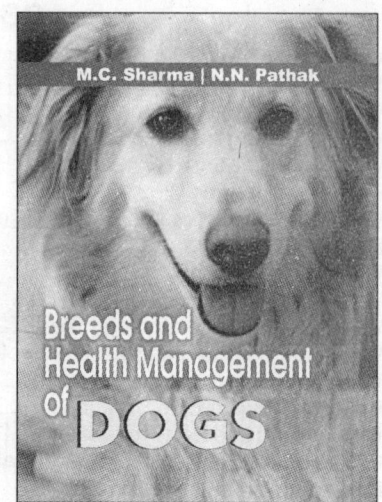

M.C. Sharma | N.N. Pathak

Breeds and
Health Management
of DOGS

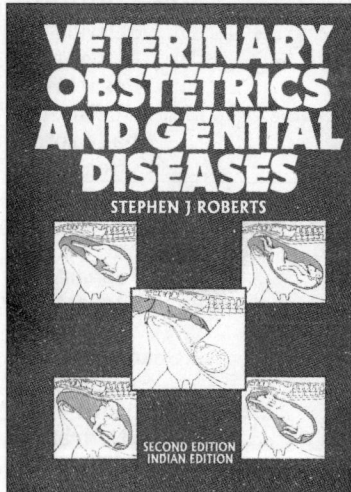

VETERINARY
OBSTETRICS
AND GENITAL
DISEASES

STEPHEN J ROBERTS

SECOND EDITION
INDIAN EDITION

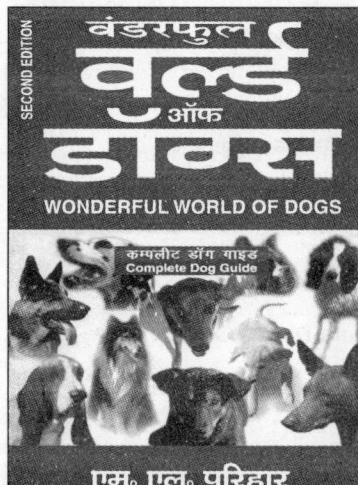

SECOND EDITION

वंडरफुल
वर्ल्ड
ऑफ
डॉग्स

WONDERFUL WORLD OF DOGS

कम्पलीट डॉग गाइड
Complete Dog Guide

एम॰ एल॰ परिहार

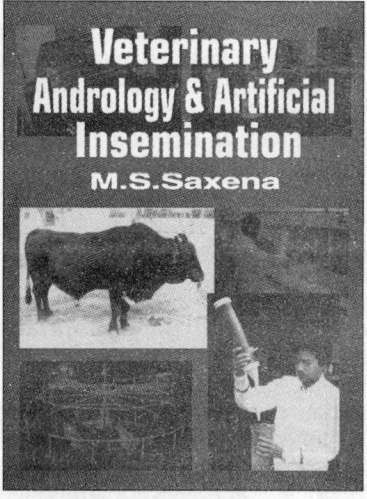

Veterinary
Andrology & Artificial
Insemination
M.S.Saxena

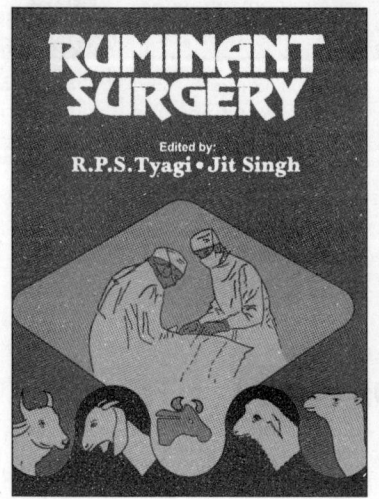

RUMINANT
SURGERY

Edited by:
R.P.S.Tyagi • Jit Singh

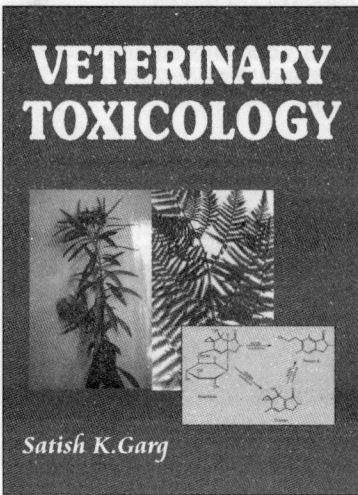

VETERINARY
TOXICOLOGY

Satish K.Garg

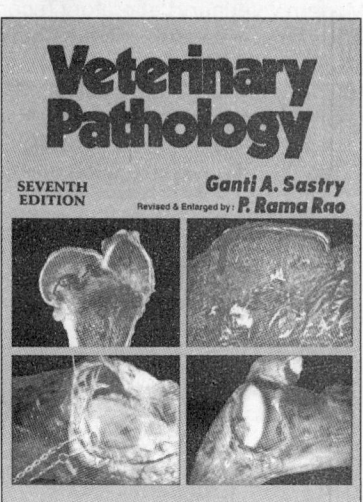

Veterinary
Pathology

SEVENTH
EDITION

Ganti A. Sastry
Revised & Enlarged by: P. Rama Rao